Cataract Surgery

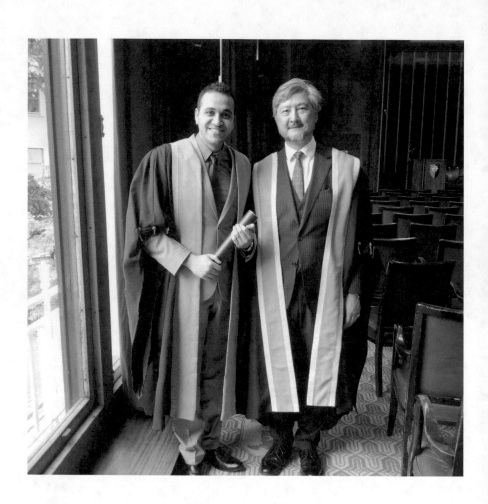

Christopher Liu · Ahmed Shalaby Bardan
Editors

Cataract Surgery

Pearls and Techniques

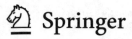 Springer

Editors
Christopher Liu
Sussex Eye Hospital, Brighton and Sussex
University Hospitals NHS Trust
Brighton, UK

Brighton and Sussex Medical School
Brighton, UK

Tongdean Eye Clinic,
Hove, UK

Ahmed Shalaby Bardan
Department of Ophthalmology
Faculty of Medicine, Alexandria University
Alexandria, Egypt

Sussex Eye Hospital, Brighton and Sussex
University Hospitals NHS Trust
Brighton, UK

ISBN 978-3-030-38236-0   ISBN 978-3-030-38234-6   (eBook)
https://doi.org/10.1007/978-3-030-38234-6

This Springer imprint is published by the registered company Springer Nature Switzerland AG
The registered company address is: Gewerbestrasse 11, 6330 Cham, Switzerland

Ahmed Shalaby Bardan dedicates this book to
Allah
from whom all wisdom and protection
emanates, his parents
Dr. Shalaby Bardan and Mrs. Amina
Elshakashah, his wife
Lamis and their children
Omar and Carma.

Christopher Liu dedicates this book
to his wife
Vivienne, their children
Sophia, George, and Henry,
his fellows and trainees past, present,
and future,
his patients, and to his
Creator the Almighty God.

Foreword

There is no shortage of textbooks on cataract surgery. However, ophthalmologists will find *Cataract Surgery-Pearls and Techniques* provides a very different and fresh perspective on our most common ophthalmic procedure. Professor Christopher Liu is an internationally recognized expert in cataract and anterior segment surgery. Over his long and prolific career, Christopher has distinguished himself as a clinician, researcher, innovator, and teacher. Dr. Liu is the President of the Brighton and Sussex Medico-Chirurgical Society, and he has been active in the leadership of the Royal College of Ophthalmologists, the United Kingdom and Ireland Society of Cataract and Refractive Surgeons, and the British Society for Refractive Surgery. Professor Liu has also provided valued mentorship to many clinical fellows, including his co-editor, Dr. Ahmed Shalaby Bardan, a rising star among anterior segment surgeons. Together, these two editors have produced a thoughtful and creative guide to cataract surgery that extends well beyond the transfer of basic and advanced surgical skills.

Cataract Surgery-Pearls and Techniques provides a uniquely holistic approach to the procedure, by exploring topics such as patient safety, surgical timing, anaesthesia options, risk assessment, surgical workflow and efficiency, and carbon footprint and sustainability. This textbook also strives to more deliberately consider the cataract patient's perspective. How can we best understand and address our patients' fears and expectations, optimize their comfort, and improve their overall experience? Finally, exploring the best ways to learn cataract surgery impacts how we can individually improve, as well as how we should be training the next generation of cataract surgeons. The editors have selected an outstanding faculty of international experts to write about each of these subjects. Many of these authors are past fellows and colleagues of Professor Liu. Like symphony conductors, the editors orchestrate these components into a comprehensive and purposeful roadmap for cataract surgeons.

Overall, this insightful textbook captures the essence and the many benefits of doing a surgical fellowship with a leading mentor. Clinical fellows not only learn surgical tips and pearls, but get to observe how the expert counsels and communicates with patients, how they organize their operating room schedule and workflow, and how they make decisions such as when to operate, what refractive IOL to use, and how to assess surgical risk. ***Cataract Surgery-Pearls and Techniques*** is a thought-provoking and practical resource for both novice and advanced cataract surgeons alike. Most importantly, it will help us to become not only better surgical technicians, but also better physicians.

Los Altos, CA, USA,   David F. Chang, MD

Preface

The story of this book started when I received an email from Elizabeth Pope after a long association with Springer publisher. We met at the rooftop café of Hilton Diagonal Mar in Barcelona during the SOE meeting to discuss four initial Ophthalmology book proposals on a sunny morning in June 2017. The first, a primer for undergraduate medical students and allied healthcare workers, and this, the second, on cataract are now complete. The third on keratoprostheses is in progress and the fourth on demystifying age-related macular degeneration to follow. Since that meeting, there has been a further agreement in principle of a *Master Ophthalmic Surgeon* series of books.

Blending my 40 years of thoughts and experience in cataract surgery (clinical, surgical, research, and managerial) with Ahmed Bardan's 10 years of practice and vigour of youth, we set out to take a fresh look at old issues with soul searching questions to redefine established practice. Rather exacting briefs were sent to our unsuspecting, expert chapter authors.

This is not just a surgical textbook. It is much more than that, or at least we have aimed so. A cataract is attached to a patient, a fellow human being with fears and emotions, with expectations of outcome, and desire for knowledge of what the process of surgery and recovery will be like. We need to demystify cataract surgery for patients. It is not a skin growing on the eye to be peeled off (that is a pterygium!), and it bears risk of permanent sight loss. The risk is proportional to the complexity of eye factors and patient factors (risk stratification) and can be reduced by careful planning of methods, techniques, team building and allowing sufficient time. A surgeon must learn not just how to operate (more on that later), but also when, and finally when not to (despite pressure from patient or relatives, or even from commercial pressure).

A question that needed answering was how do we train the next generation of surgeons? To put it simply, by book knowledge, skills lab, simulation, graded challenge, practice, inculcating the concept of a thinking surgeon, understanding that to err is human, and understanding the importance of apprenticeship and tutelage. In the final analysis, a surgeon whilst they have to be confident, needs to have some self-doubt and remain humble.

There are many things we can do to help ease the anxiety and discomfort of patients going through cataract surgery, from imparting them with information to showing them what they will experience, and from appropriate anaesthesia to inspiring confidence. All the above is covered and permeates the many chapters of this book. Simplifying patient journey, Safety, and Sustainability are also issues we have placed great importance upon. We cannot just continue do more of the same. On recovery from the COVID-19 pandemic, we suspect *Cataract Surgery by Appointment* and *Immediate Sequential Bilateral Cataract Surgery* will be viewed in a positive light. We also cannot keep wanting the best for ourselves and be wasteful, looting planet earth and short changing future generations.

Thank you for your interest in this book. We hope you will enjoy reading and rereading it. Sometimes the messages do not come through immediately and you will have to think about them. We thank our authors who have worked very hard to produce wonderful chapters. We thank them for putting up with pernickety editors. We thank Springer for accommodating our tardiness in our quest for perfection. We thank our proofreaders (Mrs. Sue Cooper, Drs. Larry Benjamin, Tommy Chan, Sharmina Khan, Pei Lin, and Vincenzo Maurino). All errors remain our fault.

Brighton, UK   Prof. Christopher Liu
December 2020   OBE, FRCOphth, FRCSEd, FRCP, CertLRS

Contents

About the Editors

Prof. Christopher Liu was born in Hong Kong to a medical family and attended a UK boarding school in the West Country. He first wanted to become an ophthalmologist when he became short-sighted at the age of 13. His undergraduate studies at Charing Cross Hospital Medical School and subsequent postgraduate training posts in London at Charing Cross, Western Ophthalmic, and Moorfields Eye Hospitals and Higher Surgical Training at Addenbrooke's in Cambridge, Norwich, and Rome led to his appointment as a Consultant with an interest in Cornea, External Eye Disease, and Cataract in Brighton at the Sussex Eye Hospital. He is a world-leading expert in the osteo-odonto-keratoprosthesis (OOKP), with patients seeking his expertise from across the globe. He also serves as an Honorary Clinical Professor and Undergraduate Ophthalmology Lead for the Brighton and Sussex Medical School and has designed the curriculum as well as supervising medical students, registrars, and fellows in research. His research interests are in the anterior segment of the eye with over 250 publications, over a dozen inventions, and a number of patents.

He is an active member in the scientific field, having served as president of the Medical Contact Lens and Ocular Surface Association, British Society for Refractive Surgery, Southern Ophthalmological Society and is the current president of Brighton and Sussex Medico-Chirurgical Society. He is also a Past Honorary Secretary of United Kingdom and Ireland Society of Cataract and Refractive Surgeons, and Council member and Trustee of the Royal College of Ophthalmologists. He holds honorary academic and clinical positions past and present in Japan (Kindai University, Osaka), Hong Kong (Chinese University of Hong Kong), Singapore, India, and Alexandria University in Egypt.

Christopher held a Silver National Clinical Excellence Award. He was Hospital Doctor of the Year in 2005. He is a Member of Merit of the Barraquer Institute in Barcelona, Spain. He was made honorary fellow of the Royal College of Surgeons, Edinburgh, and honorary fellow of the Royal College of Physicians, London, in 2018. He delivered the Kersley Lecture in 2018. He was appointed OBE in 2018 New Year's Honours list for Services to Ophthalmology.

Professor Liu established the Anterior Segment Fellowship at the Sussex Eye Hospital in 1998 and also has honorary fellows who attend for observership. His fellows have followed on his footsteps, becoming clinical and academic consultants in teaching hospitals globally. His passion for education has continued throughout his career; he is frequently invited as an international speaker at conferences and runs training courses for Ophthalmologists. He is also an active philanthropist, supporting young musicians and artists. Outside work, his passion is in music, travel, haute cuisine, cross-cultural understanding, and freemasonry. He is married to Vivienne and they have three grown-up children.

Ahmed Shalaby Bardan was born in Egypt to a medical family and attended medical school at Alexandria University, Egypt. He decided to pursue a career in Ophthalmology whilst studying the subject as a 4th-year medical student. In 2010, he graduated in medicine, and came first amongst his cohort of 1,200 graduates. He was immediately offered postgraduate training in Ophthalmology at the Faculty of Medicine, Alexandria. Following basic and higher specialty training in Egypt, he moved to the United Kingdom for a two-and-a-half-year fellowship in Cornea and Anterior Segment at the Sussex Eye Hospital in Brighton. He is currently a Consultant Ophthalmologist with subspecialty interests in Cornea, the External Eye, and Cataract at the Birmingham and Midlands Eye Centre, Birmingham, UK.

He has contributed to national and international courses and workshops on cataract surgery, immediate sequential bilateral cataract surgery, delivery of cataract service, and anterior lamellar and endothelial keratoplasty techniques. Aside from having a wide range of experience in the management of complex and challenging cases of cataract, he is also an experienced laser and lens refractive surgeon.

Mr. Bardan is an enthusiastic Ophthalmologist who has excelled in the field at a young age, being 32 years old. He continues to serve as a Lecturer of Ophthalmology at the Faculty of Medicine, Alexandria University, Egypt and was previously an Honorary Clinical Lecturer at the Brighton and Sussex Medical School, Brighton, UK.

What Do Cataract Patients Want?

Alfonso Vasquez-Perez and Christopher Liu

Cataract formation is inevitable with ageing and remains the leading cause of blindness worldwide [1]. Cataract surgery is one of the oldest surgical procedures in human history and was first documented in the fifth century BC. However, cataract surgery has not always enjoyed good levels of success. For centuries patients were doomed to be subject to dangerous procedures like dislodging of the lens or "couching" using sharp instruments with a risk of blindness. These interventions, often performed by "quacks", incurred a high risk of complications. Among the unfortunates was the famous 18th century composer Johann Sebastian Bach, who was not only left blind in both eyes but died shortly after surgery, due to complications of the procedure [2].

Developments in ophthalmic surgery during recent decades such as antibiotics, operating microscopes, sutures, intraocular lenses and phacoemulsification have positioned cataract surgery as one of the safest interventions in medicine. Modern cataract extraction by phacoemulsification and a suture-less technique is performed worldwide and successfully restores sight with a short recovery period, overcoming the adverse impact this disease has had on societies and cultures.

Despite all these surgical advances, patients may enquire about possible modalities other than surgery to treat their cataracts which of course is not possible. Also, once they accept the necessity of surgery, they may express their wish for a risk-free procedure, guaranteed instantaneous outcome and full restoration of focusing at all distances as if cataract surgery were not only a treatment to restore but to rejuvenate vision. These enquires may be the result of constant advances

A. Vasquez-Perez (✉)
Moorfields Eye Hospital, London, UK
e-mail: alest99@gmail.com

C. Liu
Sussex Eye Hospital, Brighton, UK

Tongdean Eye Clinic, Hove, UK

and misinformation by the media, making consumers more demanding for a perfect, risk free outcome. We thus need to give accurate information to our cataract patients and be able to anticipate their concerns and queries. It is the authors' wish to equip the reader with such skills and knowledge.

Anxiety and Surgical Fear

Patients always have preoperative anxiety and fear regardless of the level of intrusion and success rates of a proposed operation [3, 4]. Fear of permanent loss of vision can be found in most patients who are told they require eye surgery. Fear has been associated with increased intraoperative and postoperative pain, increased use of analgesia and poor postoperative recovery [3]. Studies have demonstrated that delivering easy-to-understand patient information alone is highly effective in reducing anxiety. Assessing and addressing surgical fear should be one of the first steps in any pre-operative workup [4–6].

Studies that examined what patients want before consenting for surgical procedures (including cataract surgery), have found patients considered it most important to meet their surgeon and secondly to receive information regarding risks, type of complications and the operative technique [7]. It is therefore the clinician's duty to anticipate patient anxiety, give reassurance and deliver understandable information in a well conducted face-to-face consultation.

Patients may express their concerns about the difficulty in keeping their head or eyes still and that making sudden movements may result in complications especially if topical anaesthesia alone is used. Asking them in advance to keep looking as much as possible at one direction (usually the operating microscope lights) will be helpful in maintaining the correct position but will also keep their mind focused on a target. Others might also be afraid to see instruments approaching their eye during the operation and they should be informed that shadows and lights are seen rather than needles and sharp edged knives. This applies for the majority of cases with the exception of high myopes who can focus objects at very near distance. For all types of patients maintaining reassurance and short explanations of what is currently happening and what they should expect to see and feel as the surgery progresses have proved to help to reduce anxiety [4]. There are however patients who would prefer not to have a running commentary. When the likelihood of poor intraoperative cooperation is predicted such as patients with known anxiety disorder or claustrophobia, a nurse or volunteer to hold their hand has proved to reduce anxiety and is recommended. In addition, cases which are predicted to have poor cooperation for topical anaesthesia, sedation (oral or intravenous) and or subtenons/peribulbar block should be considered. For even more anxious patients, general anaesthesia should be considered during preoperative planning.

Preoperative explanation of what the patient will experience (see, feel and hear), as opposed to details of surgical technique could make the experience more bearable and contribute to reducing patient anxiety [4, 6]. Patients need to know that their eyes will be "numb" with either drops or a small injection and after that they will be required to lay flat and still for the operation which usually takes between 20 and 30 minutes. Their face will be covered to allow the operation to be done under sterile conditions and they should also be informed regarding the importance of keeping their eyes open for draping and placement of the speculum (Fig. 1). It is important to explain that there will be a strong light which they will get used to, plenty of fluid or water running, and sensations of touch and pressure, rather than an empty reassurance that they will feel nothing (Fig. 2). Once the operation is finished a pad and/or shield will be placed over the eye, after which patients are moved to the recovery area. Finally, a nurse will inform patients when to remove the pad and start post-operative eye drops before they are discharged home preferably accompanied. Information on eye protection (Cartella shield, not touching the eye, keeping it dry) and the post-operative eye drops regime will further add to patient preparedness.

Supporting Information on Cataract Surgery

Information presented to patients needs to be consistent and simple to ensure their comprehension and satisfaction. The following key points must be included in the core information: despite there being no 100% guarantee of a successful result, with modern techniques the chance of severe or complete permanent loss of vision in the operated eye is less than 1 in 1000 and that more than 95% of patients have no complications at all [8, 9]. Also it is important to reassure patients that most complications are manageable although it may mean that further procedures might be required and that the recovery period may be longer than usual.

The volume of cataract surgery is increasing, and hospitals have implemented protocols to facilitate patient flow. Specialised high-volume cataract units have all the necessary arrangements and biometry completed in the first visit avoiding the need for an extra preoperative appointment [5, 10]. In this context patients might have a shorter time to weigh up the information provided. Therefore, written information (informative leaflets) usually given at the beginning of the consultation, could also be provided in advance by community opticians, general practitioners or be available online. These measures will allow patients time to formulate questions and will ensure all their concerns and doubts will be dealt with at the consultation.

Similarly, educational videos of cataract surgery are becoming more widely used and popular as they allow important and consistent information to be provided audio-visually and understood easily [6]. A well-produced short video (4–5 minutes) has been shown to offer an appealing advantage regarding the ability to deliver the necessary information about the risks and benefits of surgery [11–13]. The use of digital media will never replace the face-to-face counselling with the surgeon but offers an additional method of educating patients. It can also help to avoid misunderstandings that could otherwise occur during the informed

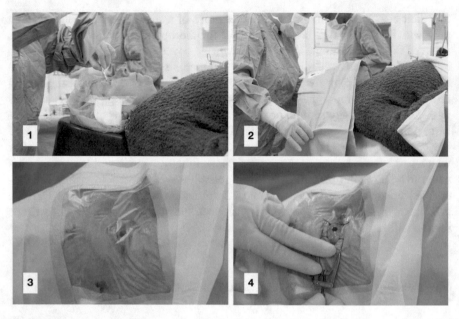

Fig. 1 Draping of a patient for cataract surgery. This stage can generate stress in patients with anxiety but good communication regarding the steps focusing on what the patient will feel is required. It is important to reassure patients and ask them to keep their eyes open for effective draping

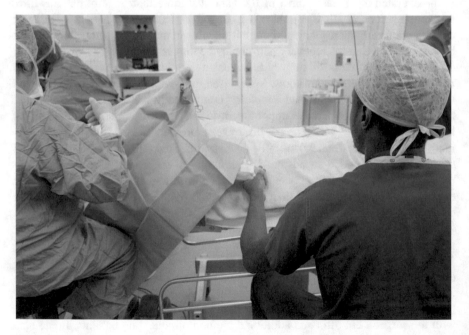

Fig. 2 Holding the hand of a staff member during cataract surgery can significantly decrease patient anxiety

consent process. It may have additional value in academic settings where trainees have not yet adequate experience with appropriately guiding patients through the informed consent process.

In addition, a telephone hotline should be implemented which could be dedicated to postoperative queries and concerns and/or similarly an email address that staff monitor regularly to reply and advise patients in accordance with their symptoms. These measures would decrease unnecessary visits in emergency and outpatient clinics improving efficiency of cataract units.

Disclosure of Cataract Surgery Training

Most cataract operations worldwide are performed in the public sector many of them at teaching hospitals. Another factor that may contribute to surgical fear is the involvement of trainees [14]. Some patients could be aware of the potential involvement of residents in their surgery and feel that the risk of complications will be higher. Surgical training, especially in cataract surgery, is a necessary facet of Ophthalmology training programmes [14, 15]. This should be accomplished through graded responsibility and surgical challenge, where trainee surgeons perform supervised increasingly complex tasks appropriate for their level of experience and competence [16]. Patients might not fully understand that the Ophthalmologist is still in training and very often the trainee's role is not fully disclosed. While some studies show most trainees and consultants feel disclosure would increase patient's anxiety levels [17], others suggest that the factors contributing to a patient's decision for resident involvement are modifiable [14]. Disclosure of resident involvement increases transparency and could allow trainees and patients to interact more openly. When patients trust their consultants, they are more likely to trust their advice on trainee involvement. In a similar manner transparency and patient's trust would decrease the anxiety of residents improving their surgical performance. Consideration should be given as to whether a patient wants to know who will be operating.

Recovery Time and Return to Work

Patients will ask about the recovery time and the postoperative need for review.

During the past two decades of phacoemulsification cataract surgery, the experience of problem-free recovery after uneventful surgery has translated into decreasing numbers of recommended postoperative check-up visits. Already in the year 1995 Tufail et al. [18] concluded that routine check-up of symptomless patients on the first day after cataract surgery is inefficient. In the majority of specialised cataract units a post-op review by the Ophthalmologist would be required only for cases with intraoperative complications, patients who received toric intraocular lenses or patients with coexisting eye conditions like diabetic retinopathy, Fuchs' dystrophy, advanced glaucoma, chronic uveitis, and previous refractive surgery.

There is no consensus regarding the time at which patients will be able to return to work or their usual daily activities following cataract surgery. Although patients have to use drops for one month, studies evaluating clear corneal incisions have found that these had spontaneously sealed by day four [19]. As the incidence of postoperative intraocular inflammation with modern sutureless phacoemulsification is low, most patients could be advised to return to their work or usual activities after one or two weeks and these could include driving if the contralateral eye has good vision or return to exercises like yoga, running or even swimming. Passive sexual activity could also resume in this sort of time frame.

Because most patients are over sixty years old and therefore not actively payroll workers, time for recovery may not have a significant economic impact on wider society but impact their families who require their support as carers for example. In reality most patients presenting for surgery have bilateral cataracts which makes it necessary to have both eyes operated on for full visual rehabilitation. In this scenario immediately sequential bilateral cataract surgery (ISBCS) offers the fastest recovery and therefore fastest return to work or activities but also offers significant financial advantages including more efficient use of operating theatres and a reduced number of clinical visits [20, 21]. Despite its advantages the most serious allegation against ISBCS is the risk of potential bilateral endophthalmitis. Only four cases of simultaneous bilateral endophthalmitis have been reported in the literature following ISBCS but none of the operations were done according to the protocol published later by the International Society of Bilateral Cataract Surgeons [22]. In fact, suitable patients willing to undergo simultaneous bilateral cataract surgery should be informed that no case of bilateral simultaneous endophthalmitis occurred in more than 95,000 ISBCS collected operated according to this guideline in a multi-centre study [23]. There are also claims that obtaining refraction from the first operated eye allows improved outcome from the second eye, however with the introduction of optical biometry the predictability for refractive outcomes has significantly improved making it unnecessary to wait for the refraction of the first eye. Another advantage of ISBCS is that it mitigates the period of anisometropia which can be a significant problem occurring after unilateral cataract surgery [24]. With ISBCS even if there is a small lapse from a target refraction the stereoscopic vision is immediately restored. With improvements of the technique and increasing demand for cataract surgery, providing surgeons with guidelines and tools to support ISBCS would increase their confidence in the adoption of ISBCS for suitable patients in the near future.

Refractive Outcome and Presbyopia Management

Predicted refractive outcome has improved significantly with the introduction of optical biometry and new generation formulae. In addition, the constant development of multifocal intraocular lenses is directing cataract surgery to evolve into a refractive procedure. In recent years, patients have also become more interested in having a treatment which can provide a spectacle-free life. Despite all improvements, presbyopia remains an obstacle in cataract surgery and achieving high quality full range of vision has become one of the greatest goals of modern cataract surgery. Patients should know that even though multifocal intraocular lenses (IOLs) are effective at improving near vision relative to monofocal IOLs, there is still uncertainty as to the size of the effect, and that there is not yet a perfect replacement compared to a young crystalline lens [25].

The main problems reported in patients receiving multifocal IOLs are dysphotopsia (glare and halos). It is known that they tolerate less residual ametropia and require earlier YAG laser capsulotomy [26]. Lifestyle, occupation and expectations must be questioned as patient selection is crucial in order to avoid dissatisfaction. Patients who drive at night, demand a perfect outcome, halos already present, have large pupils or who have ocular conditions like maculopathy, glaucoma, amblyopia, dry eye, corneal dystrophies, previous keratorefractive surgery are not good candidates for multifocal lenses [25, 26].

A different approach to treat presbyopia using monofocal IOLs is monovision. This is a low-cost option that corrects distance vision in the dominant eye and the non-dominant eye focuses intentionally for near to mid-range vision. Full monovision requires to aim for a refractive error of -2.50 D or more in the non-dominant eye but the resultant anisometropia induces loss of stereopsis and one third of patients can present with intolerance [27]. In order to improve tolerance beyond two thirds of patients, a modified approach known as "mini-monovision" requiring a smaller interocular difference power (-0.75 to -1.75 dioptres) has been described with good outcomes and thus gained popularity [27]. Monovision and mini-monovision have proved to be safe alternatives, have similar grade of patient satisfaction and have less dysphotopsia symptoms than multifocal IOLs [28]. It has been reported that patients with mini-monovision are less likely to undergo IOL exchange due to dissatisfaction when compared with multifocal IOLs [29]. Patients should be carefully counselled and warned that a period of adaptation is needed and there can be more dependence on glasses compared with multifocal IOLs [27]. Generally, patients who are used to monovision contact lens wear are particularly good candidates for this approach but they should also be warned about less predictable outcomes after surgery. This could be secondary to loss of minor residual accommodation of the crystalline lens which can be present even in middle-aged patients. A contact lens monovision trial would provide valuable information regarding prediction of postoperative tolerance but it has limitations in the presence of cataracts.

Second Eye Surgery Syndrome

Another common concern for patients is whether the second eye experience would be similar to their first operated eye. For patients who had an unpleasant experience during the first surgery a change in the anaesthetic planning may be considered. This would consist of performing either subtenons or peribulbar block instead of topical and/or using sedation (oral or intravenous). For patients who had an uneventful first cataract surgery, surgeons usually repeat the same plan for the second eye if the case is similar, however there are some issues we have to consider.

Even though patient anxiety declines for the second surgery, a meta-analysis has shown that patients experience more pain and discomfort during their second eye cataract surgery [30]. The mechanism for this phenomenon remains unknown but a few theories have been proposed. Firstly, patients who had successfully undergone first cataract surgery feel less anxiety while paying more attention to the pain perception during their second eye surgery [31, 32]. Secondly, drug tolerance may have developed to the analgesic or even the sedative after surgery of the first eye. Thirdly, the first eye surgery was regarded to give rise to sympathetic irritation making the contralateral eye prone to painful stimuli [31]. This last theory has been supported by recent studies that showed an increase of a pain related inflammatory chemokine MCP-1 in the aqueous humour in the second eye subsequent to the first eye cataract surgery which also suggests that there might have been a sympathetic ophthalmic type uveitis in the second eye prior to the first eye surgery [33]. Based on this observation patients should be informed of the possibility of increased sensation for the second eye and where necessary increased anaesthesia or sedation might be considered independently of the experience of the first eye. Through personal experience, we have found patients feel more discomfort during second eye surgery even in immediately sequential bilateral cataract surgery (ISBCS) (unpublished data). Our routine practice for ISBCS is therefore to use topical and intracameral anaesthesia in the first eye, and a sub-tenons anaesthetic for the second.

Alteration in Appearance Following Cataract Surgery

A change in appearance can be noticed and has been reported by patients after intraocular surgery. In most cases patients can notice asymmetry in their eyelids and typically upper eyelid ptosis that can develop independently of the level of difficulty of cataract surgery. Less commonly patients can present with changes in iris colour, pupil shape or size which are usually related to intraoperative trauma. The incidence of upper eyelid ptosis following cataract surgery has been reported from 7.3 to 21% [34] and in the majority of cases it resolves spontaneously during the following weeks. The causes of transitory ptosis might include eyelid oedema, indirect infiltration of the levator palpebrae superioris (LPS) by retrobulbar or peribulbar anaesthesia and ocular surface disturbance. A minor percentage can present postoperative ptosis due to disinsertion of the LPS aponeurosis with its precise aetiology remaining elusive. It has been postulated that contraction of the orbicularis oculi against the speculum may cause dehiscence of the LPS aponeurosis and also that the speculum may compress the lid against the orbital rim causing inflammation and oedema which may result in weakening of the aponeurosis [35, 36]. It has also been observed that patients with smaller palpebral apertures were more likely to develop ptosis and it would be advisable that a rigid speculum should be avoided in these particular eyes [34]. In most of the cases with postoperative upper eyelid ptosis observation initially would be recommended, however in the event of LPS aponeurosis disinsertion patients should be informed that corrective eyelid surgery can successfully restore the upper eyelid normal position. Finally some patients may notice a reflective sparkle in their eyes which is due to light reflection from the anterior surface of the intraocular lens. These patients are usually asymptomatic otherwise and need only receive reassurance.

Double Vision After Cataract Surgery

New onset diplopia after cataract extraction is uncommon with an estimated incidence between 0.17 and 0.75% [37]. Its development is an unexpected event for the patient and often a source of confusion for the physician. Moreover, its rarity inherently engenders unfamiliarity with the evaluation and has implications for identification of proper underlying disease that can result in medical litigations.

Both binocular and monocular diplopia can develop following cataract surgery and differentiating the two is the first work up in these patients. Monocular diplopia can be secondary to lens decentration or retained lens fragments and further corrective surgery for these complications eliminates diplopia. On the other hand, binocular diplopia is by far the most common postoperative acquired strabismus and vertical deviations represent 98% of its total.

Postoperative strabismus and diplopia can be related to anaesthetic procedures or pre-existing conditions unmasked by cataract surgery [38]. Whilst retrobulbar anaesthesia can induce direct needle trauma to an extraocular muscle, the anaesthetic agent itself also used in peribulbar or sub-tenons block can cause myotoxicity of the extraocular muscles and therefore strabismus [38, 39]. The use of hyaluronidase has been proposed to decrease the potential for myotoxicity due to its function as a digestive agent allowing anaesthetic dispersal through tissue preventing its accumulation in one area and damage of nearby muscles [39]. Therefore, in cases not suitable for topical anaesthesia and when ophthalmoparesis is required the addition of hyaluronidase to either retrobulbar, peribulbar or subtenons block would be recommended.

Pre-existing misalignments have been described as the most commonly identified cause of diplopia following cataract surgery [38]. Because cataract development is an insidious process and subnormal vision, which some patients may endure, can mask even long term and marked misalignments, it is then of prime importance to conduct a thorough assessment of the patient's efferent visual system prior to cataract extraction, both by history and examination. Documentation of preoperative strabismus is also helpful in the decision to operate on the dominant eye first to prevent "fixation-switch diplopia" seen when patients with a long-standing strabismus are forced to take up fixation with their non-dominant eye [40]. A cataract can occlude the vision of a deviated eye and improve symptoms of difficult or intractable diplopia. In these cases, consideration should be taken regarding the option of not removing the cataract. Finally, if a patient develops strabismus post cataract surgery, it is necessary not to obviate the need to consider other less common aetiologies of a vertical misalignment such as skew deviations, third and fourth nerve palsies, and myasthenia gravis.

Post-cataract surgery strabismus can be successfully treated with prismatic glasses and in more severe cases with corrective surgery. However, because myotoxicity or traumatic myopathies are dynamic processes patients typically need several months for the condition to become stable before strabismus surgery can be performed. In some cases, botulinum toxin injection can bring the eyes back into permanent alignment [37, 38].

Floaters and Retinal Detachment Following Cataract Surgery

Floaters can become more apparent following cataract surgery as patients see more clearly. A preoperative evaluation of the vitreous is recommended in order to identify patients without posterior vitreous detachment (PVD). In these individuals the onset of floaters following cataract surgery requires careful examination regarding the possibility of retinal tears and retinal detachment. Patients with previous PVD on the other hand should be warned regarding the increasing degree of their symptoms following surgery. Increased perception of floaters can cause significant distress, but patients should be reassured that improvement is usually seen in the following months.

Cataract surgery can also induce posterior vitreous detachment (PVD) and therefore represent a risk factor for retinal detachment [41]. The incidence of this complication is however very low and has been estimated to range from 0.3 to 0.5% for phacoemulsification [42]. Intraoperative vitreous loss and high myopia are known risk factors associated with increased incidence of retinal detachment post cataract surgery. High myopes have 6.5 times higher incidence than emmetropes [42]. These patients should be carefully assessed preoperatively and advised to seek urgent review in the onset of PVD symptoms following cataract surgery. Besides high myopes, patients with history of retinal detachment in the same or contralateral eye and those with family history of RD should be offered a follow up visit in which presence of and prophylactic treatment for predisposing retinal lesions like lattice degeneration or abnormal vitreoretinal adhesions should be evaluated.

References

1. Bourne RRA, Stevens GA, White RA, Smith JL, Flaxman SR, Price H, et al. Causes of vision loss worldwide, 1990–2010: a systematic analysis. Lancet Glob Health. 2013;1(6):e339–49.

2. Zegers HCR. The eyes of Johann Sebastian Bach. Arch Opthalmol. 2005;123:1427–30.
3. Theunissen M, Jonker S, Schepers J, et al. Validity and time course of surgical fear as measured with the Surgical Fear Questionnaire in patients undergoing cataract surgery. PLOS One. 2018.
4. Ramirez D, Brodie F, Rose-Nussbaumer J, et al. Anxiety in patients undergoing cataract surgery: a pre- and postoperative comparison. Clin Ophthalmol. 2017:11.
5. Moinul P, Ligori T, MD, Qian J, et al. Evaluating patient preparedness for cataract surgery and satisfaction with preoperative care. Can J Ophthalmol. 2019;4:54.
6. Vo TA, Ngai P, Tao JP. A randomized trial of multimedia-facilitated informed consent for cataract surgery. Clin Ophthalmol. 2018:12.
7. Elder MJ, Suter A. What patients want to know before they have cataract surgery. Br J Ophthalmol. 2004;88:331–2. https://doi.org/10.1136/bjo/2003.020453.
8. Endophthalmitis Study Group, European Society of Cataract & Refractive Surgeons. Prophylaxis of postoperative endophthalmitis following cataract surgery: results of the ESCRS multicenter study and identification of risk factors. J Cataract Refract Surg. 2007;33(6):978–88.
9. Jaycock P, Johnston RL, Taylor H, Adams M, Tole DM, Galloway P, et al. The Cataract National Dataset electronic multi-centre audit of 55 567 operations: updating benchmark standards of care in the United Kingdom and internationally. Eye. 2007;23(1):38–49.
10. Alboim C, Kliemann RB, Soares LE, Ferreira MM, Polanczyk CA, Biolo A. The impact of preoperative evaluation on perioperative events in patients undergoing cataract surgery: a cohort study. Eye. 2016;30:1614–22.
11. Tan JF, Tay LK, Ng LH. Video compact discs for patient education: reducing anxiety prior to cataract surgery. Insight. 2005;30(4):16–21.
12. Zhang Y, Ruan X, Tang H, Yang W, Xian Z, Lu M. Video-assisted informed consent for cataract surgery: a randomized controlled trial. J Ophthalmol. 2017;2017:9593631.
13. American Academy of Ophthalmology. Phaco cataract surgery with monofocal lens. Cataract and refractive surgery patient education Video Collection. 2017.
14. Corwin A, Rajkumar J, Markovitz B, et al. Association of Preoperative Disclosure of Resident Roles With Informed Consent for Cataract Surgery in a Teaching Program JAMA Ophthalmology. Published online July 25, 2019.
15. Rogers GM, Oetting TA, Lee AG, et al. Impactof a structured surgical curriculum on ophthalmic resident cataract surgery complication rates. J Cataract Refract Surg. 2009;35(11):1956–60.
16. Randleman JB, Wolfe JD, Woodward M, Lynn MJ, Cherwek DH, Srivastava SK. The resident surgeon phacoemulsification learning curve. Arch Ophthalmol. 2007;125(9):1215–9.
17. Aminlari A, Greenberg P, Scott I. Ophthalmology residents perspectives regarding disclosure of resident involvement in ophthalmic surgery. J Acad Ophthalmol. 2014;7(1).
18. Tufail A, Foss AJE, Hamilton AMP. Is the first day postoperative review necessary after cataract extraction? Br J Ophthalmol. 1995;79:646–8.
19. Chee S, Ti S, Lim L, et al. Anterior segment optical coherence tomography evaluation of the integrity of clear corneal incisions: a comparison between 2.2-mm and 2.65-mm main incisions. Am J Ophthalmol. 2010;149:768–76.
20. Smith GT, Liu CS. It is time for a new attitude to "simultaneous" bilateral cataract surgery? Br J Ophthalmol. 2001;85:1489–96.
21. O'Brien JJ, Gonder J, Botz C, Chow KY, Arshinoff SA. Immediately sequential bilateral cataract surgery versus delayed sequential bilateral cataract surgery: potential hospital cost savings. Can J Ophthalmol. 2010;45(6):596–601.
22. Haynes AB, Weiser TG, Berry WR. A Surgical Safety Checklist to Reduce Morbidity and Mortality in a Global Population. N Engl J Med. 2009;360(5):491–9.
23. Arshinoff SA, Bastianelli PA. Incidence of postoperative endophthalmitis after immediate sequential bilateral cataract surgery. J Cataract Refract Surg. 2011;37(12):2105–14.
24. Kontkanen M, Kaipiainen S. Simultaneous bilateral cataract extraction: a positive view. J Cataract Refract Surg. 2002;28(11):2060–1.

25. De Silva SR, Evans JR, Kirthi V, et al. Multifocal versus monofocal intraocular lenses after cataract extraction. Cochrane Database Syst Rev. 2016;12:12.
26. Alio JL, Plaza-Puche AB, Fernandez-Buenaga R, Maldonado M. Multifocal intraocular lenses: An overview. Surv Ophthalmol. 2017;62:611–34.
27. Labiris G, Toli A, Perente A, et al. A systematic review of pseudophakic monovision for presbyopia correction. Int J Ophthalmol. 2017;10:992–1000.
28. Wilkins MR, Allan BD, Rubin GS, et al. Randomized trial of multifocal intraocular lenses versus monovision after bilateral cataract surgery. Ophthalmology. 2013;120:2449–55.
29. Wang S, Stem M, Oren G, et al. Patient-centered and visual quality outcomes of premium cataract surgery: a systematic review. Eur J Ophthalmol. 2017;27:387–401.
30. Shi C, Yuan J, Zee B. Pain perception of the first eye versus the second eye during phacoemusification under local anaesthesia for patients going through cataract surgery: a systematic review and metanalysis. J Ophthalmol. 2019; 23: article 4106893.
31. Ursea R, Feng MT, Zhou M, Lien V, Loeb R. Pain perception in sequential cataract surgery: comparison of rst and second procedures. J Cat&Refract Surg. 2011;37:1009–14.
32. L.Jiang,K.Zhang,W.Heetal.Perceived pain during cataract surgery with topical anesthesia: a comparison between first-eye and second-eye surgery. J Ophthalmol. 2015;2015: Article ID 383456, 6 pages.
33. Zhu X, Wol D, Zhang K, et al. Molecular inflammation in the contralateral eye after cataract surgery in the first eye. Investigative Opthalmology & Visual Science. 2015;56(9):5566–73.
34. Crosby NJ, Shepherd D, Murray A. Mechanical testing of lid speculae and relationship to postoperative ptosis. Eye (Lond). 2013;27(9):1098–101.
35. Singh SK, Sekhar GC, Gupta S. Etiology of ptosis after cataract surgery. J Cataract Refract Surg. 1997;23:1409–13.
36. Paris GL, Quickert MH. Disinsertion of the aponeurosis of the levator palpebrae superioris muscle after cataract extraction. Am J Ophthalmol. 1976;81(3):337–40.
37. Bouffard & Dean M. Cestari (2018) Diplopia after Cataract Extraction, Seminars in Ophthalmology, 33:1, 11–16. https://doi.org/10.1080/08820538.2017.1353806.
38. Nayak H, Kersey JP, Oystreck DT, Cline RA, Lyons CJ. Diplopia following cataract sugery: A review of 150 patients. Eye. 2008;22:1057–64. https://doi.org/10.1038/sj.eye.6702847.
39. Dempsey GA, Barrett PJ, Kirby IJ. Hyaluronidase and peri- bulbar block. Br J Anesthes. 1997;78:671–4.
40. Samuel Williams G, Radwan M, Menon J. Cataract surgery planning in amblyopic patients—which eye first? Awareness of the potential for post-operative diplopia amongst consultant ophthalmic surgeons in Wales. Ulster Med J. 2013;82(2):82–4.
41. Norregaard JC, Thoning H, Andersen TF, et al. Risk of retinal detachment following cataract extraction: results from the International Cataract Surgery. Outcomes Study. Br J Ophthalmol. 1996; 80:689–693.
42. Coppé AM, Lapucci G. Posterior vitreous detachment and retinal detachment following cataract extraction. Curr Opin Ophthalmol. 2008;19(3):239–42.

Timing of Cataract Surgery

Alfonso Vasquez-Perez, Christopher Liu and John Sparrow

Cataract surgery not only improves quality of life, reduces risk of falling and car crashes but also reduces the long-term mortality risk by 40 percent compared to those not undergoing surgery [1–4]. While the only treatment for cataracts is surgical intervention, the right time to have surgery depends on the visual requirements of individual patients. It is the clinician's responsibility to educate and give patients enough knowledge to make an independent and well-informed decision regarding a cataract operation. The decision to have cataract surgery comes down to whether the benefits of having the operation sufficiently outweigh the small risk attached.

When Should Patients Be Offered Cataract Surgery?

Timing of cataract surgery is different for everyone and this question does not have a single answer, but in addition to clinical examination, obtaining information from patients is essential to elucidate the best plan for each person. One example would relate to driving, a patient who drives may need cataract surgery

A. Vasquez-Perez (✉)
Moorfields Eye Hospital, London, UK
e-mail: alest99@gmail.com

C. Liu
Sussex Eye Hospital, Brighton, UK

Tongdean Eye Clinic, Hove, UK

J. Sparrow
Bristol Eye Hospital, Bristol, UK

J. Sparrow
Bristol University, Bristol, UK

© Springer Nature Switzerland AG 2021
C. Liu and A. Shalaby Bardan (eds.), *Cataract Surgery*,
https://doi.org/10.1007/978-3-030-38234-6_2

13

earlier than someone who does not. Traditionally visual acuity has been the main criterion used for making a decision whether or not to offer surgery. This approach is not ideal as patients have different levels of tolerance for visual impairment which do not necessarily correspond with visual acuity.

In an attempt to guide clinicians and patients the American Academy of Ophthalmology has developed a list of four questions which patients should also ask themselves to help determine if they are ready for cataract surgery as listed below [5]:

1. **Are your cataracts impacting your daily or occupational activities?**

   The lack of contrast and clarity can be difficult for those who need clear vision for work, driving or who enjoy hobbies like reading, cooking or sewing.

2. **Are your cataracts affecting your ability to drive safely at night?**
   Cataracts can cause halos around lights and difficulty seeing in low-light settings, impacting the ability to safely drive at night. More advanced cataracts can cause vision loss sufficient to fail the vision test required for a driver's licence.

3. **Are your cataracts interfering with the outdoor activities you enjoy?**
   Cataracts can increase sensitivity to glare, which can be especially troublesome for those who enjoy skiing, surfing and many other outdoor activities. Cataracts can also cause visual differences between the eyes which can affect the distance vision golfers need.

4. **Can you manage your cataracts in other ways?**
   People who decide to delay cataract surgery can make certain adjustments to improve their vision, such as installing brighter lighting and contrasting colours in their home or office, wearing polarized sunglasses and a wide-brimmed hat to reduce glare, and using magnifying glasses to make reading easier.

These few basic queries will help to determine if seeking surgical aid for cataracts is appropriate for individual people. For those who are drivers it is accepted that surgery can wait if visual acuity still remains within legal requirements (20/40 in the best eye in most countries) and they feel that the condition is not disrupting their lives. These patients should be advised to continue regular monitoring that can be once or twice a year and to seek an earlier consultation if they notice their vision decreases (Fig. 1).

Stage of Cataract Development

Some patients might have the perception that surgery is only possible after a certain stage of cataract development. This belief comes from the fact that prior to modern phacoemulsification, cataract surgery (either intracapsular or extracapsular lens extraction) was associated with much higher risks and less predictable outcomes. Surgeons previously advised delaying surgery until advanced stages [6]. This approach is no longer in practice, as with modern surgery the cataractous lens

Fig. 1 Pictures that simulate the impact of different stages of cataract in a driver.On the top (1) vision of the road without any cataract present. In the middle (2) mild to moderate stage of cataract but vision still remains over legal driving requirements, surgery at this stage can be delayed. Bottom image (3) showed an advance stage of cataract and now the vision is under legal driving requirements, surgery in this case is required

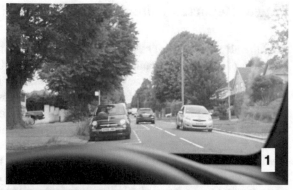

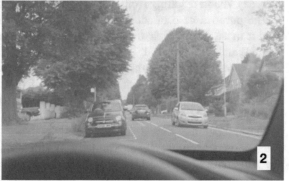

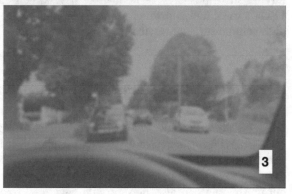

can be removed at any stage. In fact, even a transparent crystalline lens can be removed safely as is done for angle closure glaucoma (clear lens extraction) [7]. Once a cataract develops there is a case to not delay surgery too long as very dense cataracts (rock-hard, brunescent, black) are more difficult for phacoemulsification and are associated with an increased risk of complications. In addition, there are certain cataract types which can develop faster such as posterior subcapsular or intumescent, and patients should be informed that significant dropping in vision may occur over just a few months.

Patient Reported Outcome Measures (PROMs)

Traditionally visual acuity (VA) has been used as a measure of the impact of cataract on a person's vision and a guide or even determinant of the need for surgery. VA charts were developed for purposes of assessing and correcting refractive error and the limitations of VA in the context of cataract assessment are well recognised [8]. One important limitation is that VA is a measure of the performance of only one eye at a time, VA measured with both eyes open being mostly a reflection of the VA in the better eye. In a complex and mobile real-world visual environment, the 100% black on white contrast target of VA fails to capture: losses of contrast sensitivity; disturbances of colour perception; losses of stereopsis; interference to everyday vision resulting from one eye having poor vision; and glare.

The purpose of cataract surgery is to improve vision for patients where they need it most, i.e. in their own everyday environments. In the contexts of 'patient centred' and 'value based' care, a whole-person measure is required for capture of the impact of cataract on people's everyday 'lived experience' of their vision. To capture this information a structured set of questions formulated as a patient reported outcome measure or PROM is needed. Visual difficulty can be measured both before and after surgery using PROMs, allowing measurement of self-reported preoperative visual difficulty and its relief from surgery, i.e. morbidity, outcome and benefit gained. Similarly, health economic analyses which underpin value-based care and justify expenditure of public money on cataract surgery rely on such measures. A number of psychometrically well performing cataract PROMs exist and constitute a key requirement for service improvement in busy high-volume surgical services [8–10].

Age and Unilateral Versus Bilateral Surgery

Other factors to consider when offering surgery are age and status of the contralateral eye. With an increasingly ageing population it is important to recognise the benefits to very elderly people of undergoing cataract surgery, there is ample evidence of favourable outcomes to support this practice [11]. Young patients without presbyopia can also present with cataracts, frequently secondary to trauma, uveitis, steroids, post retinal detachment surgery, and previous congenital cataracts that have progressed. In individuals leading an active life, who may also have demanding work requirements, surgery may be required at earlier stages of cataract development. Despite the possibility of relatively good visual acuity, the impact of cataracts on their activities can be significant. When planning surgery in young patients (either unilateral or bilateral), thorough counselling regarding the loss of accommodation with monofocal intraocular lenses should be provided. When dealing with unilateral cataracts using a monofocal lens, it is common practice to aim for mild myopia (−0.5 to −1.0 dioptres) to compensate the lack of accommodation. This approach may work similarly to mini-monovision when the healthy eye is emmetropic or patients are able to wear a unilateral contact lens. Mini-monovision has proved to be effective in presbyopics for tasks like computer work or looking at a mobile phone screen, without compromising stereopsis [12]. Unilateral multifocal intraocular lenses remain controversial, although successful reports exist following careful selection and counselling regarding glare and halos to prevent dissatisfaction [13, 14]. In the presence of bilateral cataracts, the threshold for second eye surgery independently of age is usually lower than the first eye due to the need to restore binocular balance and to correct anisometropia. Surgery for the second eye is normally performed a few weeks after the first eye once recovery of the first operated eye has been confirmed. In most centres, patients require only one preoperative assessment when surgery is planned for both eyes and in uncomplicated cases postoperative follow-up can be made by a trained ophthalmic nurse or optometrist instead of an ophthalmologist. Immediately sequential bilateral cataract surgery (ISBCS) offers the shortest visual rehabilitation however it has not been adopted as a standard treatment mainly due to concerns regarding the theoretical risk of bilateral endophthalmitis [15, 16].

Timing of Surgery in the Presence of AMD

Many patients are afflicted by both cataracts and age-related macular degeneration (AMD). While both conditions decrease visual acuity, cataracts can be "cured" by surgery. Exudative neovascular AMD can also be treated nowadays by intravitreal anti-vascular endothelial growth factor injections (Anti-VGEF) with effective results compared with the pre anti-VGEF era [17, 18]. Dry AMD however has no effective treatment but progression until geographic atrophy is usually very slow. In AMD patients, cataract surgery can equally be offered when cataracts become visually significant, but patients should be warned regarding realistic visual prognosis according to their stage of macula disease. Multiple studies have demonstrated that cataract surgery can improve visual acuity significantly in patients affected by AMD [18–20]. Even in wet AMD accompanied by retinal fluid on OCT cataract surgery has been shown as effective without worsening of the underlying neovascular process [20, 21]. Therefore surgery can be offered to AMD patients who are undergoing intravitreal treatment and additionally removal of the opaque lens will improve visualisation of the retina. Similarly, this applies to other retinal conditions like diabetic retinopathy or choroidal tumours when adequate visualisation is paramount for diagnosis and treatment. Cataract surgery in patients undergoing anti-VGEF therapy is recommended to be done at least two weeks apart from intravitreal injections [19, 20].

Narrow Angles and Angle Closure Glaucoma

Angle closure disease is recognised as a significant health issue particularly in China and Asian countries. These populations are prone to develop occludable angles. An increase of more than 50% in the incidence of angle closure glaucoma (ACG) is predicted by 2040 [22]. Crystalline lens thickness increases as part of ageing and angle closure becomes more likely in predisposed eyes with narrow angles. Cataract surgery deepens the anterior chamber and mechanically opens the iridocorneal angle, simultaneously lowers the intraocular pressure by increasing aqueous outflow [23, 24]. The benefits of early cataract surgery and clear lens extraction (CLE) in early glaucoma have been documented in various studies [24–27]. CLE has also been proved to be superior to laser peripheral iridotomy (PI) in angle closure both for ocular pressure control and patient reported quality of life [26]. However, in patients with clear lens and narrow angles without the presence of glaucoma or a pressure above 30 mmHg the benefit of clear lens extraction (CLE) against traditional laser peripheral iridotomy has not been clearly demonstrated [25]. Among the drawbacks for CLE in this group of patients is the unpredictable refractive outcome as large deviations from the target refraction have been reported [26]. Emmetropia becomes more difficult to achieve in these eyes because of the anatomical features including short axial length, shallow anterior chamber and an anteriorly positioned lens. On these grounds, patients with narrow angles and glaucoma who present with cataracts can be considered for early removal.

Fuchs Corneal Endothelial Dystrophy

The presence of a cataract in patients with Fuchs endothelial corneal dystrophy (FECD) introduces a challenge as cataract surgery which is expected to improve vision can also trigger corneal decompensation. In addition, blurred vision, glare and loss of contrast sensitivity may be caused by corneal deterioration but can also be simply signs of cataract development. Traditionally central corneal thickness (CCT), endothelial cell density and less commonly corneal back scatter which correlate with disease severity have been proposed as factors that can help identify risk of corneal decompensation when cataract surgery is required. However, the predictive value of these data has not been found to be satisfactory for clinical decision making [28–30]. Moreover recent improvement in endothelial corneal transplantation techniques, specially Descemet membrane endothelial keratoplasty (DMEK), and the higher expectations for postoperative visual outcomes have motivated earlier interventions in these patients.

The decision whether to perform phacoemulsification alone versus a combined/staged procedure including endothelial keratoplasty is a common challenge as currently there are no simple indicators for prediction of corneal failure. In clinical practice the prognosis in these patients is frequently based on subjective clinical judgement. The American Academy of Ophthalmology preferred practice pattern identified among others a CCT greater than 640 microns as a risk factor for corneal decompensation following cataract surgery in FECD [31]. This criterion still remains a commonly adopted cut-off value for decision making whether to perform cataract surgery alone or in combination with keratoplasty despite emerging novel scoring systems based on Scheimpflug imaging [30, 32]. But regardless of the corneal thickness, the presence of central confluent guttata with an undulating posterior corneal surface can degrade visual quality significantly and combined/staged surgery with endothelial keratoplasty could be recommended in these cases [29].

As there is also a correlation between endothelial cell loss and surgical time, lens density and ultrasound power, in the presence of visually significant cataract early intervention is often advocated in FECD [33]. Clinicians should however remember that even patients in whom only cataract surgery is planned must be warned about the possibility of requiring endothelial keratoplasty to obtain full visual rehabilitation. In order to minimise the risk of corneal decompensation a cohesive-dispersive soft-shell technique may be helpful when cataract surgery is performed in patients with FECD [34].

Previous Corneal Transplantation

Patients with cataracts and previous corneal transplantation should have a similar approach for those with FECD or other conditions with low endothelial cell density [35, 36]. Because endothelial keratoplasty is uncommon in phakic patients, most corneal graft patients requiring cataract surgery may have previously had either penetrating keratoplasty (PK) or deep anterior lamellar keratoplasty (DALK). Multiple studies have shown that phacoemulsification and intraocular lens implantation in patients with well-functioning grafts is similarly safe and effective as in eyes without grafts [36, 37]. History of previous rejection episodes (which in DALK endothelial rejection is absent), as well as central corneal thickness and endothelial cell density should be assessed in order to determine the risk of postoperative graft failure and the impact on long-term graft survival.

In any type of corneal graft if the transparency is good enough for safe phacoemulsification, earlier rather than late-stage cataract intervention would allow for lower phaco power. Incisions that compromise graft host junction should be avoided in which case scleral tunnel incisions should be constructed. Low bottle height is preferable as it has been shown that lower IOP intraoperatively is less harmful to the corneal endothelium [38]. Other factors to be considered in the preoperative surgical plan include, anterior chamber depth, iris configuration, integrity of the zonules, biometry, and refractive outcome. In the presence of high cylinder or irregular astigmatism regardless of corneal transparency triple procedure with repeat PK, open sky extracapsular cataract extraction (ECCE) and IOL implantation may be preferable. Intraoperatively, viscoelastic soft-shell technique is helpful to minimise endothelial cell loss, but patients should be warned about the possibility of endothelial failure. Finally in the event of postoperative corneal graft failure, modern techniques of Decemet membrane endothelial keratoplasty (DMEK) and Descemet stripping automated endothelial keratoplasty (DSAEK) have been shown to be effective to restore the transparency of the graft [39].

References

1. Schein OD, Cassard SD Tielsch JM et al. Cataract surgery among medicare beneficiaries. Ophthalmic Epidemiol. 2012;19(5):257–64.
2. Tseng VL, Yu F, Coleman AL. Risk of fractures following cataract surgery in medicare beneficiaries. JAMA. 2012;308(5):493–501.
3. Meulernes LB, Hendrie D, Lee AH, et al. The effectiveness of cataract surgery in reducing motor vehicle crashes: a whole population study using linked data. Ophthalmic Epidemiol. 2012;19(1):23–8.
4. Fong C, Mitchell P, Rochtchina, et al. Correction of visual impairment by cataract surgery and improved survival in older persons. The Blue mountains eye study cohort. Ophthalmology. 2013;120:1720–7.
5. The American Academy of Ophthalmology. When is the right time to have cataract surgery? June 02, 2015.
6. Venkatesh R, Muralikrishnan R, Balent LC, et al. Outcomes of high volume cataract surgeries in a developing country. Br J Ophthalmol. 2005;89(9):1079–83.
7. Traverso CE. Clear lens extraction as a treatment for primary angle closure. Lancet. 2016;388(10052):1352–4.
8. Sparrow JM, Grzeda MT, Frost NA, Johnston RL, Liu CSC, Edwards L, et al. Cat-PROM5: a brief psychometrically robust self-report questionnaire instrument for cataract surgery. Eye (Lond). 2018;32(4):796–805.
9. McAlinden C, Gothwal VK, Khadka J, Wright TA, Lamoureux EL, Pesudovs K. A head-to-head comparison of 16 cataract surgery outcome questionnaires. Ophthalmology. 2011;118(12):2374–81.
10. Sparrow JM, Grzeda MT, Frost NA, Johnston RL, Liu CSC, Edwards L, et al. Cataract surgery patient-reported outcome measures: a head-to-head comparison of the psychometric performance and patient acceptability of the Cat-PROM5 and Catquest-9SF self-report questionnaires. Eye (Lond). 2018;32(4):788–95.
11. Theodoropoulou S, Grzeda MT, Donachie PHJ, Johnston RL, Sparrow JM, Tole DM. The Royal College of Ophthalmologists' National Ophthalmology Database Study of cataract surgery. Report 5: clinical outcome and risk factors for posterior capsule rupture and visual acuity loss following cataract surgery in patients aged 90 years and older. Eye (Lond). 2019;33(7):1161–70.
12. Wilkins MR, Allan BD, Rubin GS, et al. Randomized trial of multifocal intraocular lenses versus monovision after bilateral cataract surgery. Ophthalmology. 2013;120:2449–55.
13. Levinger E, Levinger S, Mimouni M, et al. Unilateral refractive lens exchange with a multifocal intraocular lens in emmetropic presbyopic patients. Curr Eye Res. 2019;44(7):726–32.
14. Alio JL, Plaza-Puche AB, Fernandez-Buenaga R, Maldonado M. Multifocal intraocular lenses: an overview. Surv Ophthalmol. 2017;62:611–34.
15. Arshinoff SA, Bastianelli PA. Incidence of postoperative endophthalmitis after immediate sequential bilateral cataract surgery. J Cataract Refract Surg. 2011;37(12):2105–14.
16. O'Brien JJ, Gonder J, Botz C, Chow KY, Arshinoff SA. Immediately sequential bilateral cataract surgery versus delayed sequential bilateral cataract surgery: potential hospital cost savings. Can J Ophthalmol. 2010;45(6):596–601.

17. Bloch SB, Larsen M, Munch IC. Incidence of legal blindness from age-related macular degeneration in Denmark: year 2000 to 2010. Am J Ophthalmol. 2012;153(2):209–13. e2. https://doi.org/10.1016/j.ajo.2011.10.016.

18. Teh BL, Megaw R, Shyamanga Borooah S, et al. Optimizing cataract surgery in patients with age-related macular degeneration. Surv Ophthalmol. 2017;62:346–56.

19. Starr MR, Mahr MA, Barkmeier AJ, et al. Outcomes of cataract surgery in patients with exudative age-related macular degeneration and macular fluid. Am J Ophthalmol. 2018;192:91–7.

20. Kessel L, Koefoed T, Torben L, et al. Cataract surgery in patients with neovascular age-related macular degeneration. Acta Ophthalmol. 2016;94:755–60.

21. Casparis H, Lindsley K, Kuo IC, Sikder S, Bressler NM. Surgery for cataracts in people with age-related macular degeneration. Cochrane Database Syst Rev. 2017;2:CD006757. https://doi.org/10.1002/14651858.cd006757.

22. Tham YC, Li X, Wong TY, Quigley HA, Aung T, Cheng CY. Global prevalence of glaucoma and projections of glaucoma burden through 2040: a systematic review and meta-analysis. Ophthalmology. 2014;121(11):2081–90.

23. Young CE, Seibold L, Kahook M. Cataract surgery and intraocular pressure in glaucoma. Curr Opin Ophthalmol. Publish Ahead of Print, November 04, 2019. https://doi.org/10.1097/icu.0000000000000623.

24. Tarongoy P, Ho CL, Walton DS. Angle-closure glaucoma: the role of the lens in the pathogenesis, prevention, and treatment. Surv Ophthalmol. 2009;54(2):211–25.

25. Razeghinejad MR, Myers JS. Contemporary approach to the diagnosis and management of primary angle-closure disease. Surv Ophthalmol. 2018;63:754–68.

26. Day AC, Cooper D, Burr J, et al. Clear lens extraction for the management of primary angle closure glaucoma: surgical technique and refractive outcomes in the EAGLE cohort. Br J Ophthalmol. 2018;102:1658–62. https://doi.org/10.1136/bjophthalmol-2017-311447.

27. Azuara-Blanco A, Burr J, Ramsay C, et al. Effectiveness of early lens extraction for the treatment of primary angle-closure glaucoma (EAGLE): a randomised controlled trial. Lancet. 2016;388:1389–97.

28. Van Cleynenbreugel H, Remeijer L, Hillenaar T. Cataract surgery in patients with Fuchs' endothelial corneal dystrophy: when to consider a triple procedure. Ophthalmology. 2014;121(2):445–53.

29. Wacker K, McLaren JW, Amin SR, Baratz KH, Patel SV. Corneal high-order aberrations and backscatter in Fuchs' endothelial corneal dystrophy. Ophthalmology. 2015;122(8):1645–52.

30. Arnalich-Montiel F, Mingo-Botin D, Dearriba Palomero P. Preoperative risk assessment for progression to descemet membrane endothelial keratoplasty following cataract surgery in Fuchs endothelial corneal dystrophy. Am J Ophthalmol. 2019;208:76–86.

31. Olson RJ, Braga-Mele R, Chen SH, et al. Cataract in the adult eye preferred practice pattern! Ophthalmology. 2017;124(2):P1–119.

32. Patel SV, Hodge DO, Treichel EJ, et al. Predicting the prognosis of fuchs endothelial corneal dystrophy by using Scheimpflug tomography. Ophthalmology Article in Press: Corrected Proof.

33. Storr-Paulsen A, Norregaard JC, Ahmed S, et al. Endothelial cell damage after cataract surgery: divide-and-conquer versus phaco-chop technique. J Cataract Refract Surg. 2008;34(6):996–1000.

34. Arshinoff SA. Dispersive-cohesive viscoelastic soft shell technique. J Cataract Refract Surg. 1999;25(2):167–73.

35. Krysik K, Dobrowolski D, Wroblewska-Czajka E, et al. Comparison of the techniques of secondary intraocular lens implantation after penetrating keratoplasty. J Ophthalmol. 2018; Article ID 3271017, 8 pages. https://doi.org/10.1155/2018/3271017.

36. Acar BT, Utine CA, Acar S, et al. Endothelial cell loss after phacoemulsification in eyes with previous penetrating keratoplasty, previous deep anterior lamellar keratoplasty, or no previous surgery. J Cataract Refract Surg. 2011;37(2013–2017):22.

37. Den S, Shimura S, Shimazaki J. Cataract surgery after deep anterior lamellar keratoplasty in age and disease matched eyes. J Cataract Refract Surg. 2018;44:496–503.
38. Suzuki H, Oki K, Shiwa T, et al. Effect of bottle height on the corneal endothelium during phacoemulsification. J Cataract Refract Surg. 2009;35(11):2014–7.
39. Pasari A, Price MO, Feng MT, et al. Descemet endothelial keratoplasty for failed penetrating keratoplasty: visual outcomes and graft survival. Cornea. 2019;38:151–6.

Risk Stratification

Ahmed Shalaby Bardan, Christopher Liu and John Sparrow

What is risk stratification? Simply, not all cases of cataracts are the same and some cases will be more prone to develop complications because of the technical difficulty and/or structural weakness of tissues (for example, the pseudo-exfoliation cataract with poorly dilating pupil, weak zonules, and association with glaucoma). These are called high risk cases. Risk stratification is a tool for identifying or predicting which patients are at high risk of surgical complications, in this case in cataract surgery. By analysing a large database of patients undergoing cataract surgery, counting incidence of complications and studying the characteristics of affected patients and their eyes, it has been possible to quantify risks related to various risk factors [1].

The importance of being able to quantify the cumulative risk for a given risk profile is twofold. Firstly, patients can be given bespoke information regarding the risk of this complication arising during their cataract operation, so that the consent process is properly informed and patients may make better judgements on the 'risk to benefit' ratio for themselves, and secondly, surgical teams can adopt strategies to reduce the risk for high-risk individuals by ensuring, for example, that an experienced senior surgeon performs the operations for high-risk cases.

Case complexity, or case mix, in cataract surgery has become even more important in the current decade as there is a trend towards creaming off routine cases

A. Shalaby Bardan
Department of Ophthalmology, Faculty of Medicine, Alexandria University, Alexandria, Egypt

Brighton and Sussex University Hospitals NHS Trust, Brighton, UK

C. Liu (✉)
Sussex Eye Hospital, Brighton, UK
e-mail: cscliu@aol.com

Tongdean Eye Clinic, Hove, UK

J. Sparrow
Department of Ophthalmology, Bristol Eye Hospital, Bristol, UK

© Springer Nature Switzerland AG 2021
C. Liu and A. Shalaby Bardan (eds.), *Cataract Surgery*,
https://doi.org/10.1007/978-3-030-38234-6_3

for waiting list initiatives and for treatment centres. These routine cases will take less time to carry out. Surgeons operating on these could be less competent and yet would still have good outcome statistics. Traditional NHS providers may then be left with more complex cases, not just from the point of view of the eye. This will have a deleterious effect on both hospital and surgeon statistics. The cost per case also will be higher (more time, increased use of more expensive devices, higher risk of complications requiring vitrectomy equipment, higher risk of retinal detachment and endophthalmitis requiring further admission and treatment, etc.).

The same surgeon may have different statistics in different NHS hospitals and in private hospitals because of the difference in case mix. And it goes without saying that the best surgeons specialising in complex cases may have poor statistics compared with their less able peers because of the case mix. The Royal College of Ophthalmologists' National Ophthalmology Database (NOD) has partially tackled this problem by introducing case complexity adjustment models from historical data which will be reviewed every few years. It aims at adjusting for the complexity of a surgeon's or Centre's case load, so as to have as fair as possible comparisons. This will give credit for taking on complex operations and no benefit from avoidance of doing difficult cases.

NOD was established to provide national audit and research data, and to provide an evidence base for revalidation standards allowing Ophthalmologists to compare their surgical outcomes with those of their anonymised peers. The NOD audit collects data on cataract surgery performed in England and Wales and provides individual surgeons, healthcare providers and the public with benchmarked reports on performance, with the aim of improving the care provided to patients.

Risk of Posterior Capsule Rupture or Vitreous Loss or Both

Posterior capsular rupture or vitreous loss or both (abbreviated in the NOD as PCR), is the most common intraoperative complication during cataract surgery. It is important as it is associated with the need for additional surgical procedures, a greater number of follow-up visits and increased frequency of postoperative complications, which may adversely affect the final visual outcome. It is widely regarded as the benchmark complication to judge the quality of cataract surgery. As the overall rate of PCR is low, prospective identification of preoperative risk factors for PCR is difficult but, if achieved, has the potential to improve informed consent for patients and for surgeons to modify their surgical strategies.

A prospective cohort study of 55,567 participants found that those with the following preoperative characteristics had higher odds of developing PCR during cataract surgery (see Table 1) [2].

When compared with those operated on by a consultant, people who were operated on by a surgeon in training, e.g. fellow or trainees had higher odds of developing PCR during cataract surgery but could not differentiate the odds for associate specialist or staff grade surgeons.

Table 1 Preoperative characteristics and odds ratio of developing PCR

Risk factor	Adjusted OR (95% CI)
Male	1.10 (1.03, 1.18)
80–89	1.15 (1.01, 1.32)
Pupil medium	1.21 (1.09, 1.34)
Glaucoma	1.23 (1.10, 1.38)
Previous vitrectomy	1.40 (1.10, 1.79)
90+	1.56 (1.30, 1.88)
Senior trainee (Fellow and SPR)	1.71 (1.59, 1.85)
No fundal view/vitreous opacities	1.72 (1.33, 2.22)
Pupil small	1.72 (1.48, 1.99)
Other	1.83 (1.60, 2.10)
pseudoexfoliation syndrome/phacodonesis	2.51 (2.07, 3.04)
Junior trainee	2.85 (2.53, 3.20)
Brunescent/white cataract	3.36 (2.95, 3.82)

Regarding age, they found that when compared with those aged under 60 at the time of surgery, people over 70 had higher odds of developing PCR during cataract surgery but could not differentiate the odds for ages 60–69. [2]

The same study reported that people who used doxazosin or were unable to lie flat for the operation had higher odds of developing PCR during cataract surgery. [2]

Risk Stratification Tools

There exists a number of risk stratification scoring tools that use risk of PCR as the main complication related to the presence of a risk factor. Muhtaseb, et al. and Habib et al. have made an excellent start with demonstrating that a simple scoring system works for predicting per-operative complications in cataract surgery. Both systems are based on the same principle of allocating points for individual risk factors thought to increase the likelihood of a complication during surgery. The points are then summated to provide an overall score for each patient preoperative-ly-that is, a potential complication score. The points allocated to each risk factor using each system are shown in Table 1.

Both methods utilize data that is easily assessed in an outpatient setting without necessitating further investigations [3, 4] (Table 2).

Another scoring system was published by Najjar and Awwad [5]. Moderate-quality evidence from 1 retrospective cohort study of 1,883 participants found that those with a cataract risk score of >6 as determined using the Najjar-Awwad risk stratification algorithm have a clinically meaningfully increased risk of complications during cataract surgery.

Table 2 Point allocation for risk factors using Muhtaseb's [3] and Habib's [4] scoring systems

Risk factor	Score allocated	
	Muhtaseb's scoring system	Habib's scoring system
Miscellaneous risk assessed by the surgeon (e.g., poor position of eye/patient)	1	–
Unable to lie flat (spinal deformity, asthma, heart failure)	–	1
Severe anxiety	–	1
Head tremor	–	1
Previous angle closure glaucoma	–	1
History of complication in fellow eye	–	1
Previous vitrectomy	1	1
Corneal scarring/cloudiness	1	1
Shallow anterior chamber	1	1
Poor pupillary dilation and/or posterior synechiae	1	1
Pseudoexfoliation	3	1
Phacodonesis/weak zonules	3	1
High ametropia (>6 D myopia or hyperopia)	1	–
High myopia (axial length>27 mm)	–	1
High hypermetropia (axial length<20 mm)	–	1
Age>88 years	1	–
Nuclear density grade 1–2	–	1
Nuclear density grade 3	–	2
Mature/brunescent/white/dense/total cataract	3	3
Posterior capsule plaque	1	–
Posterior polar cataract	1	–

Muhtaseb et al. describe the additional step of arranging patients into risk groups, where patients scoring 0 are in group 1, patients scoring 1–2 are in group 2, patients scoring 3–5 are in group 3, and patients scoring ≥ 6 are in group 4

The NOD undertook an analysis involving around 180,000 cataract operations and identified a set of risk factors which are used to risk adjust surgeon and Centre outcomes in the National Cataract Audit. Based on these analyses risk models were produced for both intraoperative PCR (as defined above) and Vision Loss associated with cataract surgery (a doubling or worse of the visual angle from before to after the surgery) [6]. These risk models are freely available to registered surgeons on the NOD website in the form of downloadable spreadsheet calculators (https://www.nodaudit.org.uk/analysis). The advantages of their use for patients, surgeons and service providers have been noted above (Table 3).

Table 3 Risk factors used in the National Ophthalmology Database (NOD) Audit for case complexity adjustment of surgeon and Centre outcomes

PCR	VA loss
Person and eye	
Grade of surgeon	Pre-operative VA
Age	Age
Index of multiple deprivation	PCR
Not able to lie flat	
Sex	
Eye treated (1st vs. 2nd)	
Presence of an ocular co-pathology	
Amblyopia	Age-related macular degeneration
Brunescent/white cataract	Amblyopia
Diabetic retinopathy	Corneal pathology
High myopia	Diabetic retinopathy
No fundal view/vitreous opacities	Glaucoma
Optic nerve/CNS disease	High myopia
Other macular pathology	Inherited eye disease
Previous trabeculectomy	Other macular pathology
Psuedoexfoliation/phacodenesis	Other retinal pathology
Unspecified other co-pathology	Previous vitrectomy surgery
	Unspecified other co-pathology

Shortcomings of the Current Risk Stratification Tools

Scoring systems available use binary questions for individual risk factors rather than a grading system. There are time consuming factors which can increase the time needed for surgery but not the difficulty, like difficult patient positioning for example which can push up theatre time as opposed to actual surgical time and difficulty.

The surgical ability is an important factor not entirely dependent on the surgeon's grade. Some trainees have very high surgical skills that surpass some of the consultants.

It is also noteworthy that other factors can affect outcomes of cataract surgery for example; quality of biometry, pre-assessment, experience, caliber and harmony of ward and theatre staff, the standard of equipment, adequate maintenance of equipment, quality of devices, cleaning and sterilisation, and so on.

Recommendations

Consider using a validated risk stratification algorithm for people who have been referred for cataract surgery, to identify people at increased risk of complications during and after surgery.

Explain the results of the risk stratification to the person and discuss how it may affect their decisions.

To minimise the risk of complications during and after surgery, ensure that surgeons in training are closely supervised in terms of case selection and operative oversight. More experienced trainees should have their case complexity gradually increased towards higher complexity surgery in line with their skills development. Extreme caution should be adopted in regard to people for whom the impact of complications would be especially severe (for example, people with only one functional eye).

Assign the more difficult cases to a more experienced consultant and allocate extra time in the operating theatre. Using case complexity adjustment models will ensure fair comparisons.

Explain to people who are at risk of developing a dense cataract that there is an increased risk of complications if surgery is delayed too long and the cataract becomes very dense.

References

1. Liu C. Risk stratification for the humble cataract. Br J Ophthalmol. 2004;88(10):1232–3.
2. Narendran N, Jaycock P, Johnston RL, et al. The Cataract National Dataset electronic multi-centre audit of 55,567 operations: risk stratification for posterior capsule rupture and vitreous loss. Eye (Lond). 2009;23(1):31–37.
3. Muhtaseb M, Kalhoro A, Ionides A. A system for preoperative stratification of cataract patients according to risk of intraoperative complications: a prospective analysis of 1441 cases. Br J Ophthalmol. 2004;88(10):1242–6.
4. Habib MS, Bunce CV, Fraser SG. The role of case mix in the relation of volume and outcome in phacoemulsification. Br J Ophthalmol. 2005;89(9):1143–6.
5. Najjar DM, Awwad ST. Cataract surgery risk score for residents and beginning surgeons. J Cataract Refract Surg. 2003;29(10):2035–6.
6. The National Ophthalmology Database (NOD). https://www.nodaudit.org.uk/. Accessed 20 Nov 2019.

Choice of Anaesthesia

Richard M. H. Lee and Tom Eke

The term 'anaesthesia' is used to describe techniques to control the patient's pain and unwanted movement during surgery. For the eye surgeon, the main components are *analgesia* (reduction or elimination of pain) and *akinesia* (reduction or elimination of movement). General anaesthesia techniques (involving loss of consciousness, and amnesia) were first discovered in the mid 1800s, and local anaesthesia (allowing painless surgery with the patient awake) in the late 1800s. Prior to this, surgeons (including cataract surgeons) needed strong assistants to hold the patient as still as possible, and relied on alcohol and/or plant extracts in an attempt to minimise surgical pain and its associated movements. The first recorded modern use of local anaesthetic was in 1884, with cocaine extract used for eye surgery. By the end of 1884, eye surgeons had already described using cocaine for retrobulbar, peribulbar, sub-Tenon's, topical and topical-intracameral anaesthesia [1]. These techniques have been refined and improved, though the principles remain the same. Patient anxiety, if present, can be controlled with anxiolytic medications and/or intravenous sedation.

In the United Kingdom (UK) and many other countries, the vast majority of cataract surgery is done using local anaesthesia (LA) techniques. However, there will always be patients who are unsuitable for standard LA, and these patients may need general anaesthesia (GA), or intravenous (IV) sedation, or specialized LA techniques. The process of preparing a patient for surgery should include the choice of anaesthesia, and this process should be a team effort involving the surgeon, nursing and theatre staff. An anaesthetist (anesthesiologist) is mandatory for

R. M. H. Lee (✉)
Chelsea and Westminster Hospital, London, UK
e-mail: richard.lee1@chelwest.nhs.uk

T. Eke
Norfolk and Norwich University Hospital, Norwich, UK

© Springer Nature Switzerland AG 2021
C. Liu and A. Shalaby Bardan (eds.), *Cataract Surgery*,
https://doi.org/10.1007/978-3-030-38234-6_4

cataract cases requiring GA or IV sedation, and many other LA cases will benefit from (or require) the assistance of an anaesthetist. The choice and provision of anesthesia is the subject of UK national guidelines on cataract surgery and intraocular surgery [2–4]. Some other countries have national guidelines for cataract surgery that include mention of anaesthesia, but the UK is presently the only country to have a national guideline dedicated to LA for intraocular surgery [3].

Brief Description of Techniques

The techniques are described in brief, as there is no substitute to hands-on learning from an experienced practitioner.

General anaesthesia (GA). For much of the 20th century, GA was used for the majority of cataract surgery. General anaesthesia should give 'perfect' operating conditions, in that the patient is unconscious with no memory of the surgery (amnesia) and the globe is free of movement (akinetic). For surgical training, GA allows free conversation between trainer and trainee, because the patient cannot overhear the discussions. For example, the trainer can point out the dangers of a surgical manoeuvre, without risk of causing the patient distress. However, a GA approach uses a large amount of resources, in terms of time, personnel, and use of hospital beds and has its own risk profile including life threatening complications. Improved surgical techniques have therefore allowed LA to become the default anaesthetic technique for cataract surgery nowadays [3].

General anaesthesia is now reserved for cataract patients who really need it—for example children, patients with severe psychological/emotional problems, patients with learning difficulties or dementia who cannot co-operate, extreme anxiety, uncontrolled movement disorders, etc. While many GA cataract patients can now be managed as day-cases, it is often necessary to keep a GA patient in hospital overnight following surgery. Discussion of the necessary preparation and technique of GA is beyond the scope of this chapter.

Retro-bulbar anaesthesia (RBA). This technique tends to be mentioned first in lists of LA techniques, partly because it was the main LA technique used for the first part of the 20th century. RBA provides good analgesia, and the extra-ocular muscles are blocked, thereby providing good akinesia in addition. However, RBA is also considered to be the LA technique that carries the highest risk of sight-threatening or life-threatening complications. Serial national surveys show that RBA has largely fallen out of use for cataract surgery in the UK [5] although RBA is still widely used in some other countries. In 2017, the UK National Institute for Health and Care Excellence (NICE) published a guideline on Cataract in Adults, which stated 'do not offer RBA for people having cataract surgery' [4].

The technique of RBA involves using a sharp needle to inject the LA into the orbit, behind the eyeball [6]. Another term for RBA is the 'intra-conal' LA block, because the needle tip is aimed behind the eyeball, within the 'cone' of the four rectus muscles. The technique gives good analgesia and akinesia, albeit with a small risk of serious complications. The main 'sight-threatening' complications are needle damage to the globe or optic nerve, or severe arterial bleeding into the orbit. The risk of globe perforation is much increased with larger (myopic) eye-balls, posterior staphyloma, abnormal globe-orbit relationship, longer needles, and gaze directed away from the needle. Needle damage to the optic nerve may also cause partial or complete blindness. Vision may be lost due to a vascular occlusion or without obvious cause ('wipe-out'). Inadvertent injection of LA under the coverings of the optic nerve will allow the LA to track back to the brain. This 'brainstem anaesthesia' can present within seconds or minutes of RBA, with loss of consciousness, apnoea, epileptic fitting, labile blood pressure and hypotension. With immediate life support and transfer to an intensive care unit, most patients will recover [3].

Peri-bulbar anaesthesia (PBA). In this technique, a sharp needle is also used for orbital injection but unlike with RBA, the needle is aimed away from the eye-ball and muscle cone—an 'extraconal' injection [6]. Again, there is a good sensory and motor 'block', providing good analgesia and akinesia. Some practitioners suggest using two injections, one from the infero-temporal orbit and another medially. However, the volume of the first injection may push the globe medially, and increase the likelihood of a globe perforation [7]. Many clinicians believe that PBA is less likely to cause severe complications, compared to RBA, though all of the sight-threatening and life-threatening complications of RBA have also been reported with PBA. A 1996 survey found that 2% of UK ophthalmologists had experienced a patient death due to LA—at that time, almost all LA had been either RBA or PBA [8].

For those few cataract patients who require a needle block to the orbit, PBA is preferred to RBA. The UK guidance from NICE is that most adult cataract patients should have either sub-Tenon's or topical LA (see sections below), but 'if both sub-Tenon's and topical (with or without intracameral) anaesthesia are contraindicated, consider peribulbar anaesthesia' [4]. Current advice for administering PBA is to use a short needle and to administer only one injection, which should be in the far infero-temporal quadrant or (preferably) via the medial canthal area [9].

Sub-Tenon's anaesthesia (STA). This technique uses a blunt cannula (non-needle approach) to deliver the LA to the retrobulbar space, thereby avoiding the risks inherent to needle LA blocks. Again, there can be a good block with analgesia and akinesia though larger volumes of LA (around 3.5 ml or more) are needed for akinesia. Many cataract surgeons feel that STA gives the best balance of globe akinesia, analgesia and patient satisfaction together with a low risk of anaesthetic complications. The 2013 UK national survey showed that STA was used for over 50% of LA cataract operations in the UK [5]. The 2017 NICE guideline states that UK surgeons should 'offer sub-Tenon's or topical (with or without intracameral) anaesthesia for people having cataract surgery' [4].

Most clinicians will use a specially designed metal sub-Tenon's cannula (e.g. Stevens or Eagle type), though it is possible to use other types of blunt metal cannulae, or the plastic part of an intravenous cannula. The blunt cannula means that the risks of needle blocks appear to be much reduced though not completely eliminated [10]. Cases of globe perforation have been described e.g. eyes with thin sclera, or attempted dissection in eyes with Tenon's scarring. If the metal cannula is directed very posteriorly, it can damage the short posterior ciliary arteries near to the optic nerve insertion, and cause ischemia of the optic nerve head or choroid. Advancing the metal cannula a little further still will risk optic nerve trauma and even brainstem anaesthesia: deaths have been reported with STA, as well as with sharp needle blocks.

Most clinicians will use spring-scissors to make a small 'snip' in the conjunctiva and Tenon's layer, in order to pass the cannula into the sub-Tenon's space. A good technique is to make the snip about 5 mm posterior to the limbus in the infero-nasal quadrant, exposing the bare sclera, and to pass the cannula just behind the equator before slowly injecting [11] (Fig. 1). Instead of using scissors, it is possible to make the initial hole with a pencil-point type instrument (e.g. lacrimal dilator or a 'conjunctival probe' (Blink Medical, Solihull, UK). Experienced clinicians may employ a 'no snip' STA technique, in which the metal cannula is pushed directly through conjunctiva and Tenon's, without the need for scissors or probe [12].

Topical anaesthesia (TA) and Topical-intracameral anaesthesia (TA-ICA). This means administering the LA topically, to the front of the eye. Most clinicians use LA eye-drops although it is also possible to use an LA gel [6]. Topical anesthesia means that all the risks of needle or STA blocks are avoided. However, there is no akinesia with TA, meaning that the eye may be mobile and this could potentially cause a surgical complication.

Topical anaesthesia is frequently augmented with additional LA that is placed into the anterior chamber at the start of surgery [13]. This is termed intra-cameral anaesthesia (ICA). The ICA can be given as a solution of lidocaine (which must be without preservative), or it can be combined with viscoelastic (e.g. Visthesia®, Carl Zeiss Meditec, Jena, Germany). Despite initial concerns, studies have shown that intracameral lidocaine is safe for the corneal endothelium [13].

Some practitioners will use a LA injection to block the facial nerve, in order to minimize lid squeezing with TA. With a modern lid speculum, a facial nerve block is usually unnecessary and many TA practitioners never use lid blocks. If a lid block is felt to be necessary, it is preferable to use the 'van Lint' block, which involves injection to the orbicularis muscle, behind the lateral orbital rim. More proximal blocks to the facial nerve (nearer to the ear) are more likely to have serious complications than the van Lint block.

If using gel for TA, then it is important to think about the efficacy of the pre-operative iodine solution. Iodine (or equivalent) is routinely used to sterilize the conjunctiva prior to surgery. However, if gel is used for TA then it may form a physical barrier to commensal bacteria and prevent the iodine from reaching them. Therefore, if using gel TA it is important to instill iodine prior to the gel, or alternatively one should rinse the gel carefully from the conjunctival fornices before applying the iodine. Most practitioners find it most expedient to simply use LA drops prior to instilling iodine and not use gel LA at all.

Fig. 1 Sub-Tenon's anaesthesia. **a** Instruments are round-ended spring scissors (e.g. Westcott) and conjunctival forceps (e.g. Moorfields). Local anaesthetic and iodine drops are instilled; a lid speculum may be used. A small cut (snip) is made in the conjunctiva & Tenon's layer, about 5mm behind the limbus, in the infero-nasal quadrant. This will expose the bare sclera and allow access to the sub-Tenon's space (**b**, **c**) the sub-Tenon's cannula is advanced, following the curvature of the sclera, to just behind the equator **d** local anaesthetic is slowly injected, and the cannula is withdrawn

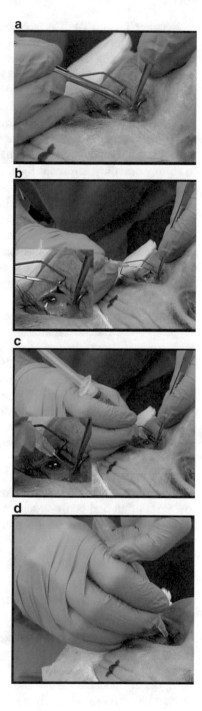

Because TA and TA-ICA techniques do not affect the extra-ocular muscles, it is possible for the eye to move during surgery. Surgeons can use this to their advantage by instructing the patient to keep looking toward the microscope light and this will help to minimise kinesia while keeping the eye 'on axis', facilitating the operation. This 'mobile eye' can be particularly useful for patients who cannot adopt a standard position under the operating microscope e.g. those with orthopnea or kyphosis. However, a small proportion of patients are unable to keep the eye still and in these rare cases it is possible to give additional anaesthesia via STA 'on the table'. If a TA patient complains that the light is too bright, it is usually adequate to simply dim the microscope light, then brighten it again after a minute or so.

There has been some debate as to whether TA may be associated with an increased rate of surgical complications, because of the potentially 'mobile eye'. Proponents of TA may argue that TA makes surgery easier, because a 'block' LA from STA or PBA may contribute to vitreous bulge, and the immobile eye may not be on axis. A review of publications that compared 'block' LA with TA or other 'kinetic' LA found no difference in posterior capsule rupture rates [14].

Subconjunctival LA. A subconjunctival injection of 0.5–1 ml of LA can be given by the surgeon at the start of cataract surgery. This technique was reasonably common when scleral tunnels were used for phacoemulsification. Now that most surgeons use clear corneal incisions, subconjunctival LA is rarely required for cataract surgery. The technique is useful for glaucoma surgery (e.g. trabeculectomy), in cases where akinesia is not required.

Anxiolytics, and intravenous sedation. It is to be expected that most or all patients will have a degree of anxiety regarding their cataract surgery. In most cases, this anxiety can be much reduced by a careful pre-operative explanation of the process of cataract surgery. Most patients appreciate having a person's hand to hold during the surgery, with instructions to 'squeeze my hand if you have any discomfort or concerns'.

Most patients can be managed with explanation, but some will need pharmacological anxiolysis or sedation. For anxiety, many patients will be happy with a low dose of an oral benzodiazepine (e.g. diazepam 5 mg). If intravenous sedation is required, then an anaesthetist must give this, with appropriate backup measures in place [3].

What Anaesthetic Drugs Can Be Used?

Lidocaine (previously known as lignocaine) is the mainstay drug for LA in eye surgery. It can be given as an injection for STA or PBA block. If used for ICA it is important that the lidocaine should be a preservative-free solution. Standard strengths of lidocaine are 1% and 2%. Bupivacaine has a longer period of action, so may be useful for blocks in cases that are expected to take a long time although this is rarely the case for cataract surgery. For TA, surgeons can use proxymetacaine (proparacaine), lidocaine, oxybuprocaine or tetracaine. However there is a risk of corneal epitheliopathy with tetracaine that may require surgery being post-poned to a later date [5].

Historically, adrenaline (epinephrine) was frequently added to the LA mixture for needle blocks. However, this gives no real advantage and could potentially cause ischaemia in vulnerable globes (e.g. some types of glaucoma, risking 'wipe-out') and therefore adrenaline is best avoided. Hyaluronidase is an enzyme that aids penetration of the LA mixture through the orbital tissues. It allows faster onset of akinesia, and appears to reduce the likelihood of extra-ocular muscle damage and diplopia following 'block' LA. However, patients can occasionally develop a severe orbital inflammation following the use of animal-derived hyaluronidase, and this can be sight-threatening [15]. In some countries (e.g. USA) it is possible to obtain hyaluronidase that is made with recombinant DNA technology, and this appears to have a much lower risk of hyaluronidase orbitopathy. The NICE guideline on cataract surgery [4] states 'Consider hyaluronidase as an adjunct to sub-Tenon's anaesthesia, particularly if trying to stop the eye moving during surgery' [4].

Intracameral lidocaine will dilate the pupil, though the effect is not sufficient to replace the pre-operative mydriatic drops in routine cataract surgery. Mixtures of lidocaine and mydriatics are more effective, though they take time to work (up to 90 s) and the pupil may not be as large as with standard pre-operative drops. A commercially available solution, Mydrane® (Thea Pharmaceuticals, Clermont-Ferrand, France), comprises lidocaine 1%, tropicamide 0.02% and phenylephrine 0.31% [16]. Some clinicians use Mydrane instead of pre-operative dilating drops and standard ICA, others use it in the management of small pupil and intra-operative floppy iris syndrome.

Complications of LA Techniques and Reducing the Risk

The main complications of LA have been discussed above: sharp needles can cause sight-threatening complications by needle penetration of globe or optic nerve, or severe arterial bleeding, known as orbital haemorrhage or retrobulbar haemorrhage [6]. Blunt-cannula STA will reduce but not eliminate this risk [6, 10]. Vascular occlusions have been reported with both PBA and STA [17]. Brainstem anaesthesia has been reported with sharp needle blocks but also with STA and deaths have occurred [18, 8]. LA techniques may also cause diplopia from direct damage to the muscle or toxicity towards the LA agent used. There are some patient characteristics that may increase the risk of sight-threatening LA complications and the clinician should be aware of these when choosing the anaesthesia for the patient.

Severe arterial bleeding (orbital haemorrhage) may occur with needle blocks. It presents as an increasing proptosis and hard orbit, usually with some obvious bleeding into the orbit or under the conjunctiva. Milder cases can be managed with counter-pressure to the orbit and observation. Some give osmotic agents such as acetazolamide or mannitol. More severe cases may require a lateral canthotomy and/or cantholysis [19]. This complication occurs almost exclusively with needle blocks, though it appears to be less likely if the needle is used in the far infero-temporal or medial approach [3]

Myopic eyes are usually significantly larger than average, as evidenced by the axial length measurement in the biometry printout. Clinicians should remember that these eyes are also wider than average and very myopic eyes are highly likely to have a posterior staphyloma [20]. These staphylomas are often in the infero-temporal part of the globe, meaning that highly myopic eyes are at a much greater risk of globe perforation when needle LA is used [21]. Therefore it would be preferable to avoid using a needle block for these eyes and if absolutely necessary, the medial canthal approach with a short needle should minimize the risk of perforation [9].

Eyes with scleral thinning and/or conjunctival scarring may be unsuitable for STA because of the risk of globe perforation. In eyes with progressive scarring problems (e.g. pemphigoid), STA should be avoided because it may exacerbate the scarring. Thin sclera (e.g. patients with rheumatoid disease or scleritis) could potentially be ruptured by a metal sub-Tenon's cannula [22]. If there has been previous squint surgery or retinal surgery, particularly if there has been a plomb or encircling band, it may be difficult or impossible to dissect the layers to give a STA block. Globe perforation has been described when attempting to dissect past an encircling band [23]. An encircling band may make the eyeball more 'hourglass shaped', mimicking or exacerbating the effect of a posterior staphyloma: thus eyes with previous encircling band may be 'higher risk' for sight-threatening complications of any type of 'block' LA.

One should also consider the relationship of the globe to the orbit. Older cataract patients may have a degree of enophthalmos, due to age-related atrophy of the orbital fat. Long-term glaucoma treatment with prostaglandin eye-drops can also cause this effect. Marked enophthamos, or any significant abnormality of the orbit, may make it difficult or impossible to give a sharp-needle LA safely via the traditional infero-nasal approach.

Patients with ocular movement disorders (e.g. nystagmus) may need a 'block' LA, in order to obtain globe akinesia during surgery. Some patients with congenital nystagmus may have a 'null position' of gaze that would allow TA but otherwise a 'block' LA may be necessary. If the patient has a significant head tremor or other movement disorder (e.g. Parkinson's disease) it may be possible to schedule LA surgery at the time of day that the tremor is minimal, or alternatively it may be necessary to use GA.

Orbital injections of LA could potentially cause orbital infection, by inoculating bacteria into the orbit through the LA needle/cannula. It is standard practice to instil iodine or similar bacteriocidal into the eye prior to cataract surgery to minimize the risk of endophthalmitis: to minimize the risk of orbital infection, this iodine should be instilled prior to any trans-conjunctival LA. In practice, severe orbital inflammation after LA appears to be more commonly associated with the use of animal-derived hyaluronidase in the LA mixture, therefore a 'hot orbit' post-operatively may need treatment with oral steroid in addition to antibiotics.

Conjunctival granulomatous inflammation may occur after sub-Tenon's LA. Smaller incisions and minimal dissection will probably make this less likely to occur.

The term 'wipe-out' is used to describe unexplained visual loss following surgery. Glaucoma patients may be at higher risk. It is possible that anaesthesia technique may account for some cases of wipe-out. Possible mechanisms include direct optic nerve damage from a needle or cannula, vascular occlusion caused by a needle or cannula, vasoconstriction from adrenaline (epinephrine) in the mixture, or prolonged compression of the optic nerve from a large volume of LA and/or use of orbital compression after the LA. Thus, careful attention to LA technique is required to minimise incidences of wipe-out [6, 17]

In summary, one should remain vigilant, anticipate the possibility of serious LA complications, choose the right technique for the patient and eye, and have processes in place to deal with any potential problems. The 2012 Royal Colleges' national guideline on LA for ophthalmic surgery points out that any cataract patient can potentially have a life-threatening problem, though this may not be attributable to anaesthesia. The Guideline states that *'Ideally, an anaesthetist should be available in the theatre complex, particularly when needle blocks such as peribulbar, retrobulbar, and sub-Tenon's blocks for difficult cataracts, or when complex or long cases are being performed. If an anaesthetist is not available in the hospital or ophthalmic unit, peribulbar or retrobulbar techniques should only be used if appropriately skilled staff are immediately available in the operating theatre. A clear, agreed and regularly tested pathway to enable the patient to receive appropriate advanced medical care, including intensive care, should be in place for isolated units"* [3].

Preparing the Patient

When preparing a patient for cataract surgery, one should consider what type of anaesthesia would be appropriate for the patient. For most patients LA is appropriate and is the best choice [3]. The exact technique of anaesthesia may depend on features of the cataract, the eye, the orbit, the patient, the surgical team and the place where the surgery is done. For cataract surgery, the commonest techniques are either STA or TA/ICA. However, a significant proportion of patients will require an anaesthetic technique that is different to the department's 'default' technique, for reasons outlined above. Thus, pre-operative assessment should include explanation of the surgery, and an assessment of patient anxiety level and ability to cooperate with LA [3]. A frequently asked question is whether or not the patient is 'able to lie flat and still for 20 min'. A significant proportion of patients are unable to do this for a large variety of reasons. Depending on the reason for inability to lie flat and/or still, most of these patients can have LA for cataract surgery [24].

In the UK, pre-operative assessment are normally conducted by specially trained nurses, with input from surgical and anaesthetic teams as needed. The

2012 Guideline on LA for Ophthalmic Surgery states that the patient's medical history should be recorded, in order to plan safe surgery and also to facilitate the safe management of any emergency that might occur. The main aspects that should be recorded are past and present illnesses, medications and allergies, past surgery and anaesthesia (and any complications), communicable diseases, ability to lie flat and still, psychosocial issues (anxiety, confusion, panic attacks, claustrophobia, etc.) and communication issues.

The Guideline states that, for a routine patient with no special concerns, examination should be limited to: pulse (rate and rhythm), blood pressure, hearing/comprehension/cooperation, and tremor/abnormal movements. Examination by a doctor should only be needed for those who need input from an anaesthetist for general anaesthesia, intravenous sedation, or if the nurses' assessment indicates that a medical examination would be appropriate, whether or not the patient was due for cataract surgery. Axial length is of relevance to anaesthesia choice, particularly if needle blocks are to be considered—of course, this is routinely measured for cataract patients. Where clinically indicated, the Guideline recommends: pulse oximetry if patient is breathless, examination for sepsis elsewhere in the body, assessment of ability to position appropriately for surgery [3].

Special tests are not necessary for most patients prior to LA cataract surgery. Historically, cataract patients would have a pre-operative physical examination, blood tests (full blood count, renal function tests) and electrocardiogram. There is now good evidence, from well-designed large prospective randomized trials, that these tests are not necessary for routine cataract patients [25, 13]. The Royal Colleges' Guideline states that *'for the patient with no history of significant systemic disease and no abnormal findings on examination at the nurse-led assessment, no special investigations are indicated. In general, tests should only be considered when the history or physical findings would have indicated the need for an investigation even if surgery had not been planned'* [3]. There are some special cases, as follows. For patients on anticoagulants (particularly warfarin), the clotting profile/INR should be assessed within 24 h of surgery. For patients on dialysis, the electrolytes should be assessed on the day of surgery. Screening for infection should be in line with local protocols. The Guideline has advice on the management of patients with diabetes, ischaemic heart disease, hypertension, anticoagulants, renal and pulmonary disease. The Guideline pre-dates the common usage of direct oral anti-coagulants (DOACs) - these, and other agents such as aspirin, should normally be continued for routine cataract surgery.

Consent

Patients must sign a consent form for cataract surgery. At the time of writing this (2018), there is no requirement for a specific consent form to be signed for the anaesthesia. The 2012 Guideline states that the process of surgery should be explained to the patient, and that there should be some mention of anaesthesia.

Written information should be provided. '*Consent must be obtained in the full knowledge of both general and special risks relevant to the operation and anaesthesia. It is the responsibility of the individual administering the anaesthetic to discuss possible complications of the anaesthetic. A separate consent form for the anaesthetic per se is not required, although it is advisable to record the discussion in the patient records*' [3].

More recently, the case of Montgomery versus Lanarkshire [26] has highlighted the need for specific discussions about the likelihood of complications. The court ruled that the surgical consent process should be a dialogue, with risks discussed not just in percentages but also in terms of significance of those risks. The explanation should be comprehensible (i.e. in plain language), and the doctor should discuss all significant risks of the proposed procedure, and also the risks of any reasonable alternatives or variants. The test of 'material risk' is whether in the particular case, 'a reasonable person in the patient's position would be likely to attach significance to the risk, or the doctor is or should reasonably be aware that the particular patient would be likely to attach significance'. In the context of anesthesia for cataract surgery, this means that the clinician should discuss the relative risks of the proposed anaesthesia technique (and the risks of alternative anaesthesia techniques) as part of the process of agreeing which anaesthetic technique to use, and obtaining formal consent.

The discussions of relative risk are made more difficult because of the controversies in ophthalmic anaesthesia, and the lack of hard data on relative risk. The relative risks of sight-threatening and life-threatening complications for the different LA techniques are not fully understood. To ascertain this information would need a prospective randomised trial so large that it could probably never be organised. However, it does appear that needle blocks are more likely to cause sight-threatening or life-threatening complications; blunt-cannula STA lowers this risk and TA/ICA should not have any of these risks. Using TA/ICA avoids these risks, but the potentially 'mobile eye' means that there may possibly be an increased likelihood of surgical complications in certain cases. The evidence-based NICE guideline on cataract surgery in adults [4] advises to use TA/ICA or STA as the default, and that PBA should only be considered if both these techniques are contraindicated. This implies that if needle LA for cataract surgery is required, the reasons for doing so should be explicitly recorded, and the risks discussed with the patient.

Which Anaesthetic to Use, When?

Every patient is different and while surgical teams will often have their preferred 'default' anaesthesia technique, there will always be patients who are unsuitable for the default anaesthesia approach. The following is a guide only and the advice may not apply to your particular patient.

Previous LASIK or other refractive surgery. These patients were usually myopic prior to their corrective procedure. Thus the patient may not need spectacles, yet the globe will remain 'myopic' with a long, wide eye and possible posterior staphyloma. Needle LA is best avoided for these eyes although one could use a single medial peribulbar LA if strictly necessary. Preferred techniques would be STA or TA/ICA.

Myopic eye. See above

Previous explant surgery for retinal detachment. Eyes with an encircling band may become somewhat 'hourglass shaped' giving the same effect as a posterior staphyloma. Thus an encircling band may increase the likelihood of a perforation from a needle LA. The band or explant means that it may be difficult or impossible to pass the cannula for STA. Thus, TA/ICA would be preferable, though in some circumstances it may be appropriate to consider a single medial peribulbar LA

Anxious patient. The patient should be asked why they are anxious about the surgery pre-operatively. Often, all that is needed is explanation and reassurance. Many patients worry that they will not be able to breathe under the drapes, or that they will not be able to keep the eyelids open or stay still. A reclining surgical chair, a hole in the surgical drape, and a person to hold the patient's hand with an agreed method of communication if the patient wishes to request more analgesia is often all that is needed. With good pre-operative assessment and explanation, sedation may be avoided. Others consider mild anxiolytics such as benzodiazepines (e.g. Diazepam 5 mg) IV sedation or general anaesthesia.

Claustrophobia. Again, this issue should be picked up at the pre-operative assessment and not during surgery. Explanation and reassurance may be all that is needed. A 'trial' of positioning and draping in the surgical chair as part of the pre-operative assessment may help patient decide whether their level of claustrophobia enables them to cope with the draping process. Many patients will appreciate having the surgical drape held away from the mouth and nose and/or a large hole in the paper surgical drape. Some patients may require a translucent drape, removal of most of the paper drape, or a 'turban' type drape with cloth wrapped around the head and the face exposed, save for a 20×20 cm transparent sticky drape over the surgical area. Again, a hand-holder and reassurance will be helpful. The surgeon should ensure that the patient is happy to proceed, prior to commencing surgery.

Patient cannot lie flat. There are many reasons why a patient would be 'unable to lie flat and still for 20 minutes'. Often there is an element of anxiety and/or claustrophobia. There are several approaches that can be taken, depending on the reason that the patients cannot lie flat [27]. For orthopnoeic patients with a flexible neck, it may be possible for the patient to sit upright with neck extended, facing the overhead microscope—the surgeon will usually need to stand rather than sit. If there is significant spinal curvature or rigidity, it may be necessary to adopt the 'face to face upright seated position', with the surgeon facing the patient and the microscope rotated toward the horizontal. In this technique, it is preferable to use TA/ICA, in order to ensure that the eye is 'on axis'. Face to face positioning can be very useful for 'extreme' cases such as those patients who need to be very upright, or are unable to transfer from wheelchair to operating chair [28].

Cataract surgery on both eyes on the same day. It would not be desirable to have a 'block' LA for both eyes, because this may mean that both eyes need to be padded and/or the vision may be poor for some hours, until the block wears off. Often these patients are GA patients, but if LA is used then it would be preferable to use TA/ICA for one or both eyes.

Which Technique is Best for Cataract Surgery?

The above discussion has explained that there is no such thing as a 'best technique of anaesthesia that is perfect for all cataract patients'. Most patients will be suitable for LA, and most patients would be suitable for either TA/ICA or STA. Neither of these LA techniques is absolutely perfect and neither would be suitable for 100% of eyes, 100% of patients or 100% of surgeons. As explained above, each technique has its own risk profile although needle blocks appear to be inherently more prone to sight-threatening or life-threatening complications. Therefore the decision-making process should involve a proper assessment of the patient and discussion of the relative risks of the different anaesthesia techniques. As explained by NICE guidelines, *'If both sub-Tenon's and topical (with or without intracameral) anaesthesia are contraindicated, consider peribulbar anaesthesia. Do not offer retrobulbar anaesthesia for people having cataract surgery'* [4].

How Can I Find Out More About Eye Anaesthesia?

We hope that this short chapter will stimulate the reader to take an interest in eye anaesthesia. Modern books on ophthalmic anaesthesia explain more about techniques [29, 6], but there is no substitute for hands-on learning from experts. Some centres of excellence offer training in ophthalmic anaesthesia techniques, and several societies worldwide also offer practical training as part of scientific meetings. The British Ophthalmic Anaesthesia Society was formed in the mid 1990s, and has annual meetings that include practical hands-on training (www.boas.org). The original Ophthalmic Anesthesia Society (USA) had its first scientific meeting in 1987, and meets annually in Chicago (www.eyeanesthesia.org). In India, the Ophthalmic Forum of Indian Society of Anaesthesiologists (OFISA) meets every two years (ofisa.sankaranethralaya.org). At the time of writing, a new European Society of Ophthalmic Anaesthesia is being set up (link via www.boas.org). Every four years, the World Congress of Ophthalmic Anaesthesia (WCOA) provides a global forum for ophthalmologists and anaesthetists to meet and exchange ideas. Refining and improving anaesthesia techniques should lead to fewer complications and better outcomes for our cataract patients.

References

1. Knapp H. On cocaine and its use in ophthalmic and general surgery. Arch Ophthalmol. 1884;13:402.
2. Cataract Surgery Guidelines. The Royal College of Ophthalmologists. 2010.
3. Local anaesthesia for ophthalmic surgery. Joint guidelines from the Royal College of Anaesthetists and the Royal College of Ophthalmologists. 2012.
4. Cataracts in adults: management. National Institute for Health and Care Excellence (NICE). 2017.
5. Lee RMH, Thompson JR, Eke T. Severe adverse events associated with local anaesthesia in cataract surgery: 1 year national survey of practice and complications in the UK. Br J Ophthalmol. 2016;100:772–6.
6. Jaichandran VV, Kumar C. Jagadeesh. Principles and Practice of Ophthalmic Anaesthesia: Jaypee Brothers Medical Publishers; 2017.
7. Ball JL, Woon WH, Smith S. Globe perforation by the second peribulbar injection. Eye. 2002;16:663–5.
8. Eke T, Thompson JR. The National Survey of Local Anaesthesia for Ocular Surgery I. Survey methodology and current practice. Eye. 1999;13:189–95.
9. Kumar CM. Needle-based blocks for the 21st century ophthalmology. Acta Ophthalmol. 2011;89:5–9.
10. Kumar CM, Eid H, Dodds C. Sub-Tenon's anaesthesia: complications and their prevention. Eye. 2011;25:694–703.
11. Guise P. Sub-Tenon's anesthesia: an update. Local and regional anesthesia. 2012;5:35–46.
12. Allman KG, Theron AD, Byles DB. A new technique of incisionless minimally invasive sub-Tenon's anaesthesia. Anaesthesia. 2008;63:782–3.
13. Minakaran N, Ezra DG, Allan BDS. Topical anaesthesia plus intracameral lidocaine versus topical anaesthesia alone for phacoemulsification cataract surgery in adults. Cochrane Database of Systematic Reviews 2020, Issue 7. Art. No.: CD005276. https://doi.org/10.1002/14651858.CD005276.pub4
14. Lee RM, Foot B, Eke T. Posterior capsule rupture rate with akinetic and kinetic block anesthetic techniques. J Cataract Refract Surg. 2013;39:128–31.
15. Silverstein SM, Greenbaum S, Stern R. Hyaluronidase in Ophthalmology. J Appl Res. 2012;12.
16. Labetoulle M, Findl O, Malecaze F, Alio J, Cochener B, Lobo C, Lazreg S, Hartani D, Colin J, Tassignon MJ, Behndig A. Evaluation of the efficacy and safety of a standardised intracameral combination of mydriatics and anaesthetics for cataract surgery. Br J Ophthalmol. 2016;100:976–85.
17. Creese K, Ong D, Sandhu SS, Ware D, Alex Harper C, Al-Qureshi SH, Wickremasinghe SS. Paracentral acute middle maculopathy as a finding in patients with severe vision loss following phacoemulsification cataract surgery. Clin Exp Ophthalmol. 2017;45:598–605.
18. Quantock CL, Goswami T. Death potentially secondary to sub-Tenon's block. Anaesthesia. 2007;62:175–7.
19. Burkat C, Lemke B. Retrobulbar hemorrhage: anterolaterateral anterior orbitotomy for emergent management. Arch Ophthal. 2005;123:1260–2.
20. Ohno-Matsui K. Proposed classification of posterior staphylomas based on analyses of eye shape by three-dimensional magnetic resonance imaging and wide-field fundus imaging. Ophthalmology. 2014;121:1798–809.
21. Edge R, Navon SE. Scleral perforation during retrobulbar and peribulbar anesthesia: risk factors and outcome in 50,000 consecutive injections. J Cataract Refract Surg. 1999;25:1237–44.
22. Faure C, Faure L, Billotte C. Globe perforation following no-needle sub-Tenon anesthesia. J Cataract Refract Surg. 2009;35:1471–2.

23. Frieman BJ, Friedberg MA. Globe perforation associated with subtenon's anesthesia. Am J Ophthalmol. 2001;131:520–1.
24. Injarie A, Clancy GP, Eke T. Prevalence, surgical management, and complication rate in patients unable to lie flat for cataract surgery. J Cataract Refract Surg. 2013;39:1120–2.
25. Schein OD, Katz J, Bass EB, Tielsch JM, Lubomski LH, Feldman MA, Petty BG, Steinberg EP. The value of routine preoperative medical testing before cataract surgery. Study of Medical Testing for Cataract Surgery. N Engl J Med. 2000;342:168–75.
26. UK Supreme Court. Montgomery v Lanarkshire Health Board (Scotland). UKSC 11, 2015.
27. Rentka A, Kemeny-Beke A. Factors to be considered when performing cataract surgery in patients unable to recline flat. Semin Ophthalmol. 2018;33:443–8.
28. Sohail T, Pajaujis M, Crawford SE, Chan JW, Eke T. Face-to-face upright seated positioning for cataract surgery in patients unable to lie flat: Case series of 240 consecutive phacoemulsifications. J Cataract Refract Surg. 2018;44:1116–22.
29. Kumar C, Dodds C, Gayer S, editors. Ophthalmic anaesthesia. OUP Oxford; 2012.

Novel Methods of Delivery

Mehran Zarei-Ghanavati

Introduction

Cataract surgery is the most commonly performed operation in ophthalmology. It is predicted that the need for cataract surgery will increase sharply in the coming decades due to increase in life expectancy. This presents a significant burden on eye services and health economy in general. The technique of cataract surgery has been revolutionised since the invention of phacoemulsification. It yields a high success rate with a low risk of complications [1]. Although the application of femtosecond in cataract surgery brings hope for improvement in outcomes of cataract surgery, future studies and improvements will be needed. It seems that optimising delivery of cataract surgery is one way to promote the efficiency of cataract surgery units. One promising approach is immediately sequential bilateral cataract surgery (ISBCS). There is clear evidence that cataract surgery of second eye improves vision-related quality of life. Although surgical and rehabilitation time is short and risk of surgical complications is low in comparison to intra-capsular and extra-capsular cataract surgery, ophthalmologists in most countries prefer delayed sequential bilateral cataract surgery (DSBCS) regardless of technique and complexity of cataract surgery. However, ISBCS is done for a considerable percentage of cataract surgery in countries like Finland and Sweden. There is also a growing trend toward ISBCS especially since the onset of the COVID-19 pandemic. Another approach is to develop new systems to improve efficacy of referral for cataract surgery and patient flow from pre-assessment before cataract surgery to discharge afterwards.

M. Zarei-Ghanavati (✉)
Farabi Eye Hospital, Tehran University of Medical Sciences, Qazvin Square, Tehran, Iran
e-mail: mehran_zarei@yahoo.com

© Springer Nature Switzerland AG 2021
C. Liu and A. Shalaby Bardan (eds.), *Cataract Surgery*,
https://doi.org/10.1007/978-3-030-38234-6_5

Bilateral Surgery in Ophthalmology

Lids and strabismus operation are routinely performed bilaterally. Infection is easier to manage and less vision threatening in these operations. Further, corneal refractive surgery (LASIK and PRK) is also done on both eyes at the same sitting despite the risk of infective keratitis [2, 3]. Phakic IOLs are also implanted bilaterally on the same day by some surgeons. Intravitreal injection of anti-VEGF is commonly done bilaterally. Therefore, the concept of doing bilateral extraocular and intra-ocular surgery is not only common; it is well-acceptable in the field of ophthalmology. Unexpectedly, considering modern cataract surgery as less invasive operation, bilateral cataract surgery is still viewed as a taboo by some ophthalmologists in several countries.

Suggested Protocol for ISBCS

A patient with clinically significant cataract in both eyes may be considered for ISBCS. All necessary examinations should be done including visual acuity, refraction, IOP measurement, optic disc and retinal examination. Surgeons should exclude patients who have:

- Higher risk for infection e.g.

  - Diabetes/immunosuppression
  - Iodine allergy

- Risk of corneal decompensation
  - Fuchs endothelial dystrophy, previous corneal pathologies, scarring, HSK, corneal grafts
- Cataract type and lenticular abnormalities
  - pseudoexfoliation, subluxation, phacodonesis, previous trauma, posterior polar cataract, mature cataract, dense nuclear cataract
- History of glaucoma
- Risk of RD

  - High myopia
  - Retinal break
  - History of retinal laser or vitrectomy

- Risk of biometry error

  - Axial length of <20 mm or >26 mm
  - Previous history of corneal refractive surgery
  - Irregular cornea

- Risk of intraocular inflammation.

It is estimated that about half of patients may be suitable for ISBCS [4]. If a patient with bilaterally significant cataract is suitable for ISBCS, they should have been clearly informed about the possible advantages and disadvantages of this method. The final decision to choose between delayed or simultaneous cataract surgery should be done by the patient with unbiased guidance of the surgeon.

The surgeon can choose these types of anaesthesia: topical, subtenons or general anaesthesia. One common combination is topical and intracameral for the first eye, and subtenons for the second eye. ISBCS should only be offered by an experienced surgeon and team in an operating room with good track record and low rate of complications including endophthalmitis.

In the event of a complication occuring during the first eye surgery, it would be wise to not proceed with the second eye at the same setting. This should be explicitly explained to the patient preoperatively. Surgeons and assistants should change gloves and gowns and redo draping for the second eye operation. A new trolley of instruments should be used for the second eye. Ideally a phaco set packed a week previously should be used for one eye as that would have been of proven sterility following the week's operations using instruments from the same sterilisation cohort. This may reduce the error in the sterilization cycle on a single day putting both eyes at risk. If IOL power for both eyes are the same, it is better to use implants with different lot numbers, or use an implant of 0.5 dioptre less or more in power for one of the two eyes in order to be sure that they have not been manufactured on the same day. For any solution entering the eye e.g balanced salt solution (BSS), ophthalmic viscosurgical devices (OVDs), anaesthetic, antibiotic, etc. different manufacturers or different lot numbers should be used. Any unfamiliar device or material should be avoided. Manufacture-packed right eye and left eye sets of instruments would decrease workload in theatre and chances of error. Disposable instruments are also preferable if possible.

Health Economy and ISBCS

DSBCS mandates second preoperative assessment and patients' preparation in operating room. Therefore, it imposes more steps and is less time-efficient than ISBCS. There are several reports that ISBCS is more cost-effective for both patients and health system. National savings by implementation of ISBCS is substantial. For instance, it is estimated to be of €5.7 million annually in Finland [5]. In a US-based study, it is reported that Medicare and patients would save approximately US$522 million, and US$261 million annually by implementation of ISBCS; respectively [6]. One study found that ISBCS is 14% less expensive compared to DSBCS in Sweden [7]. Another study in Finland reported savings of €449 for each patient in medical costs and this amount increased to €849–€1631 when non-healthcare costs were included [5]. This saving to society can be invested in other fields of ophthalmology or medicine. This economical advantage of ISBCS will be a big drive for prompting ISBCS by healthcare commissioners.

Patient Quality of Life After ISBCS

Both DSBCS and ISBCS improve patients' quality of life [11]. Patients after DSBCS will experience short term anisometropia, loss of stereopsis and delay in new eyeglass prescription that cause a delay in visual rehabilitation. Furthermore, these patients will need more postoperative visits, pre-assessment and admission for surgery. Patients' daily activity and life enjoyment will be affected by eye surgery and coexisting perioperative stress. The increased number of total leave days and its consequences is also noticeable. ISBCS will ease all these issues for patients. A combination of these factors may provide better short term quality of life after ISBCS. Qualitative analysis will be need to evaluate these issues in future studies.

Barriers and Concerns About ISBCS

Ethics

There is no evidence that ISBCS is not as safe as DSBCS [8, 9]. Therefore, ISBCS observes the principle of non-maleficence. After all information about ISBCS given to patients, they should be free to choose between immediate or delayed cataract surgery if they meet all criteria for ISBCS. The autonomy of patients is therefore respected. As ISBCS is more cost-effective, it should be considered a valid approach for conserving resources for patients and society.

Tariff and Reimbursement Rate

In many countries, the tariff for second eye surgery in simultaneous bilateral fashion is less than first eyes [9]. The US Medicare will pay 50% for second eye. It is the same in Australia. In some countries like Japan, no fee will be paid for the second eye. Therefore; although ISBCS saves money for health systems, it brings financial penalties to ophthalmologists and hospitals. This issue can explain differences in popularity of ISBCS among countries to some extent.

Presumed Risk of Bilateral Complications

One of the main concerns about ISBCS is the possibility of bilateral complications. Robust inclusion criteria and protocol for ISBCS decrease the likelihood of bilateral or any complications. Systematic reviews reported no difference in improvement of best spectacle corrected visual acuity (BSCVA) after ISBCS or DSBCS [10, 11].

Postoperative Refractive Error

There is some evidence that input of first eye refraction can be used to adjust second eye IOL power to improve refractive outcomes [12]. However, patients who are at higher risk of IOL power calculation errors like short or long axial lengths and history of previous refractive surgery are excluded from ISBCS. Moreover, optical biometry and modern IOL calculation formula have improved the results of post cataract surgery refraction. Also, it is not clear that what percentage of ophthalmologists routinely optimise second eye IOL powers based on refractive result of the first eye. Therefore; further studies will be needed to compare clinical significance of postoperative refractive error difference between ISBCS and DSBCS by applying recent improvement in IOL power calculation.

Toxic Anterior Segment Syndrome (TASS)

Toxic Anterior Segment Syndrome (TASS) is an acute toxic inflammatory reaction which is due to several etiologies, including intraocular lens materials and several toxic substances enter inside eyes during cataract surgery. It may also be caused by a deficit in the sterilization process. The International Society of Bilateral Cataract Surgeons' (iSBCS) strict guideline to use different sterilization cycle for instruments and different brands or lot numbers for right and left eye would theoretically make the risk of TASS for any eye independent of the other. It is of note that there is one report of bilateral TASS in the literature after DSBCS [13].

Cystoid Macular Oedema

Cystoid macular oedema (CMO) is the most common complication of cataract surgery with incidence rate of 1–2% for clinically significant CMO [14]. The peak incidence of CMO is 4–6 weeks postoperatively. Therefore, DSBCS would not have many advantages over ISBCS when there is a gap of less than six weeks between first and second eyes. Although previous studies have not reported an increase in CMO after ISBCS, there is a real concern about bilateral CMO. It seems that a more effective protocol for prevention and diagnosis of CMO should be designed for ISBCS.

Endophthalmitis

Bilateral visual loss from bilateral endophthalmitis is a great concern with ISBCS. Surgeons have reported this as the main reason why they do not offer ISBCS [15]. It seems that strict guidelines from ISBCS to completely separate the two operations should be effective to decrease the theoretical chance of bilateral endophthalmitis to a very low level [18]. Due to the proven effectiveness of intracameral antibiotics to decrease the risk of endophthalmitis, the use of intracameral antibiotics for ISBCS is highly recommended [16].

To calculate the probability of bilateral endophthalmitis, the risk of unilateral endophthalmitis should be squared and multiplied by a linkage factor (that shows how much risk of second eye infection is linked to the first eye). Although different rates of endophthalmitis have been reported, the main issue is that there is no agreement about the estimation of average linkage factors. It is also different for each individual. There are four cases of bilateral endophthalmitis in the literature but iSBCS' guidelines were not followed in these cases [17]. There is no report of bilateral endophthalmitis in recent studies about ISBCS [10, 11, 18]. More studies with larger sample sizes would be needed to estimate this risk. Recently, the risk of endophthalmitis after intravitreal injection among more than one hundred thousand eyes in office-based setting was 0.026%; quite the same rate as post-cataract surgery endophthalmitis [19]. They did not report any case of bilateral endophthalmitis. There is no guarantee for zero risk of bilateral endophthalmitis but following iSBCS' guidelines and use of intracameral antibiotics will decrease it to a very low level. It is estimated that the cost of avoiding the possibility of bilateral endophthalmitis would be around 3 billion Euros. On the other hand, due to advances in the treatment of endophthalmitis by vitrectomy, endophthalmitis does not necessarily result in blindness and considerable percentage of patients with endophthalmitis will achieve vision of $\geq 6/12$. A difficult question is what level of risk of bilateral endophthalmitis is acceptable given the many advantages of ISBCS.

Retinal Detachment

Retinal detachment rate increases after cataract surgery [20]. There are two major risk factors of this complication, axial myopia and vitreous loss. Axial myopia is excluded from ISBCS and surgery of second eye will be avoided in a case of posterior capsular tear and vitreous loss in the first eye. However, retinal detachment is a late postoperative complication. Therefore, usual separation of two eyes' surgery by several weeks in DSBCS cannot be helpful for prevention of retinal detachment.

Road Toward ISBCS

In some countries like Finland or Sweden it is not difficult to start ISBCS. In many others, surgeons who would like to do ISBCS may find few colleagues to support them. ISBCS is taboo in many ophthalmology communities. The starting step for developing ISBCS is talking about it to colleagues in local or national gatherings. It will help both sides to discuss their opinions and concerns and to build up a more robust system for ISBCS. It is pivotal to get some sort of support from national ophthalmology councils or health authorities. It will decrease concern about medico-legal issues for surgeons wishing to do ISBCS. There is also a need for consensus statements, guidelines and protocols for ISBCS developed by national and international workshops. Negotiation with insurance or government payers for more fair reimbursement rate will help to overcome one important obstacle for ISBCS in many countries. More well-designed studies should be done to answer our questions about possible advantages and disadvantages of ISBCS. Mixed methods research will be necessary to compare issues like short-term postoperative quality of life between ISBCS and DSBCS.

Other Aspects of Cataract Surgery Delivery

There is a drive to boost quality of service provided to customers in service industries. Health systems that offer cataract surgery should follow this example. All aspects of the service from pre-operative to post-operative period should be looked at. There are dissimilar models for delivery of cataract surgery by healthcare providers in different countries. Although there is no robust evidence about which model is the best, different aspects of these models should be considered by ophthalmologists. The Way Forward published by the Royal College of Ophthalmologists is a good example for more thoughts and debates about cataract surgery delivery in the future [21]. It is essential to redesign cataract delivery systems to be more efficient but at the same time not jeopardizing patient safety. It is also vital to consider socioeconomic aspects and national policies of health authorities for the system to evolve. The rise in burden of cataract and limited resources will compel ophthalmology communities and health system managers to seek more efficient pathways for provision of cataract surgery. Robust supervision strategy is needed to monitor outcomes of newly designed systems.

Other Strategies for More Cost-Efficient Cataract Surgery Delivery

Referral System

Improvement in referral system for cataract surgery will boost efficacy of eye care units. It will reduce wastage of time and money. Visual acuity should not be considered a sole criterion for being eligible for cataract surgery. In some models, referral is done by optometrists or general practitioners. Although over-referral is a big concern, any referral system should be watchful for systematic under-referral of any specific group of patients.

Task Delegation to Health Care Professionals

Health care professionals (HCPs) including optometrists and nurses are recently participating in preoperative assessment, biometry and obtaining informed consent [21]. There are different pathways for deploying HCPs to improve flow of patients. Although these models save time for ophthalmologists, they still have the responsibility of taking a final decision for operation and confirmation of consent in any preoperative pathway. On the other hand, the traditional first-day postoperative visit by ophthalmologists is fading [22]. It is mostly done by HCPs, often by telephone, rather than by ophthalmologists in the UK [21].

Presence of Anaesthetist

Nowadays, routine cataract surgery is done under local anaesthesia rather than general anaesthesia. In some settings, anaesthetists do not attend cataract list without any patient requiring general anaesthesia or intravenous sedation. There should be staff who are trained for cardiopulmonary resuscitation. Reducing or consolidating lists into LA only or anaesthetic cover required may reduce the need and expense of an anaesthetist.

Number of Staff and Cataract Cases Per List

There is a drive to improve productivity of cataract services by doing higher numbers of cataract cases per list. Various factors should be considered in this regard: training surgeon or consultant, number of staff in theatre and level of case complexity (risk stratification system would be helpful). However, employing extra staff may be challenging for some health systems. Finally, it is pivotal to find solutions for rewarding surgeons and theatre staff in addition to avoiding burnout.

References

1. Jaycock P1, Johnston RL, Taylor H, Adams M, Tole DM, Galloway P, Canning C, Sparrow JM. UK EPR user group. The cataract national dataset electronic multi-centre audit of 55,567 operations: updating benchmark standards of care in the United Kingdom and internationally. Eye (Lond). 2009;23(1):38–49.

2. Garg P, Bansal AK, Sharma S, Vemuganti GK. Bilateral infectious keratitis after laser in situ keratomileusis: a case report and review of the literature. Ophthalmology. 2001;108(1):121–5.

3. Karimian F, Baradaran-Rafii A, Javadi MA, Nazari R, Rabei HM, Jafarinasab MR. Bilateral bacterial keratitis in three patients following photorefractive keratectomy. J Refract Surg. 2007;23(3):312–5.

4. Shah V, Naderi K, Maubon L, Jameel A, Patel DS, Gormley J, et al. Acceptability of immediate sequential bilateral cataract surgery (ISBCS) in a public health care setting before and after COVID-19: a prospective patient questionnaire survey. BMJ Open Ophthalmol. 2020;5(1):e000554.

5. Leivo T, Sarikkola AU, Uusitalo RJ, Hellstedt T, Ess SL, Kivelä T. Simultaneous bilateral cataract surgery: economic analysis; Helsinki simultaneous bilateral cataract surgery study report 2. J Cataract Refract Surg. 2011;37(6):1003–8. https://doi.org/10.1016/j.jcrs.2010.12.050.

6. Neel ST. A cost-minimization analysis comparing immediate sequential cataract surgery and delayed sequential cataract surgery from the payer, patient, and societal perspectives in the United States. JAMA Ophthalmol. 2014;132(11):1282–8.

7. Lundström M, Albrecht S, Roos P. Immediate versus delayed sequential bilateral cataract surgery: an analysis of costs and patient value. Acta Ophthalmol. 2009;87(1):33–8.

8. Herrinton LJ, Liu L, Alexeeff S, Carolan J, Shorstein NH. Immediate sequential vs. delayed sequential bilateral cataract surgery: retrospective comparison of postoperative visual outcomes. Ophthalmology. 2017;124(8):1126–35.

9. Singh R, Dohlman TH, Sun G. Immediately sequential bilateral cataract surgery: advantages and disadvantages. Curr Opin Ophthalmol. 2017;28(1):81–6.

10. Kessel L, Andresen J, Erngaard D, Flesner P, Tendal B, Hjortdal J. Immediate sequential bilateral cataract surgery: a systematic review and meta-analysis. J Ophthalmol. 2015;2015:912481.

11. Malvankar-Mehta MS, Chen YN, Patel S, Leung AP, Merchea MM, Hodge WG. Immediate versus delayed sequential bilateral cataract surgery: a systematic review and meta-analysis. PLoS One. 2015;10(6):e0131857.

12. Olsen T. Use of fellow eye data in the calculation of intraocular lens power for the second eye. Ophthalmology. 2011;118(9):1710–5.

13. Kim SY, Park YH, Kim HS, Lee YC. Bilateral toxic anterior segment syndrome after cataract surgery. Can J Ophthalmol. 2007;42(3):490–1.

14. Yonekawa Y1, Kim IK. Pseudophakic cystoid macular edema. Curr Opin Ophthalmol. 2012;23(1):26–32.

15. Amsden LB, Shorstein NH, Fevrier H, Liu L, Carolan J, Herrinton LJ. Immediate sequential bilateral cataract surgery: surgeon preferences and concerns. Can J Ophthalmol. 2018;53(4):337–41.

16. Gower EW, Lindsley K, Tulenko SE, Nanji AA, Leyngold I, McDonnell PJ. Perioperative antibiotics for prevention of acute endophthalmitis after cataract surgery. Cochrane Database Syst Rev. 2017;2:CD006364.

17. Lansingh VC, Eckert KA, Strauss G. Benefits and risks of immediately sequential bilateral cataract surgery: a literature review. Clin Exp Ophthalmol. 2015;43(7):666–72.

18. Arshinoff SA, Bastianelli PA. Incidence of postoperative endophthalmitis after immediate sequential bilateral cataract surgery. J Cataract Refract Surg. 2011;37(12):2105–14.

19. Borkar DS, Obeid A, Su DC, Storey PP, Gao X, Regillo CD, Kaiser RS, Garg SJ, Hsu J. Wills post injection endophthalmitis (PIE) study group. Endophthalmitis rates after bilateral same-day intravitreal anti-vascular endothelial growth factor injections. Am J Ophthalmol. 2018;194:1–6.

20. Day AC, Donachie PHJ, Sparrow JM, Johnston RL. Royal college of ophthalmologists' national ophthalmology database. United Kingdom national ophthalmology database study of cataract surgery: report 3: Pseudophakic retinal detachment. Ophthalmology. 2016;123(8):1711–5.

21. The Way Forward Cataract—The Royal College of Ophthalmologists. https://www.rcophth.ac.uk/wp-content/uploads/2015/10/RCOphth-The-Way-Forward-Cataract-300117.pdf. Accessed 14 March 2019.
22. Grzybowski A, Kanclerz P. Do we need day-1 postoperative follow-up after cataract surgery? Graefes Arch Clin Exp Ophthalmol. 2018.

Refractive Aim and Choice of Intraocular Lens

Tommy C. Y. Chan, Sharon S. W. Chow and John S. M. Chang

Introduction

In recent decades, there have been revolutionary changes to the design and material of intraocular lenses (IOLs), resulting in a wide diversity of choices available in the market. Different IOLs have different properties and it is important to understand each IOL to assist for the best selection for our patients. IOL materials can be rigid, flexible or foldable. Rigid IOLs are made from polymethyl methacrylate (PMMA), foldable IOLs can be made from Silicone, hydrophilic acrylic or hydrophobic acrylic. IOL designs can be one piece or three piece, square edged or rounded, planar or angulated haptics, they can also be open loop or plate haptic designed as well as short wavelength filtered or ultraviolet filtered. As for its optical properties, it can be monofocal, multifocal or of extended depth of focus, it can also be spherical or toric, depending on the need for each patient. IOL selection is an individualised process and is largely based on the patient's visual requirements and expectations. An ideal IOL should be able to provide a satisfactory visual outcome with good visual quality to the patient, and to the surgeon, it should be easy to handle and insert, with low rates of complications and a long-term safety profile.

T. C. Y. Chan (✉) · J. S. M. Chang
Department of Ophthalmology, Hong Kong Sanatorium and Hospital, Hong Kong, Hong Kong
e-mail: tommychan.me@gmail.com

S. S. W. Chow
Department of Ophthalmology, Grantham Hospital, Hong Kong, Hong Kong

© Springer Nature Switzerland AG 2021
C. Liu and A. Shalaby Bardan (eds.), *Cataract Surgery*,
https://doi.org/10.1007/978-3-030-38234-6_6

IOL Biomaterials

IOL materials can be rigid, flexible or foldable. Rigid IOLs are made from PMMA, which is a transparent material with a refractive index of 1.49. Flexible IOLs can be made from silicone, which consists of polymers of silicone and oxygen, with a refractive index of 1.41–1.46. Foldable IOLs include hydrophobic acrylic and hydrophilic acrylic. Hydrophobic or hydrophilic depends on its interaction with water. Hydrophobic acrylic IOLs consists of acrylate and methacrylate with a refractive index of 1.54, whereas hydrophilic acrylic IOLs are composed of poly-hydroxyethyl-methylacrylate (HEMA) and hydrophilic acrylic monomer with a refractive index of 1.47.

PMMA

PMMA is the first material used for IOLs. It is rigid, non foldable and hydrophobic with an optical diameter of 5–7 mm. It has been shown that implantation of a foldable or rigid IOL gives similar excellent results with the advantage of being inexpensive [1]. However, due to its lack of flexibility, it requires a large corneal incision for insertion, which has caused it to grow out of favor. PMMA IOLs are also reported to have a significantly higher rate of posterior capsule opacification (PCO) than silicone or acrylic IOLs [2]. Heparin surface modified PMMA IOLs have also been used, theoretically it can reduce postoperative inflammation, and its use in uveitis patients was shown to have good results [3]. PMMA IOLs are currently considered when performing extracapsular cataract extraction, and due to their overall rigidity resulting in good centration and resistance to tilt, it is used for scleral fixating IOLs. PMMA material is also used in anterior chamber IOLs as well as iris fixated IOLs due to its inert property with minimal inflammation.

Silicone

Silicone material is flexible and hydrophobic. Because of this property, it allows a smaller corneal incision for IOL implantation. In 1980s, silicone IOLs have come into place, it is a flexible IOL with an optical diameter of 5.5–6.5 mm [4]. However, since 1990s, several case studies have reported an interaction between silicone oil used in vitreoretinal surgeries with silicone IOLs. The strong adherence of silicone droplets on the IOL have caused significant visual loss and in some cases, resulted in the need for IOL exchange [5–8]. Therefore, it is not considered in potential cases for vitreoretinal surgeries such as high myopia or eyes with proliferative diabetic retinopathy. Silicone IOLs are also not easy to handle, as they become slippery when wet, which is almost unavoidable during a cataract surgery. Another disadvantage is its rapid unfolding. Surgeons have reported unexpected posterior capsule rupture in apparently uneventful phacoemulsifications until the IOL was injected [9].

Hydrophobic Acrylic

Hydrophobic acrylic materials are a series of copolymers of acrylate and methacrylate derived from rigid PMMA, which makes it both durable and foldable. Hydrophobic acrylic foldable IOLs were first presented in 1993 and have quickly dominated the market ever since their introduction. They have an optical diameter between 5.5 and 7.0 mm and are available in one piece or three piece designs. They have a higher refractive index, therefore allows for thinner lenses and they also have a very low water content. Although being foldable, they have a slower and more controlled unfolding rate as compared to silicone IOLs. Meta-analysis and different studies have also reported a lower PCO rate when compared with hydrophilic acyclic IOLs [10–12]. Other studies have also shown a lower incidence of Nd:YAG laser capsulotomy in hydrophobic acrylic IOLs than PMMA or silicone IOLs [13]. However, they have a disadvantage of having intralenticular changes where small water inclusions cluster together and this has been reported to cause significantly greater level of glistening than silicone and PMMA [14], leading to visual disturbance.

Hydrophilic Acrylic

Hydrophilic acrylic materials are composed of a mixture of poly-HEMA and hydrophilic acrylic monomer. They are foldable, soft, with high water content and have excellent biocompatibility due to the hydrophilic surface. They also have a slower unfolding rate as compared with silicone IOLs and are easy to handle and relatively more resistant to instrumental damage or Nd:YAG laser [15]. Postoperatively, hydrophilic acrylic IOLs have been shown to have minimal inflammatory cells on the anterior surface of the IOL, which indicates a high uveal biocompatibility [16]. The best IOL should provide optimal uveal and capsular biocompatibility, which can be determined by examining the cellular reaction on the anterior and posterior surface of the IOL [17]. The cellular reaction consists of foreign body giant cell reaction to the IOL, which is an indicator of the uveal biocompatibility. As for capsular biocompatibility, this can be determined by the proliferation of lens epithelial cells (LEC) after contact between the capsule and the IOL. When comparing with hydrophobic acrylic IOLs, hydrophilic acrylic IOLs are also shown to have better biocompatibility [18]. However, case reports have shown the presence of calcium deposition on IOL optics (under certain circumstances), which leads to decrease in visual acuity and the need for IOL exchange [19–21]. Hydrophilic acrylic material was also shown to carry a higher risk of

PCO than hydrophobic material [22], this may be explained by the higher water content which attracts LEC migration. Furthermore, hydrophilic IOL is considered contraindicated in patients with asteroid hyalosis.

IOL Optical Design

IOL evolution was driven by efforts to improve its surgical handling as well as optical performance. There is a large variety of different designs available aiming at different purposes to improve visual outcome.

Three Piece or One Piece?

Since the introduction of hydrophobic acrylic IOLs, they have become the most popular foldable IOL worldwide. In 1993, the first hydrophobic acrylic model was introduced into the market—three piece Alcon AcrySof. It quickly gained popularity due to its stable clinical results, excellent biocompatibility and low rate of PCO [23]. In 2000, Alcon introduced the one piece AcrySof (Fig. 1), aiming to allow a easier insertion through a smaller incision. Three piece IOL are made of different materials, the optic can be made of PMMA, silicone or acrylic, while the

Fig. 1 Alcon® AcrySof one piece IOL

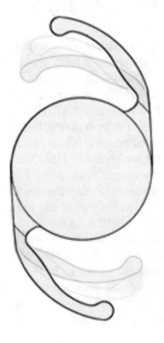

highly elastic haptics tend to be made of PMMA (Fig. 2). For a one piece IOL, it is entirely made out of one material and is usually acrylic. When compared with the three piece IOL, the one piece IOL has similar overall length and optic diameter, the optic edge is slightly thicker due to broad haptic shoulders at the transition from the optic, also, it has a flat configuration as oppose to a slight angulation in the haptics of a three piece IOL.

The first clinical comparison of the two AcrySof designs was published in 2003, the retrospective study showed similar visual acuity, centration and refractive stability between the two IOLs [24]. However, one piece IOLs were shown to have more PCO than three piece IOLs. The higher incidence of PCO was thought to be due to a lack of a sharp posterior edge, which is present in three piece IOLs, to indent the posterior capsule for a barrier to prevent migration of LEC. However, further prospective, randomized comparison showed equal stability and degree of opacification between three piece and one piece IOLs [25].

With regards to implantation, due to more rigid haptics, three piece IOLs require a larger corneal incision to reduce risk of damage to the haptics, they also carry a higher risk of posterior capsule rupture during insertion and unfolding. Therefore, in current practice, they are mainly considered when there is a need for sulcus implantation, due to better stability in the sulcus and a lower chance of iris chafing by slightly thinner haptics [26]. Indeed, the ASCRS recommended a 13.5 mm three piece IOL with posteriorly angulated haptic and rounded anterior optic edge to be inserted in the sulcus with optic capture at the anterior capsulotomy for best results.

Fig. 2 Precision Lens®
AR40 three piece IOL

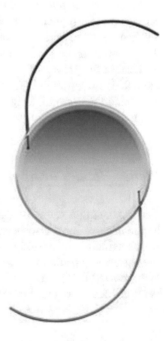

Square Edged or Round Edged?

The incidence of PCO with AcrySof IOLs was noted to be significantly lower. Studies have been carried out to determine whether the material or the design contributes to the reduction of PCO. An animal study showed the inhibition of LEC proliferation by creating a sharp capsular bend from using square edged acrylic IOLs [27]. Another prospective study implanted otherwise identical acrylic IOLs with or without a square edge in alternate eyes and found that the eyes receiving square edged design developed less PCO [28]. Further studies have also found that PMMA or silicone IOLs with square edged designs also significantly prevents PCO [28, 29]. These findings conclude that it is the square edge rather than the IOL material that is the primary factor in reducing the formation of PCO. The rationale being that any IOL with a squared edge, regardless of the material, is able to indent the posterior capsule, which forms a mechanical barrier to prevent LEC migration and PCO formation. A meta-analysis comparing square and round edged IOLs also showed a clear beneficial effect of square edged IOLs in PCO prevention [30].

However, it is well documented that square edged designs have their specific drawbacks. Edge glare phenomenon or unwanted optical images have been reported in square edged designs [31, 32]. These unwanted images contribute to symptoms of dysphotopsia, which can be positive or negative. Positive dysphotopsia is characterized by brightness or light streaks radiating from a central source of light. Negative dysphotopsia is characterized by darkness or shadows at the temporal peripheral field of vision [33]. Dysphotopsia symptoms are thought to be due to distribution of intensified edge glare rays to the peripheral retina. Round edges provide a great reduction in potential glare by disbursing reflected edge glare rays and reducing the intensity on the retina. Edge rounding can significantly reduce the potential for unwanted optical images, however it loses the ability for a capsular bend in the prevention of PCO. As both square edged and round edged designs have their own tradeoff, further refinements in edge design will be necessary to determine the optimal design that can both minimize edge glare phenomenon and PCO.

Planar Haptics or Angulated Haptics?

Besides having a squared edge as a barrier to prevent the formation of PCO, IOL haptic designs have also been considered in PCO prevention. Haptics with a forward angulation of roughly 5–10 degrees aim to push the optic backwards against the posterior capsule to cause a barrier effect for LEC migration. However, studies have showed that angulated haptic designs do not seem to have a better PCO prevention effect than those with planar haptics [34].

Loop Haptic or Plate Haptic?

Capsule contraction syndrome was defined as a reduction in equatorial diameter of the capsular bag, fibrosis of the anterior capsule and shrinkage of its opening [35]. Shrinkage of capsule is due to an imbalance between centrifugal and centripetal forces on the capsular bag. The size of the continuous curvilinear capsulorrhexis (CCC), zonular stability, IOL material and IOL design may play a role in the formation of capsular contraction syndrome. The smaller the CCC, the greater the sphincter effect on the IOL. The weaker the zonules, the more imbalance between the forces and the capsulorrhexis perimeter. As for the IOL design, excessive capsular fibrosis has been observed more commonly with silicone IOLs, this was attributed to the chronic low grade inflammation that was seen after the implantation of silicone material intraocularly as well as a relatively flexible material which is less resistant to capsular tension [36, 37]. On the other hand, haptic design - loop haptic (Fig. 3) versus plate haptic (Fig. 4) - was shown to have a major effect on the causation of capsular contraction syndrome. A study compared a loop haptic design with a plate haptic design with almost identical optics in terms of material, diameter and thickness, the study reported a marked constriction of the CCC in the plate haptic design [38]. The authors proposed three reasons for the causation of such. Firstly, it can be explained by the large area of contact of the plate haptic with the anterior capsule that may stimulate cell proliferation and fibrosis. Secondly, the large size of the plate haptic may have prevented fusion between the

Fig. 3 Zeiss® CT Lucia loop haptic IOL

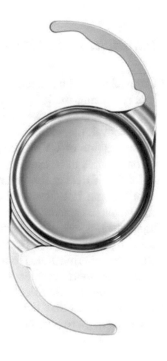

Fig. 4 Zeiss® CT Asphina
plate haptic IOL

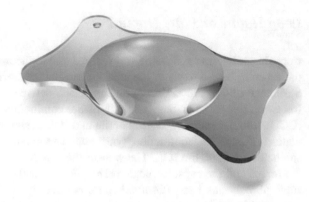

anterior and posterior capsules, such that capsule bending is not possible and this allows for LEC migration. Thirdly, the plate haptic has a small arc of contact with the fornix of the capsular bag and may inhibit the proliferation of LEC less than loop haptics.

With regards to optical performances, there have been contrasting evidences when comparing loop haptic to plate haptic designs. Studies have showed that due to a better stability, plate haptic designs result in better optical performances than loop haptic designs [39]. However, recent studies have showed similar optical performances and rotational stability when using plate haptic or loop haptic toric IOLs [40, 41].

Ultraviolet Light Filtered or with Blue Light Filtered?

Ultraviolet (UV) has been proven to be toxic to the retina due to short wavelength energy causing oxidative stress to the retina [42]. Retinal protection against UV and blue visible light is usually done by the cornea and crystalline lens. After cataract removal, the amount of light transmission to the retina increases, which leads to the creation of UV filtering IOLs (Fig. 5), and subsequently, by adding yellow chromophores to it, blue light filtering IOLs were introduced. Blue light filtering IOLs (Fig. 6) were also referred to as yellow tinted IOLs. The rationale for blue light filtering IOL is to imitate the human crystalline lens. With ageing, yellow chromophores accumulate in the lens and decrease the transmission of visible blue light which is one of the factors in the pathogenesis of age related macular degeneration (ARMD) [43]. Theoretically, with the addition of yellow chromophores, blue light filtering IOL reduces chromatic aberration, provides protection against phototoxic short wavelength light and also reduces cyanopsia, which is when patients notice a blue tinge to their vision post operatively [44, 45]. Studies have also suggested other benefits including improvement in contrast sensitivity and reduction in glare [46, 47].

Fig. 5 Alcon® AcrySof
SN60WF blue light filtered
IOL

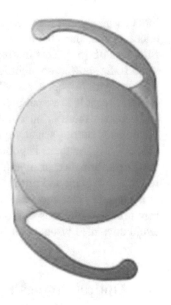

Fig. 6 Bausch+Lomb®
enVISTA MX60 UV light
filtered IOL

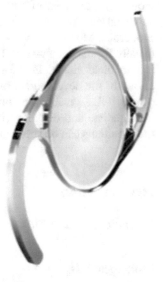

Although blue light filtering IOLs have been suggested to be retinal protective and prevent the development of ARMD, firm clinical evidence is still lacking. There has been contrasting evidence on the photoprotective effect of blue light filtered IOLs. A recent small study showed strong support of a photoprotective role of blue light filtered IOL on the progression of geographical atrophy in ARMD [48]. Blue light filtering IOLs were also shown to significantly reduce blue light induced apoptosis to the RPE cells [49, 50]. However, others reported no differences in macular changes between an ultraviolet filtering IOL and a blue light filtering IOL [51]. This finding was also supported in another study where blue filtered IOLs showed no significant clinical or optical coherence tomography (OCT) findings with respect to ARMD [52].

With regards to visual performance, recent systematic review and meta analysis showed that there is no clinically meaningful difference in visual acuity, colour vision and contrast sensitivity, both IOLs demonstrated similar visual performance [51, 53, 54]. As there is good evidence in the literature to support a similar good visual performance of blue filtering IOLs with definite and theoretical benefits of reduction in glare and filtration of short wavelength light, using blue filtering IOLs is a sensible precaution especially in cases with high risk of ARMD [55]. In current practice, surgeons opt to match the IOL with the one used in the fellow eye to avoid unwanted visual disturbances and imbalance between both eyes.

IOL Optical Properties

Nowadays, the goal of cataract surgery is to provide good visual acuity as well as visual quality preferably at all distances. Different IOLs have different optical properties. Monofocal IOLs aim at providing clear vision at one distance, which is usually for distance vision. Therefore, reading glasses will be needed for near and intermediate vision. In the last decade, many improvements have been made to allow for the development of a wide spectrum of IOLs beyond the standard monofocal IOLs. Presbyopia-correcting IOLs aim at providing clear vision for near, intermediate and distance vision, which is limited in monofocal IOLs, such that these patients can be spectacle independent at all times.

IOL Selection

Spherical Correction

Monofocal IOL

Monofocal IOL is the most common type of IOL used in cataract surgery. It has one focusing distance and it can be set to focus for near, intermediate or distance vision depending on the targeted refractive error. Most patients opt for low myope or even emmetropia to set for clear distance vision so they will be spectacle independent most of the day, however, they will need reading glasses for near and intermediate work.

Presbyopia

Presbyopia-Correcting IOLs

After cataract extraction, there is a loss of accommodation, which was present in the native lens in younger patients. The implantation of the standard monofocal IOLs can only provide clear vision at one distance, therefore, patients will still need to rely on glasses for other distances. Presbyopia-correcting IOLs were developed to combat the loss of accommodation and they can be subdivided into multifocal IOLs, accommodative IOLs and extended depth of focus IOLs.

Multifocal IOL

Multifocal IOL functions by generating different foci by either a diffractive or a refractive design, this addresses the visual limitation in monofocal IOLs. Diffractive IOLs are created by the use of concentric rings of decreasing height on the posterior surface of the IOL, which causes diffraction of light at both near and distance [56]. Diffractive IOLs can be subdivided into apodized or non apodized (Figs. 7 and 8). Apodization causes optical properties of the IOL to change

Fig. 7 Optical profile in Apodization

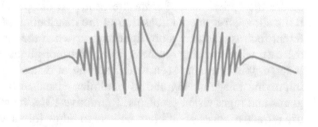

Fig. 8 Apodized Diffractive IOL

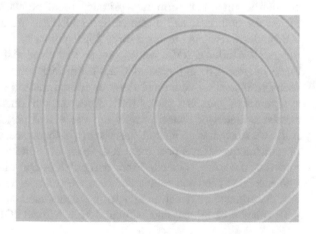

Fig. 9 Alcon® AcrySof
Restor Multifocal IOL

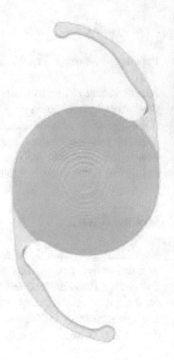

across the optical surface from the centre to the periphery. Apodized diffractive IOLs allow for a smooth transition of the distribution of light energy between different foci, so allowing more light to near when the pupil is small, this is usually the case when carrying out near tasks, and more light to distance when the pupil is large, this is usually seen when looking at distance [57]. Apodization helps in improving image quality and to minimize visual disturbances such as halos and glares and night vision problems. Refractive IOLs function by the use of concentric refractive zones of different powers to allow for viewing at all distances [58].

Multifocal IOLs (Fig. 9) can be bifocal or trifocal. Bifocal IOLs are made of concentric rings that form two primary focal points, aiming at providing clear vision for both near and distance. Trifocal IOLs are a newer type of multifocal IOL and are designed to form three focal points to provide a better intermediate vision than bifocal IOLs, while preserving clear vision for both near and distance ranges. Although trifocal IOLs seem ideal, the addition of an intermediate focus results in an additional defocus image instead of one, which may lead to symptoms of glare and haloes [59]. Since the introduction of trifocal IOLs, it has caused a matter of concern regarding the visual performances between the two IOLs. A study has compared the visual performance after bilateral implantation of a diffractive bifocal or trifocal IOL from the same manufacturer using the same material, the study concluded that trifocal IOL can provide a significantly better intermediate vision and equivalent distance and near vision as bifocal IOL without any disturbance in visual quality [60]. Recent meta-analysis compared the visual performance of bifocal and trifocal IOLs, trifocal IOLs have a clear advantage over bifocal IOLs in intermediate vision, however, both IOLs have similar near and distance visual performance, spectacle independence and postoperative satisfaction [61, 62].

Despite aiming to provide good vision at all distances, multifocal IOLs have their own drawbacks. Multifocal IOLs have been shown to cause a decrease in near contrast sensitivity under both mesopic and photopic conditions, and a decrease in distance contrast sensitivity under mesopic conditions [63]. This may be due to redirection of light from the other focal points causing coexisting images and a lower contrast sensitivity. A recent systematic review and meta-analysis compared multifocal IOLs to standard monofocal IOLs. With multifocal IOLs, a higher proportion of patients were able to achieve spectacle independence but at a greater risk of unwanted visual phenomena, these includes symptoms of halo and glare [64].

When comparing diffractive and refractive IOLs, diffractive IOLs can provide a slightly better near vision and less halo and glare, however they have a slightly worse intermediate vision. Refractive IOLs are more dependent on pupil diameter which may lead to night vision problems, and this is probably due to the zonal design of the IOL [58, 65]. With an attempt to incorporate the best of both diffractive and refractive IOLs, mix-and-match method has been introduced. Mix-and-match method functions by bilateral implantation of diffractive in one eye, and refractive multifocal IOLs into the fellow eye in attempt to achieve better visual outcomes. A few studies on the mix-and-match method have shown safe and good results at all distances, an increase in contrast sensitivity, a high level of patient satisfaction and a high rate of spectacle independence [66–68].

The decision to implant multifocal IOLs should be based on consideration of a patient's motivation to achieve spectacle independence, if so, pre operative counseling is of vital importance. Patients should be notified on the possible side effects such as decrease in contrast sensitivity, halos, glares, starburst, night vision problems and the need for visual adaptation.

Supplementary IOL

Refractive surprises or undesirable visual outcomes happen occasionally after multifocal IOL implantation. To address for this problem, many methods have been discussed, these include IOL exchange, refractive corneal surgery and supplementary piggyback IOLs. A retrospective analysis showed multifocal retreatment rate was 10.8%, of which supplementary piggyback IOLs consists of 89% [69]. Supplementary IOLs are implanted into the ciliary sulcus for refractive correction, Sulcoflex® IOL (Fig. 10) is one such lens. Recent studies evaluated the implantation of Sulcoflex® IOL for post operative negative dysphotopsia, these studies concluded that Sulcoflex® IOL can successfully treat negative dysphotopsia and symptoms resolved completely in all cases [70, 71]. Sulcoflex® IOL has been shown to be an effective treatment option with predictable outcome in the correction of post operative refractive surprises, it also reduces spectacle dependence and is well tolerated by implanted eyes [72].

Fig. 10 Rayner Sulcoflex®
Trifocal IOL

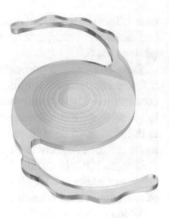

Accommodative IOL

Accommodative IOL is designed by simulating the natural accommodative process by changing optical power in response to ciliary muscle contraction [73]. A recent systematic review and meta-analysis confirmed that accommodative IOLs can provide better distance corrected near visual acuity and results in higher levels of spectacle independence than standard monofocal IOLs [74]. Accommodative IOLs also produce minimal unwanted visual disturbances such as halos and glares and contrast sensitivity is preserved when compared with multifocal IOLs.

There are mainly two types of accommodative IOLs, the single optic and the dual optic IOLs. After a single optic accommodative IOL is placed into the capsular bag, the anterior capsule fibroses and induces pressure on the optic plate, which cause it to vault posteriorly. When the ciliary muscle contracts, it moves the optic forward and causes an axial positional change in the IOL thus adjusting its optical power. Approximately 1 mm of movement is equivalent to a 2 diopters power change [75]. The main drawback of this design is that it is very dependent on the function of the capsular bag. With time, anterior capsule fibrosis may develop, this may limit the axial movement of the IOL and progressively loses its accommodative ability. Also, the degree of refractive change differs according to the axial length in each eye, which may lead to unpredictable outcome. The dual optic accommodative IOL functions by a spring system comprising a high plus power anterior optic coupled to a compensatory minus power posterior optic. When the dual optic accommodative IOL is implanted in the capsular bag, it is compressed due to capsular tension. During accommodation, the zonules relax and the capsular tension is released, leading to an expansion of the capsular bag. Due to the spring system design, it causes a forward axial displacement of the optic and a dynamic increase in dioptric power of the IOL [76, 77]. The dual optic system is currently the most promising generation to attempt to simulate a larger degree of accommodative effect, however, larger trials with longer follow up are necessary to support clinical usage.

Fig. 11 Tecnis® Symfony
Extended Depth of Focus
IOL

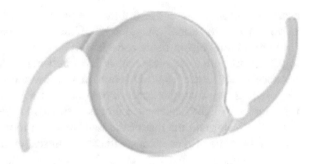

Extended Depth of Focus IOL

As multifocal and accommodative IOLs both have their own drawbacks, the goals of spectacle independence as well as optimizing visual quality have driven the development of extended depth of focus (EDOF) IOLs (Fig. 11). EDOF IOLs provides a single elongated focal point to enhance depth of focus or range of vision. The principle behind EDOF IOL is to focus light rays in an extended longitudinal plane as opposed to monofocal and multifocal IOLs, which focus light rays at one single point or multiple points respectively. This elongated focus aims to eliminate the overlapping of near and far images created by multifocal IOLs and therefore significantly reduces potential halos and glares [78]. A recent study has shown that EDOF IOLs provide better optical quality than monofocal and multifocal IOLs [79]. Due to the novelty of this design, limited studies have been carried out, but preliminary results are promising. To date, there is only one large prospective multicenter study being performed, which reported a successful visual restoration across all distances and a minimal level of disturbing halos and glares, as well as high levels of patient satisfaction [80]. Recently, the use of 'blended EDOF' has also been discussed. Blended EDOF aims at implantation of an EDOF IOL in one eye and a multifocal IOL in the fellow eye. A recent study compared visual outcomes between bilateral implantation of a diffractive multifocal IOL with blended EDOF, results showed that blended EDOF exhibited a better performance for uncorrected distance visual acuity but slightly worse in uncorrected near and intermediate visual acuity, blended EDOF also showed better contrast sensitivity under photopic conditions [81]. EDOF IOLs have promising results, however, larger clinical trials are also needed for better evidence to support clinical implantation.

Refractive Rotational Asymmetry IOL

Nowadays, patients have high visual expectations. After cataract surgery, patients not only expect to have clear vision for all distances including presbyopia correction, they also do not expect any compromise in contrast sensitivity and dislike unwanted visual symptoms. To overcome the drawbacks of multifocal IOLs, a new single piece refractive IOL has been introduced. The Lentis Mplus X IOL is a refractive rotational asymmetry IOL aiming at providing high contrast sensitivity and minimising halos and glare. The IOL provides multifocality by having 2 sectors with a seamless transition in between, there is an aspheric sector for distance vision and a +3.00 D sector in the lower IOL segment for near vision. This IOL is based on the concept of rotational asymmetry to reduce any potential sources of light scattering. Light is refracted to the near focus specifically in the lower sector and the rest of the lens acts as a monofocal IOL, this allows for more light to the distance focus without being scattered by diffraction, which then improves contrast sensitivity, causes less halo and glare and better image quality [82]. This IOL has a diameter of 11 mm and an optical zone diameter of 6 mm. A study with bilateral implantation of Lentis Mplus X IOL concluded that this new generation multifocal IOL was able to provide adequate distance, intermediate and near vision with high rates of spectacle independence [83]. Another study compared EDOF IOLs with Lentis Mplus X IOL, results showed that the Lentis Mplus X IOL had the highest higher order aberration in all cases [84]. However, although this new generation IOL was shown to provide a wide range of focus with no significant decrease in optical quality, IOL tilt in eyes are factors that limit its near vision outcomes [82]. Therefore, new haptic designs and a longer follow up period is needed to confirm the stability of this new generation multifocal IOL.

Monovision and Mini-Monovision

Monovision functions by using standard monofocal IOLs to correct distance vision in the dominant eye and to intentionally focus for near to intermediate vision in the non dominant eye. Monovision requires a process of neuroadaptation, which is how the brain adapts to use the dominant eye for distance image and the non dominant eye for near image to achieve a wide range of vision to achieve spectacle independence [85]. Monovision is usually achieved when the non dominant eye targets for roughly −2.50 D or more, but this is not always the case. Patient dissatisfaction usually arises from insufficient unaided reading capacity [86]. However, larger degrees of intended anisometropia come at a price, which causes a compromised visual function such as stereopsis and contrast sensitivity. Therefore, this technique is not appropriate for all patients. To address this, mini-monovision is a technique to aim at a smaller range of anisometropia, where the non dominant reading eye aims between −0.75 and −1.25 D, this provides a good distance and intermediate vision, better stereopsis, fewer optical side effects but requires spectacle wear for certain near tasks such as reading fine prints or computer work [87]. Studies have compared bilateral implantation of multifocal IOLs to the effect of using mini-monovision technique, multifocal IOLs demonstrated better near vision and higher spectacle independence rate but also more likely to undergo IOL exchange, whereas mini-monovision technique reported fewer visual disturbances with acceptable rates of spectacle independence

[88–90]. The greatest challenge of using monovision technique is patient selection. Ideally, potential patients should undergo a contact lens trial to ensure good neuroadaptation for the technique. Mini-monovision technique is a choice to consider, as it creates a lesser degree of anisometropia and provides a good balance between spectacle independence and better stereopsis. It is also more cost effective when compared with multifocal IOLs. However, patients should be warned of the potential need for spectacles for specific near tasks.

Astigmatism

Toric IOL

Corneal astigmastism correction has become an essential part of cataract surgery in order to provide the best visual outcome. Toric IOLs (Fig. 12) are currently one of the main options for astigmatic correction during phacoemulsification. Toric IOLs were first introduced in 1992 as a three piece non-foldable PMMA IOL which evolved into the first foldable one piece silicone toric IOL in 1994. Since then, many advancements have been made in improving its IOL material and design. Toric IOLs function by neutralizing regular corneal astigmatism by accurate axis placement against the steepest corneal axis. Current toric IOLs can correct up to 6D of astigmatism and can be used in both monofocal and multifocal IOL designs. However, toric IOLs depend on its rotational stability. A 5 degree rotation can cause a decay in image quality to up to 7% and a 10 degree rotation causes a decay in up to 11%. Rotations up to 30 degrees will lead to a 45% decay in image quality and will eliminate the correcting effect of the IOL [91, 92]. IOL biomaterial has a major influence on rotational stability. After implantation of a toric IOL into the capsular bag, the anterior and posterior capsule fuses with the IOL and prevents postoperative rotation. In vitro and animal studies have indicated acrylic IOLs to have the strongest adhesions with the capsular bag as compared with other biomaterials [93, 94].

Fig. 12 Tecnis® Toric IOL

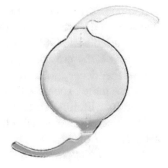

Keys to success in implanting toric IOLs depend on preoperative and intraoperative measures as well as proper patient selection. Ideal patients should have at least 1–1.5 D corneal astigmatism. Preoperatively, comprehensive ocular examination and topography should be done to rule out ocular comorbidities that may interfere with postoperative outcomes. Eyes with irregular astigmatism such as corneal scars are not preferred for toric IOL implantation, eyes with a regular bowtie astigmatism are the most suitable candidates. As a stable capsular bag IOL complex is essential for rotational stability, zonular instability and posterior capsular instability are also contraindications for implanting toric IOLs. As for preoperative investigations, accurate biometry and keratometry are needed for precise IOL power calculation. Accuracy can be enhanced by taking repeated measurements and using different devices based on different principles [95]. Intraoperatively, alignment accuracy can be improved by accurate corneal marking. Various methods have been described in axis marking, these can be done either manually or by image guided systems. Manual marking can be done by coaxial slit beam, bubble marker, pendulum marker or tonometer marker. A comparative study of the four different marking techniques showed a minimal rotational deviation with pendular marker and a least vertical misalignment with the slit lamp marking technique [96]. Manual marking should be done when the patient is sitting erect with the back resting against a wall and looking straight ahead, so as to avoid any cyclotorsion which can go up to 28 degrees when there is a change in position from sitting to supine [97]. Image guided techniques include iris fingerprinting, where the iris and limbal landmarks are captured preoperatively and intraoperative image registration are used to match the images and to calculate the distance in degrees from the targeted axis [95]. Newer advancements include intraoperative aberrometry, these devices can be used to perform real time assessment of the lens status to provide an accurate toric IOL alignment.

Before the introduction of toric IOLs, preoperative corneal astigmatism was addressed by the technique of limbal relaxing incisions (LRI) during cataract surgery. LRI involves the creation of paired incisions corresponding to the steep meridian, resulting in flattening of the cornea and reducing the astigmatic power. Although LRI is easy to perform, inexpensive and effective in reducing up to 4D of astigmatism, it carries the risk of corneal perforation. Also, LRI results are often unpredictable, as it depends on the rate and degree of corneal healing and remodeling. Moreover, LRI is unable to correct high astigmatisms as in toric IOLs. When comparing toric IOLs and monofocal IOLs with LRIs, study have showed that toric IOLs are able to provide a more effective and predictable outcome when compared to LRIs [98]. A recent systematic review and meta-analysis also showed that toric IOLs provide better uncorrected distance visual acuity, greater spectacle independence and lower amounts of residual astigmatism [99]. Although toric IOLs are more expensive than monofocal IOLs, economical analyses have demonstrated that lifetime costs are reduced with the use of toric IOLs because of the reduced need for spectacles [100]. Toric IOLs should be considered in cases with astigmatism of over 1D as it effectively neutralizes astigmatism and provides a good visual outcome.

Aniridic IOLs

Aniridia can be due to congenital conditions or it may be acquired after ocular trauma. Aniridia affects visual quality and leads to significant photophobia as well as symptoms of halo and glare, it can also lead to poor cosmesis. In aniridia cases, if lens extraction is needed, implantation of an aniridic IOL can be considered. An aniridic IOL is an IOL with a black diaphragm, manufactured by Morcher GmBH (Stuttgart, Germany) and they are available in several types. BDI consists of a clear central optic (4.5, 5 or 6.5 mm diameter), surrounded by a black diaphragm and 2 haptics (12.5 or 13.5 mm) with the latter built with a hoop in the haptic to allow for scleral fixation (Fig. 13). Due to its large optical diameter, a large corneal incision is required for BDI placement.

BDIs are shown to effectively improve visual acuity, decrease photophobia and resolve cosmetic issues in most both congenital aniridia and traumatic aniridia cases [101, 102].

BDIs can have potential complications, one being corneal decompensation from endothelial cell loss, this can be due to mechanical damage from insertion of a large IOL, postoperative persistent inflammation or high intraocular pressure [103]. A large study reported long-term follow up in eyes with congenital aniridia and identified glaucoma as a major long-term complication [104]. Although these eyes were already at risk of developing glaucoma, other contributing factors were hypothesized to be due to a direct compression onto the trabecular meshwork by the haptics, which was especially true in cases where BDIs were placed in a relatively anterior position as seen with ultrasound biometry. However, high intraocular pressure was also noted in cases with a normal BDI position. This was thought to be due to chronic postoperative inflammation or a large IOL size impairing aqueous outflow.

BDIs seem to be a safe and effective IOL in aniridic eyes, however, long-term follow up is needed for its potential complications.

Fig. 13 Morcher® Aniridic IOL

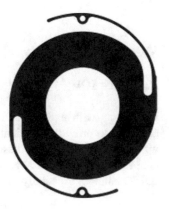

Adjustable IOLs

Nowadays, a patient who wishes to undergo cataract surgery often has high expectations and demand for accurate refractive outcomes. However, realistically, these cannot always be achieved and will often lead to patient dissatisfaction. The introduction of adjustable IOLs aims at improving refractive accuracy, visual outcome and patient satisfaction. The idea is to allow patients to choose their specific refractive outcomes and to allow for post op adjustment accordingly, so to deliver accurate results. Light adjustable lenses (LAL) consist of photosensitive silicone macromers diffused over the IOL, irradiation of the LAL with ultraviolet light causes photosensitive macromers to polymerize. This polymerization causes the formation of silicone polymers in the irradiated region, a diffusion gradient between the radiated and non-radiated portions will then be created, this allows macromers to migrate towards the irradiated portion and leads to lens swelling and refractive power increment [105]. As with other IOLs, LALs are implanted into the capsular bag with standard phacoemulsification techniques. Roughly around one month after the operation, the patient will undergo refraction, a light delivery device system will then be used to deliver ultraviolet light at the slit lamp to induce predictable and precise changes to the shape and refractive power of the IOL optic to allow for post operative fine refractive adjustments. After the new refractive power is confirmed, a lock in procedure will be carried out with the light delivery device to allow irradiation to the entire lens to polymerize all remaining macromers, this will not cause any diffusion gradient and will not result in any lens power change, thus preventing additional changes to the refractive outcome. A recent study concluded that light adjustable IOLs are able to achieve accurate refractive outcomes to around emmetropia with good uncorrected distance visual acuity, which remained stable over time [106]. Another study also concluded that light adjustable IOLs are able to reduce postoperative spherical and cylindrical errors to up to 2D. There was significant improvement in uncorrected distant visual acuity and the refractive changes were stable [107]. LALs seem to be a promising IOL with good refractive results, however, long term results are needed for evidence of a stable refractive outcome.

Special IOL Techniques

Piggyback IOL

In patients with extreme refractive errors, a single high power IOL may not be adequate to provide sufficient power, the use of piggyback IOLs help by implanting two IOLs to correct these high powers. Piggyback IOLs can also be considered in cases of undesirable optical results, the procedure carries a lower risk than IOL exchange, especially in cases when the IOL has already been fibrosed in the capsular bag, the optical result is often also more predictable and accurate [108, 109]. Piggyback IOLs are usually done with one IOL implanted into the capsular bag and a second IOL implanted in the sulcus.

In cases of extreme high powers, the image quality of piggyback IOL is superior to that of a single IOL, as with a single IOL, a steep radius is needed to provide high powers which will contribute to significant spherical abberations and will lead to severely distorted image quality [110]. The optimal image quality that can be achieved in eyes with extreme axial length was found to be by a piggyback IOL system. Piggyback IOL also provides additional benefit in terms of depth of focus. This was hypothesized to be due to the presence of a contact zone between the two IOLs being implanted, which was surrounded by concentric Newton rings [111]. The size of the contact zone depends on the curvature of the IOL and its material, and causes a pressure forcing the IOLs together. The Newton rings surrounding the contact zone are due to the presence of a very thin gap between the two IOLs, causing possible interference. Within the contact zone, the lens curvature is flatter than that outside of the zone, which then provides a lower refractive power. Therefore, this design principle simulates that of a multifocal IOL, where the central zone with less refractive power can be used for distance viewing and the non-contact zone with more refractive power can be used for near distance viewing. Defocus curves in piggyback IOLs have been shown to have a greater depth of focus than those in single IOLs.

However, piggyback IOLs have their own drawbacks. The presence of Elschnig pearls and intralenticular opacification have been reported between the interface of the piggyback IOLs [112, 113]. These membranous formations affect visual acuity and also cause late refractive surprises [114]. To prevent intralenticular opacification, meticulous polishing of the anterior capsule has been recommended to eliminate residual LEC, a large capsulorrhexis can also prevent migration of LEC into the intralenticular space [115]. Vaulting to avoid IOL-IOL contact can eliminate interlenticular opacification.

Anterior Chamber IOLs

Anterior chamber IOLs are considered in myopia correction by phakic IOLs or aphakic correction when the IOL is considered not suitable to be placed in the capsular bag. Anterior chamber IOLs can be angle supported or iris supported. Angle supported IOLs are fixed with four haptic points in the anterior chamber. Iris supported IOL is positioned in the anterior chamber and held in place by fixation to the mid-peripheral iris stroma. When comparing angle supported IOL and iris supported IOLs, although angle supported IOLs are technically easier, they have a significantly higher rate of endothelial cell loss [116], and also leads to higher rates of glaucoma. Therefore, angle supported IOLs are often not the desired choice and are contraindicated in young patients, eyes with preexisting glaucoma or corneal endothelial pathologies.

As for iris supported IOLs, they are shown to be safe, efficacious, predictable and stable in correcting high or severe myopia with significant gains in visual acuity [117, 118]. Postoperative complications include glare and halos from poor centration or from implantation in eyes with large pupil sizes, other complication includes the formation of cataract in phakic IOLs. Another important issue is also the rate of endothelial cell loss. A four year endothelial study has reported endothelial cell loss rate to be 3.85% at 6 months to 13.42% at 4 years [119]. Due to its anterior position, there are a few recommendations before considering implanting of iris supported IOLs. Firstly, an anterior chamber depth of at least 3.2 mm is required before considering its implantation. Secondly, preoperative specular microscopy is also essential in excluding eyes with preexisting compromised endothelial cell count. Lastly, extra caution has to be taken in considering the implantation in young patients due to a potential risk of corneal decompensation in the future.

Retropupillary iris supported IOLs have been designed aiming to reduce the rate of loss of endothelial cell count, however, a retrospective analysis has showed that the technique does not have a significant effect on decreasing the rate [120]. Other studies have also showed pigment dispersion to be a potential complication with retropupillary placement [121].

Scleral Fixating IOLs

In cases of inadequate capsular support after cataract surgery, choices of angle supporting IOLs, iris supporting IOLs or scleral fixating IOLs (SFIOL) can be considered. A literature review was conducted to determine the safety and efficacy between the three types of IOL fixation methods in eyes with inadequate capsular support, it was concluded that there is insufficient evidence to demonstrate the superiority of one lens type or fixation method over another [122].

Regarding scleral fixating IOLs, its surgical techniques have evolved over the past decades. Scleral fixating IOLs can be fixated to the sclera by sutures or by tunneling the haptics without the use of sutures or by the formation of terminal bulbs on the haptic ends to avoid suture usage as well. SFIOL techniques can largely be grouped into sutured or sutureless techniques.

For sutured techniques, suture was used to fix the haptics of the IOL to the sclera at 3 and 9 o'clock positioned 2 mm posterior to the limbus. As sutures are tied onto the sclera, there is a risk of suture exposure and conjunctival erosion. Symptoms of foreign body sensation have also been reported due to exposed suture ends. To improve this, scleral flaps were fashioned to cover the suture knots to avoid exposure or irritable symptoms [123]. However, scleral flap technique requires a conjunctival peritomy and can be problematic in patients requiring future glaucoma filtration surgeries. Therefore, the introduction of Hoffman's pouch aims at creating scleral pockets without the need of conjunctival peritomy and allows adequate suture knot coverage [124]. In the recent decades, the Lewis technique has been widely used, a 10-O polypropylene suture with a straight needle was passed from one scleral side to the opposite and the needle was turned around and passed back into the eye and emerged at the original scleral bed. Both sutures were withdrawn and cut and tied to the eyelet of the IOL and IOL was inserted through the corneoscleral wound. The sutures were then tied and knots rotated and covered with conjunctiva. A recent study demonstrated long-term stability with the Lewis technique, although knot erosion is not uncommon, the IOL remains stable due to a fibrotic process around the sutures and the IOL haptics [125]. To enhance durability of the sutures, thicker materials such as Gore-Tex have been used. A recent series using 7-O Gor-Tex suture reported no cases of suture breakage during a 33 months follow up period [126]. Long-term studies of sutured SFIOL have reported it to be a safe and effective technique, however potential risks include suture erosion and breakage leading to IOL dislocation or lens tilt and suture exposure causing endophthalmitis [127].

For sutureless techniques, intrascleral fixation, fibrin glue assisted or the Yamane technique have been described. Intrascleral fixation was described by Scharioth [128], which creates sclerotomies 2 mm posterior to the limbus then partial thickness scleral tunnels parallel to the limbus at the original sclerotomy sites. A three-piece IOL was inserted into the eye and the haptics were externalized through the sclerotomy incisions and placed into the scleral tunnels. The Scharioth technique was shown to provide exact centration and axial stability and prevented distortion in most cases. Fibrin glue has also been used to secure haptics to the sclera. Scleral flaps were fashioned and fibrin glue was applied to the bed of the flap to allow the haptics to be fixed in place, the scleral flap was positioned over the haptic to seal the flaps. Studies have shown one year results to be promising, however long term results are lacking [129]. The Yamane technique was recently described, the technique first introduced a three-piece IOL into the anterior chamber, then a 27-G needle was used to create a scleral tunnel posterior to the limbus, the haptic was then introduced into the lumen of the needle and externalized. Cautery was applied to the ends of the haptic to allow formation of a terminal bulb to secure the IOL in place, conjunctiva was mobilized onto the bulb ends to prevent erosion [130].

Currently, there are limited studies comparing one type of SFIOL technique with another, there is limited long-term evidence to support the superiority of any one technique.

Rare IOL Related Complication

IOL Opacification

The opacification of IOLs is a rare complication and usually occurs during the late post operative period [131]. The exact cause and mechanism is still unknown. IOL opacification may cause decreased post operative visual acuity, reduction in contrast sensitivity and symptoms of glare, in severe cases, it requires explantation and IOL exchange [132]. Explanted opacified IOLs have been sent for analysis using light and scanning electron microscopy, results revealed numerous fine, granular, crystalline like deposits on both the anterior and posterior surfaces of the IOLs [132]. A report related its cause to individual manufacturers in relation to the differences in the water content of hydrophilic acrylic materials [133]. Another report attributed IOL opacification to primary calcification which was found in a significant number of patients implanted with hydrophilic-hydrophobic acrylic IOLs and had a significant effect on their vision [134]. Other surgical interventions with injection of foreign material into the anterior chamber such as air or gas, also seem to increase the risk of IOL opacification [135]. There have been increasing reports on hydrophilic IOL opacification after endothelial keratoplasty with intra-cameral instillation of air or gas [136–139]. IOL explantation is the only treatment choice in severe cases, however it is often associated with increased complication rate [140]. A recent study even recommends to avoid hydrophilic acrylic IOLs in procedures that will require intracameral air or gas injection such as endothelial keratoplasty [141]. Although IOL opacification is a rare late post operative complication, it can lead to severe undesirable visual outcome requiring IOL explantation, which can be a high risk procedure.

Conclusion

With the evolution of IOLs, there is currently a large diversity of IOLs available in the market. IOL selection is an individualized process and should be based on the patient's motivation for spectacle independence, activities of daily living and visual expectations. Although newer IOLs seem to show favorable outcomes, they will need larger clinical trials for better evidence in support of clinical usage.

References

1. Hennig A, Puri LR, Sharma H, Evans JR, Yorston D. Foldable vs rigid lenses after phacoemulsification for cataract surgery: a randomised controlled trial. Eye (Lond). 2014;28(5):567–75.
2. Ronbeck M, Kugelberg M. Posterior capsule opacification with 3 intraocular lenses: 12-year prospective study. J Cataract Refract Surg. 2014;40(1):70–6.
3. Alio JL, Chipont E, BenEzra D, Fakhry MA, International Ocular Inflammation Society SGoUCS. Comparative performance of intraocular lenses in eyes with cataract and uveitis. J Cataract Refract Surg 2002;28(12):2096–108.
4. Habal MB. The biologic basis for the clinical application of the silicones. A correlate to their biocompatibility. Arch Surg. 1984;119(7):843–8.
5. Apple DJ, Federman JL, Krolicki TJ, et al. Irreversible silicone oil adhesion to silicone intraocular lenses. A clinicopathologic analysis. Ophthalmology. 1996;103(10):1555–61; discussion 1561–52.
6. Bartz-Schmidt KU, Konen W, Esser P, Walter P, Heimann K. Intraocular silicone lenses and silicone oil. Klin Monbl Augenheilkd. 1995;207(3):162–6.
7. Kusaka S, Kodama T, Ohashi Y. Condensation of silicone oil on the posterior surface of a silicone intraocular lens during vitrectomy. Am J Ophthalmol. 1996;121(5):574–5.

8. Wong D, Williams R, Batterbury M. Adherence of silicone oil to intraocular lenses. Eye (Lond). 1995;9(Pt 4):539.
9. Smith GT, Coombes AG, Sheard RM, Gartry DS. Unexpected posterior capsule rupture with unfolding silicone plate-haptic lenses. J Cataract Refract Surg. 2004;30(1):173–8.
10. Chang A, Kugelberg M. Posterior capsule opacification 9 years after phacoemulsification with a hydrophobic and a hydrophilic intraocular lens. Eur J Ophthalmol. 2017;27(2):164–8.
11. Duman R, Karel F, Ozyol P, Ates C. Effect of four different intraocular lenses on posterior capsule opacification. Int J Ophthalmol. 2015;8(1):118–21.
12. Li Y, Wang J, Chen Z, Tang X. Effect of hydrophobic acrylic versus hydrophilic acrylic intraocular lens on posterior capsule opacification: meta-analysis. PLoS One. 2013;8(11):e77864.
13. Pozlerova J, Nekolova J, Jiraskova N, Rozsival P. Evaluation of the posterior capsule opacification in different types of artificial intraocular lenses. Cesk Slov Oftalmol. 2009;65(1):12–5.
14. Oshika T, Ando H, Inoue Y, et al. Influence of surface light scattering and glistenings of intraocular lenses on visual function 15 to 20 years after surgery. J Cataract Refract Surg. 2018;44(2):219–25.
15. Dick B, Schwenn O, Pfeiffer N. Extent of damage to different intraocular lenses by neodymium:YAG laser treatment—an experimental study. Klin Monbl Augenheilkd. 1997;211(4):263–71.
16. Schild G, Amon M, Abela-Formanek C, Schauersberger J, Bartl G, Kruger A. Uveal and capsular biocompatibility of a single-piece, sharp-edged hydrophilic acrylic intraocular lens with collagen (Collamer): 1-year results. J Cataract Refract Surg. 2004;30(6):1254–8.
17. Pande MV, Spalton DJ, Kerr-Muir MG, Marshall J. Postoperative inflammatory response to phacoemulsification and extracapsular cataract surgery: aqueous flare and cells. J Cataract Refract Surg. 1996;22(Suppl):1770–4.
18. Richter-Mueksch S, Kahraman G, Amon M, Schild-Burggasser G, Schauersberger J, Abela-Formanek C. Uveal and capsular biocompatibility after implantation of sharp-edged hydrophilic acrylic, hydrophobic acrylic, and silicone intraocular lenses in eyes with pseudoexfoliation syndrome. J Cataract Refract Surg. 2007;33(8):1414–8.
19. Lee SJ, Choi JH, Sun HJ, Choi KS, Jung GY. Surface calcification of hydrophilic acrylic intraocular lens related to inflammatory membrane formation after combined vitrectomy and cataract surgery. J Cataract Refract Surg. 2010;36(4):676–81.
20. Park DI, Ha SW, Park SB, Lew H. Hydrophilic acrylic intraocular lens optic opacification in a diabetic patient. Jpn J Ophthalmol. 2011;55(6):595–9.
21. Cavallini GM, Volante V, Campi L, De Maria M, Fornasari E, Urso G. Postoperative diffuse opacification of a hydrophilic acrylic intraocular lens: analysis of an explant. Int Ophthalmol. 2018;38(4):1733–9.
22. Findl O, Leydolt C. Meta-analysis of accommodating intraocular lenses. J Cataract Refract Surg. 2007;33(3):522–7.
23. Hayashi H, Hayashi K, Nakao F, Hayashi F. Quantitative comparison of posterior capsule opacification after polymethylmethacrylate, silicone, and soft acrylic intraocular lens implantation. Arch Ophthalmol. 1998;116(12):1579–82.
24. Wallin TR, Hinckley M, Nilson C, Olson RJ. A clinical comparison of single-piece and three-piece truncated hydrophobic acrylic intraocular lenses. Am J Ophthalmol. 2003;136(4):614–9.
25. Nejima R, Miyata K, Honbou M, et al. A prospective, randomised comparison of single and three piece acrylic foldable intraocular lenses. Br J Ophthalmol. 2004;88(6):746–9.
26. Raskin EM, Speaker MG, McCormick SA, Wong D, Menikoff JA, Pelton-Henrion K. Influence of haptic materials on the adherence of staphylococci to intraocular lenses. Arch Ophthalmol. 1993;111(2):250–3.
27. Nishi O, Nishi K, Sakanishi K. Inhibition of migrating lens epithelial cells at the capsular bend created by the rectangular optic edge of a posterior chamber intraocular lens. Ophthalmic Surg Lasers. 1998;29(7):587–94.

28. Findl O, Menapace R, Sacu S, Buehl W, Rainer G. Effect of optic material on posterior capsule opacification in intraocular lenses with sharp-edge optics: randomized clinical trial. Ophthalmology. 2005;112(1):67–72.
29. Nishi O, Nishi K. Preventing posterior capsule opacification by creating a discontinuous sharp bend in the capsule. J Cataract Refract Surg. 1999;25(4):521–6.
30. Findl O, Buehl W, Bauer P, Sycha T. Interventions for preventing posterior capsule opacification. Cochrane Database Syst Rev. 2007;(3):CD003738.
31. Holladay JT, Lang A, Portney V. Analysis of edge glare phenomena in intraocular lens edge designs. J Cataract Refract Surg. 1999;25(6):748–52.
32. Masket S, Geraghty E, Crandall AS, et al. Undesired light images associated with ovoid intraocular lenses. J Cataract Refract Surg. 1993;19(6):690–4.
33. Davison JA. Positive and negative dysphotopsia in patients with acrylic intraocular lenses. J Cataract Refract Surg. 2000;26(9):1346–55.
34. Findl O, Drexler W, Menapace R, et al. Accurate determination of effective lens position and lens-capsule distance with 4 intraocular lenses. J Cataract Refract Surg. 1998;24(8):1094–8.
35. Davison JA. Capsule contraction syndrome. J Cataract Refract Surg. 1993;19(5):582–9.
36. Davison JA. Inflammatory sequelae with silicone-polypropylene IOLs. J Cataract Refract Surg. 1992;18(4):421–2.
37. Cochener B, Jacq PL, Colin J. Capsule contraction after continuous curvilinear capsulorhexis: poly(methyl methacrylate) versus silicone intraocular lenses. J Cataract Refract Surg. 1999;25(10):1362–9.
38. Gonvers M, Sickenberg M, van Melle G. Change in capsulorhexis size after implantation of three types of intraocular lenses. J Cataract Refract Surg. 1997;23(2):231–8.
39. Wang M, Corpuz CC, Fujiwara M, Tomita M. Visual and optical performance of diffractive multifocal intraocular lenses with different haptic designs: 6 month follow-up. Clin Ophthalmol 2014;8919–26.
40. Seth SA, Bansal RK, Ichhpujani P, Seth NG. Comparative evaluation of two toric intraocular lenses for correcting astigmatism in patients undergoing phacoemulsification. Indian J Ophthalmol. 2018;66(10):1423–8.
41. Prinz A, Neumayer T, Buehl W, et al. Rotational stability and posterior capsule opacification of a plate-haptic and an open-loop-haptic intraocular lens. J Cataract Refract Surg. 2011;37(2):251–7.
42. Boulton M, Rozanowska M, Rozanowski B. Retinal photodamage. J Photochem Photobiol, B. 2001;64(2–3):144–61.
43. Tomany SC, Cruickshanks KJ, Klein R, Klein BE, Knudtson MD. Sunlight and the 10-year incidence of age-related maculopathy: the Beaver Dam Eye Study. Arch Ophthalmol. 2004;122(5):750–7.
44. Davison JA, Patel AS, Cunha JP, Schwiegerling J, Muftuoglu O. Recent studies provide an updated clinical perspective on blue light-filtering IOLs. Graefes Arch Clin Exp Ophthalmol. 2011;249(7):957–68.
45. Margrain TH, Boulton M, Marshall J, Sliney DH. Do blue light filters confer protection against age-related macular degeneration? Prog Retin Eye Res. 2004;23(5):523–31.
46. Hammond BR, Jr., Renzi LM, Sachak S, Brint SF. Contralateral comparison of blue-filtering and non-blue-filtering intraocular lenses: glare disability, heterochromatic contrast, and photostress recovery. Clin Ophthalmol. 2010;41465–73.
47. Wolffsohn JS, Cochrane AL, Khoo H, Yoshimitsu Y, Wu S. Contrast is enhanced by yellow lenses because of selective reduction of short-wavelength light. Optom Vis Sci. 2000;77(2):73–81.
48. Pipis A, Touliou E, Pillunat LE, Augustin AJ. Effect of the blue filter intraocular lens on the progression of geographic atrophy. Eur J Ophthalmol. 2015;25(2):128–33.
49. Rezai KA, Gasyna E, Seagle BL, Norris JR Jr, Rezaei KA. AcrySof Natural filter decreases blue light-induced apoptosis in human retinal pigment epithelium. Graefes Arch Clin Exp Ophthalmol. 2008;246(5):671–6.

50. Hui S, Yi L, Fengling QL. Effects of light exposure and use of intraocular lens on retinal pigment epithelial cells in vitro. Photochem Photobiol. 2009;85(4):966–9.
51. Lavric A, Pompe MT. Do blue-light filtering intraocular lenses affect visual function? Optom Vis Sci. 2014;91(11):1348–54.
52. Kara-Junior N, Espindola RF, Gomes BA, Ventura B, Smadja D, Santhiago MR. Effects of blue light-filtering intraocular lenses on the macula, contrast sensitivity, and color vision after a long-term follow-up. J Cataract Refract Surg. 2011;37(12):2115–9.
53. Downie LE, Busija L, Keller PR. Blue-light filtering intraocular lenses (IOLs) for protecting macular health. Cochrane Database Syst Rev. 2018:5CD011977.
54. Zhu XF, Zou HD, Yu YF, Sun Q, Zhao NQ. Comparison of blue light-filtering IOLs and UV light-filtering IOLs for cataract surgery: a meta-analysis. PLoS One. 2012;7(3):e33013.
55. Downes SM. Ultraviolet or blue-filtering intraocular lenses: what is the evidence? Eye (Lond). 2016;30(2):215–21.
56. Lichtinger A, Rootman DS. Intraocular lenses for presbyopia correction: past, present, and future. Curr Opin Ophthalmol. 2012;23(1):40–6.
57. Portney V. Light distribution in diffractive multifocal optics and its optimization. J Cataract Refract Surg. 2011;37(11):2053–9.
58. Barisic A, Dekaris I, Gabric N, et al. Comparison of diffractive and refractive multifocal intraocular lenses in presbyopia treatment. Coll Antropol. 2008;32(Suppl):227–31.
59. Carson D, Hill WE, Hong X, Karakelle M. Optical bench performance of AcrySof((R)) IQ ReSTOR((R)), AT LISA((R)) tri, and FineVision((R)) intraocular lenses. Clin Ophthalmol. 2014;82105–2113.
60. Liu X, Xie L, Huang Y. Comparison of the Visual Performance After Implantation of Bifocal and Trifocal Intraocular Lenses Having an Identical Platform. J Refract Surg. 2018;34(4):273–80.
61. Jin S, Friedman DS, Cao K, et al. Comparison of postoperative visual performance between bifocal and trifocal intraocular Lens based on randomized controlled trails: a meta-analysis. BMC Ophthalmol. 2019;19(1):78.
62. Yoon CH, Shin IS, Kim MK. Trifocal versus bifocal diffractive intraocular lens implantation after cataract surgery or refractive lens exchange: a meta-analysis. J Korean Med Sci. 2018;33(44):e275.
63. Montes-Mico R, Espana E, Bueno I, Charman WN, Menezo JL. Visual performance with multifocal intraocular lenses: mesopic contrast sensitivity under distance and near conditions. Ophthalmology. 2004;111(1):85–96.
64. Khandelwal SS, Jun JJ, Mak S, Booth MS, Shekelle PG. Effectiveness of multifocal and monofocal intraocular lenses for cataract surgery and lens replacement: a systematic review and meta-analysis. Graefes Arch Clin Exp Ophthalmol. 2019; 257(5):863–75.
65. Montes-Mico R, Ferrer-Blasco T, Charman WN, Cervino A, Alfonso JF, Fernandez-Vega L. Optical quality of the eye after lens replacement with a pseudoaccommodating intraocular lens. J Cataract Refract Surg. 2008;34(5):763–8.
66. Goes FJ. Visual results following implantation of a refractive multifocal IOL in one eye and a diffractive multifocal IOL in the contralateral eye. J Refract Surg. 2008;24(3):300–5.
67. Lubinski W, Podboraczynska-Jodko K, Gronkowska-Serafin J, Karczewicz D. Visual outcomes three and six months after implantation of diffractive and refractive multifocal IOL combinations. Klin Oczna. 2011;113(7–9):209–15.
68. Gunenc U, Celik L. Long-term experience with mixing and matching refractive array and diffractive CeeOn multifocal intraocular lenses. J Refract Surg. 2008;24(3):233–42.
69. Gundersen KG, Makari S, Ostenstad S, Potvin R. Retreatments after multifocal intraocular lens implantation: an analysis. Clin Ophthalmol. 2016;10365–371.
70. Makhotkina NY, Dugrain V, Purchase D, Berendschot T, Nuijts R. Effect of supplementary implantation of a sulcus-fixated intraocular lens in patients with negative dysphotopsia. J Cataract Refract Surg. 2018;44(2):209–18.
71. Makhotkina NY, Berendschot TT, Beckers HJ, Nuijts RM. Treatment of negative dysphotopsia with supplementary implantation of a sulcus-fixated intraocular lens. Graefes Arch Clin Exp Ophthalmol. 2015;253(6):973–7.

72. Falzon K, Stewart OG. Correction of undesirable pseudophakic refractive error with the Sulcoflex intraocular lens. J Refract Surg. 2012;28(9):614–9.
73. Doane JF. Accommodating intraocular lenses. Curr Opin Ophthalmol. 2004;15(1):16–21.
74. Zhou H, Zhu C, Xu W, Zhou F. The efficacy of accommodative versus monofocal intraocular lenses for cataract patients: A systematic review and meta-analysis. Medicine (Baltimore). 2018;97(40):e12693.
75. Alio JL, Alio Del Barrio JL, Vega-Estrada A. Accommodative intraocular lenses: where are we and where we are going. Eye Vis (Lond). 2017;416.
76. McLeod SD, Vargas LG, Portney V, Ting A. Synchrony dual-optic accommodating intraocular lens. Part 1: optical and biomechanical principles and design considerations. J Cataract Refract Surg. 2007;33(1):37–46.
77. Marques EF, Castanheira-Dinis A. Clinical performance of a new aspheric dual-optic accommodating intraocular lens. Clin Ophthalmol. 2014;82289–95.
78. Akella SS, Juthani VV. Extended depth of focus intraocular lenses for presbyopia. Curr Opin Ophthalmol. 2018;29(4):318–22.
79. Gallego AA, Bara S, Jaroszewicz Z, Kolodziejczyk A. Visual Strehl performance of IOL designs with extended depth of focus. Optom Vis Sci. 2012;89(12):1702–7.
80. Cochener B, Concerto Study G. Clinical outcomes of a new extended range of vision intraocular lens: International Multicenter Concerto Study. J Cataract Refract Surg. 2016;42(9):1268–75.
81. de Medeiros AL, de Araujo Rolim AG, Motta AFP, et al. Comparison of visual outcomes after bilateral implantation of a diffractive trifocal intraocular lens and blended implantation of an extended depth of focus intraocular lens with a diffractive bifocal intraocular lens. Clin Ophthalmol. 2017;111911–16.
82. Alio JL, Pinero DP, Plaza-Puche AB, Chan MJ. Visual outcomes and optical performance of a monofocal intraocular lens and a new-generation multifocal intraocular lens. J Cataract Refract Surg. 2011;37(2):241–50.
83. Munoz G, Albarran-Diego C, Ferrer-Blasco T, Sakla HF, Garcia-Lazaro S. Visual function after bilateral implantation of a new zonal refractive aspheric multifocal intraocular lens. J Cataract Refract Surg. 2011;37(11):2043–52.
84. Camps VJ, Tolosa A, Pinero DP, de Fez D, Caballero MT, Miret JJ. In vitro aberrometric assessment of a multifocal intraocular lens and two extended depth of focus IOLs. J Ophthalmol. 2017;2017:7095734.
85. Greenstein S, Pineda R 2nd. The Quest for Spectacle Independence: A Comparison of Multifocal Intraocular Lens Implants and Pseudophakic Monovision for Patients with Presbyopia. Semin Ophthalmol. 2017;32(1):111–5.
86. Greenbaum S. Monovision pseudophakia. J Cataract Refract Surg. 2002;28(8):1439–43.
87. Hayashi K, Ogawa S, Manabe S, Yoshimura K. Binocular visual function of modified pseudophakic monovision. Am J Ophthalmol. 2015;159(2):232–40.
88. Labiris G, Giarmoukakis A, Patsiamanidi M, Papadopoulos Z, Kozobolis VP. Mini-monovision versus multifocal intraocular lens implantation. J Cataract Refract Surg. 2015;41(1):53–7.
89. Wilkins MR, Allan BD, Rubin GS, et al. Randomized trial of multifocal intraocular lenses versus monovision after bilateral cataract surgery. Ophthalmology. 2013;120(12):2449–55 e2441.
90. Mu J, Chen H, Li Y. Comparison study of visual function and patient satisfaction in patients with monovision and patients with bilateral multifocal intraocular lenses. Zhonghua Yan Ke Za Zhi. 2014;50(2):95–9.
91. Felipe A, Artigas JM, Diez-Ajenjo A, Garcia-Domene C, Alcocer P. Residual astigmatism produced by toric intraocular lens rotation. J Cataract Refract Surg. 2011;37(10):1895–901.
92. Tognetto D, Perrotta AA, Bauci F, et al. Quality of images with toric intraocular lenses. J Cataract Refract Surg. 2018;44(3):376–81.
93. Lombardo M, Carbone G, Lombardo G, De Santo MP, Barberi R. Analysis of intraocular lens surface adhesiveness by atomic force microscopy. J Cataract Refract Surg. 2009;35(7):1266–72.

94. Oshika T, Nagata T, Ishii Y. Adhesion of lens capsule to intraocular lenses of polymethylmethacrylate, silicone, and acrylic foldable materials: an experimental study. Br J Ophthalmol. 1998;82(5):549–53.
95. Browne AW, Osher RH. Optimizing precision in toric lens selection by combining keratometry techniques. J Refract Surg. 2014;30(1):67–72.
96. Popp N, Hirnschall N, Maedel S, Findl O. Evaluation of 4 corneal astigmatic marking methods. J Cataract Refract Surg. 2012;38(12):2094–9.
97. Ciccio AE, Durrie DS, Stahl JE, Schwendeman F. Ocular cyclotorsion during customized laser ablation. J Refract Surg. 2005;21(6):S772–4.
98. Leon P, Pastore MR, Zanei A, et al. Correction of low corneal astigmatism in cataract surgery. Int J Ophthalmol. 2015;8(4):719–24.
99. Kessel L, Andresen J, Tendal B, Erngaard D, Flesner P, Hjortdal J. Toric intraocular lenses in the correction of astigmatism during cataract surgery: a systematic review and meta-analysis. Ophthalmology. 2016;123(2):275–86.
100. Laurendeau C, Lafuma A, Berdeaux G. Modelling lifetime cost consequences of toric compared with standard IOLs in cataract surgery of astigmatic patients in four European countries. J Med Econ. 2009;12(3):230–7.
101. Qiu X, Ji Y, Zheng T, Lu Y. The efficacy and complications of black diaphragm intra-ocular lens implantation in patients with congenital aniridia. Acta Ophthalmol. 2016;94(5):e340–4.
102. Dong X, Yu B, Xie L. Black diaphragm intraocular lens implantation in aphakic eyes with traumatic aniridia and previous pars plana vitrectomy. J Cataract Refract Surg. 2003;29(11):2168–73.
103. Qiu X, Ji Y, Zheng T, Lu Y. Long-term efficacy and complications of black diaphragm intraocular lens implantation in patients with traumatic aniridia. Br J Ophthalmol. 2015;99(5):659–64.
104. Reinhard T, Engelhardt S, Sundmacher R. Black diaphragm aniridia intraocular lens for congenital aniridia: long-term follow-up. J Cataract Refract Surg. 2000;26(3):375–81.
105. Schwartz DM. Light-adjustable lens. Trans Am Ophthalmol Soc. 2003;101417–436.
106. Villegas EA, Alcon E, Rubio E, Marin JM, Artal P. Refractive accuracy with light-adjustable intraocular lense. J Cataract Refract Surg. 2014;40(7):1075–84.
107. Hengerer FM, Hutz WW, Dick HB, Conrad-Hengerer I. Combined correction of sphere and astigmatism using the light-adjustable intraocular lens in eyes with axial myopia. J Cataract Refract Surg. 2011;37(2):313–23.
108. Gayton JL, Sanders VN. Implanting two posterior chamber intraocular lenses in a case of microphthalmos. J Cataract Refract Surg. 1993;19(6):776–7.
109. Sales CS, Manche EE. Managing residual refractive error after cataract surgery. J Cataract Refract Surg. 2015;41(6):1289–99.
110. Hull CC, Liu CS, Sciscio A. Image quality in polypseudophakia for extremely short eyes. Br J Ophthalmol. 1999;83(6):656–63.
111. Findl O, Menapace R, Rainer G, Georgopoulos M. Contact zone of piggyback acrylic intraocular lenses. J Cataract Refract Surg. 1999;25(6):860–2.
112. Gayton JL, Apple DJ, Peng Q, et al. Interlenticular opacification: clinicopathological correlation of a complication of posterior chamber piggyback intraocular lenses. J Cataract Refract Surg. 2000;26(3):330–6.
113. Hua X, Yuan XY, Song H, Tang X. Long-term results of clear lens extraction combined with piggyback intraocular lens implantation to correct high hyperopia. Int J Ophthalmol. 2013;6(5):650–5.
114. Shugar JK, Schwartz T. Interpseudophakos Elschnig pearls associated with late hyperopic shift: a complication of piggyback posterior chamber intraocular lens implantation. J Cataract Refract Surg. 1999;25(6):863–7.
115. Fenzl RE, Gills JP 3rd, Gills JP. Piggyback intraocular lens implantation. Curr Opin Ophthalmol. 2000;11(1):73–6.

116. Aerts AA, Jonker SM, Wielders LH, et al. Phakic intraocular lens: Two-year results and comparison of endothelial cell loss with iris-fixated intraocular lenses. J Cataract Refract Surg. 2015;41(10):2258–65.
117. Budo C, Hessloehl JC, Izak M, et al. Multicenter study of the Artisan phakic intraocular lens. J Cataract Refract Surg. 2000;26(8):1163–71.
118. Silva RA, Jain A, Manche EE. Prospective long-term evaluation of the efficacy, safety, and stability of the phakic intraocular lens for high myopia. Arch Ophthalmol. 2008;126(6):775–81.
119. Menezo JL, Cisneros AL, Rodriguez-Salvador V. Endothelial study of iris-claw phakic lens: four year follow-up. J Cataract Refract Surg. 1998;24(8):1039–49.
120. Forlini M, Soliman W, Bratu A, Rossini P, Cavallini GM, Forlini C. Long-term follow-up of retropupillary iris-claw intraocular lens implantation: a retrospective analysis. BMC Ophthalmol. 2015;15143.
121. Rijneveld WJ, Beekhuis WH, Hassman EF, Dellaert MM, Geerards AJ. Iris claw lens: anterior and posterior iris surface fixation in the absence of capsular support during penetrating keratoplasty. J Refract Corneal Surg. 1994;10(1):14–9.
122. Wagoner MD, Cox TA, Ariyasu RG, Jacobs DS, Karp CL, American Academy of O. Intraocular lens implantation in the absence of capsular support: a report by the American Academy of Ophthalmology. Ophthalmology. 2003;110(4):840–59.
123. Lewis JS. Ab externo sulcus fixation. Ophthalmic Surg. 1991;22(11):692–5.
124. Hoffman RS, Fine IH, Packer M. Scleral fixation without conjunctival dissection. J Cataract Refract Surg. 2006;32(11):1907–12.
125. Cavallini GM, Volante V, De Maria M, et al. Long-term analysis of IOL stability of the Lewis technique for scleral fixation. Eur J Ophthalmol. 2015;25(6):525–8.
126. Khan MA, Gupta OP, Smith RG, et al. Scleral fixation of intraocular lenses using Gore-Tex suture: clinical outcomes and safety profile. Br J Ophthalmol. 2016;100(5):638–43.
127. Heilskov T, Joondeph BC, Olsen KR, Blankenship GW. Late endophthalmitis after transscleral fixation of a posterior chamber intraocular lens. Arch Ophthalmol. 1989;107(10):1427.
128. Scharioth GB, Prasad S, Georgalas I, Tataru C, Pavlidis M. Intermediate results of sutureless intrascleral posterior chamber intraocular lens fixation. J Cataract Refract Surg. 2010;36(2):254–9.
129. Narang P, Narang S. Glue-assisted intrascleral fixation of posterior chamber intraocular lens. Indian J Ophthalmol. 2013;61(4):163–7.
130. Yamane S, Inoue M, Arakawa A, Kadonosono K. Sutureless 27-gauge needle-guided intrascleral intraocular lens implantation with lamellar scleral dissection. Ophthalmology. 2014;121(1):61–6.
131. Werner L. Causes of intraocular lens opacification or discoloration. J Cataract Refract Surg. 2007;33(4):713–26.
132. Tandogan T, Khoramnia R, Choi CY, et al. Optical and material analysis of opacified hydrophilic intraocular lenses after explantation: a laboratory study. BMC Ophthalmol. 2015;15170.
133. Izak AM, Werner L, Pandey SK, Apple DJ. Calcification of modern foldable hydrogel intraocular lens designs. Eye (Lond). 2003;17(3):393–406.
134. Bompastor-Ramos P, Povoa J, Lobo C, et al. Late postoperative opacification of a hydrophilic-hydrophobic acrylic intraocular lens. J Cataract Refract Surg. 2016;42(9):1324–31.
135. Dhital A, Spalton DJ, Goyal S, Werner L. Calcification in hydrophilic intraocular lenses associated with injection of intraocular gas. Am J Ophthalmol. 2012;153(6):1154–60 e1151.
136. Patryn E, van der Meulen IJ, Lapid-Gortzak R, Mourits M, Nieuwendaal CP. Intraocular lens opacifications in Descemet stripping endothelial keratoplasty patients. Cornea. 2012;31(10):1189–92.
137. Mojzis P, Studeny P, Werner L, Pinero DP. Opacification of a hydrophilic acrylic intraocular lens with a hydrophobic surface after air injection in Descemet-stripping automated

endothelial keratoplasty in a patient with Fuchs dystrophy. J Cataract Refract Surg. 2016;42(3):485–8.

138. Norouzpour A, Zarei-Ghanavati S. Hydrophilic Acrylic Intraocular Lens Opacification after Descemet Stripping Automated Endothelial Keratoplasty. J Ophthalmic Vis Res. 2016;11(2):225–7.

139. Fellman MA, Werner L, Liu ET, et al. Calcification of a hydrophilic acrylic intraocular lens after Descemet-stripping endothelial keratoplasty: case report and laboratory analyses. J Cataract Refract Surg. 2013;39(5):799–803.

140. Dagres E, Khan MA, Kyle GM, Clark D. Perioperative complications of intraocular lens exchange in patients with opacified Aqua-Sense lenses. J Cataract Refract Surg. 2004;30(12):2569–73.

141. Giers BC, Tandogan T, Auffarth GU, et al. Hydrophilic intraocular lens opacification after posterior lamellar keratoplasty—a material analysis with special reference to optical quality assessment. BMC Ophthalmol. 2017;17(1):150.

Calculating the Human Eye—Basics on Biometry

Sibylle Scholtz, Alan Cayless and Achim Langenbucher

Introduction

The word "biometry" derives from the Greek words "βίος" (bíos: life) and "μέτρον" (métron: measure, measurement) and is the method of applying mathematical principles to describing the anatomical characteristics of living organisms. In our case "biometry" refers to the anatomical and refractive properties of the human eye. Before cataract surgery it is essential to gather such biometric data in order to properly calculate the IOL power which will offer the optimum post-operative refractive outcome.

Refractive errors are most probably as old as mankind. In prehistoric times, keen eyesight would have been essential for hunting or foraging, and any defect or impairment a severe disadvantage in avoiding becoming prey oneself. For thousands of years, refractive errors were often perceived as an infirmity which condemned people to passivity, reduced options for communication and orientation—and thus led to isolation. Vision was and still is the most important sensory function for humans: about 75–80% of environmental information is delivered by our eyes to our brain. Worldwide, there are around 37 million blind people, 90% of whom live in developing countries. In up to 75% of these cases, blindness could be avoided. By far the most common cause of blindness globally is cataract. In industrialised countries cataract ranks third after glaucoma and diabetes mellitus related eye diseases. Although cataract surgeries have been performed for more than 3,000 years, the history of intraocular lens implantation began as recently as

S. Scholtz (✉) · A. Langenbucher
Institute of Experimental Ophthalmology, Saarland University, Homburg/Saar, Germany
e-mail: Sibylle.Scholtz@gmx.de

A. Langenbucher
e-mail: achim.langenbucher@uks.eu

A. Cayless
School of Physical Sciences, The Open University, Milton Keynes, UK
e-mail: a.t.cayless@open.ac.uk

© Springer Nature Switzerland AG 2021
C. Liu and A. Shalaby Bardan (eds.), *Cataract Surgery*,
https://doi.org/10.1007/978-3-030-38234-6_7

1949. Invented by the military eye surgeon Harold Ridley, this procedure offered the possibility of an optical implant for cataract patients for the first time. Cataract surgery faces new challenges today: well-informed "Baby Boomer" generation and post-LASIK patients are reaching the age at which they may require cataract surgery. These highly demanding cataract patients put ophthalmologists and surgeons under pressure to deliver an optimal refractive outcome of their surgery. This leads to the need for suitable, modern biometry and IOL calculation formulae for these special cases, because former methods may no longer be adequate to the expectations of these demanding patients. The European Registry of Quality Outcomes for Cataract and Refractive Surgery (EUREQUO, funded by ESRCS) provides a global platform, which also includes data on the refractive outcome of more than 2.6 million cataract surgeries to date. Scrutiny of the data shows that 93.8% of all monitored patients achieved an outcome ±1.0 D. While this may appear quite satisfactory at first sight, it raises the question of the remaining 6.2% of patients who suffer from more than 1.0 D of post-surgical refractive error, and the extent to which these suboptimal outcomes may have been caused by incorrect or inappropriate biometry and IOL calculation. In the context of the number of cataract surgeries listed in EUREQUO this means up to 161,200 patients with poor refractive outcomes after their surgery—a significant number!

With the invention and implantation of the first intraocular lens by Harold Ridley in 1949 the question arose as to how the refractive power of such artificial lenses could be determined. Ridley initially tried to replicate the dimensions of the human crystalline lens, but this simplistic approach proved far from correct. Even with the most modern technical devices and the most advanced calculation formulae and methods available today, the accurate biometry and calculation of the corresponding IOL still represents one of cataract surgery´s ongoing challenges.

Devices and Measurement Principles

History

As early as 1905, Gullstrand's model eye quantified the refractive power of the human eye primarily from the refractive properties of the cornea, lens, ocular media and the length of the eye. In 1967, Fyodorov and his team were the first to set up a vergence formula to estimate the optical power of an IOL.

Only once ultrasound measurements of the eye using A-scans became available in the 1970s were improved vergence formulae able to allow a more accurate calculation of the IOL. By using ultrasound A-scans to measure the length of the eye, variations of these fundamental vergence formulae were derived and published in the 1980s. The first ultrasound measurements of the eye were made as applanation or indentation examination. Here, the ultrasound probe is placed directly on the corneal surface, which inevitably leads to a compression of the cornea and the anterior chamber. Depending on the manual technique of the examiner, this in turn leads to differences in measurement results and thus to incorrect calculations of the IOL. As a technical development, immersion ultrasound measurement avoids direct contact between the ultrasound probe and the cornea by coupling the ultrasound probe to the cornea via a liquid-filled cylinder, immersion gel or through the eyelids. The development of this immersion method has enabled more meaningful, accurate, and reproducible results than contact measurements.

By using ultrasound the echo time of the signal is measured in seconds and converted into distance (mm) using an average sound velocity. Proper conversion is only possible if the individual proportions of the underlying model eye and the corresponding velocities match. Depending on the respective properties of structures within the eye, these velocities can differ significantly: the overall sound velocity in the eye is ~1550 m/s, but for silicone oil filled spaces it can be as low as 900 m/s and in hard nuclei as high as 1600 m/s.

Ultrasound A-Scans measure the total length of the eye, the anterior chamber depth and the thickness of the crystalline lens. This procedure should only be performed by experienced personnel. Additional keratometry measurements are needed to calculate the corresponding IOL. However, since the development of optical techniques, ultrasound biometry is no longer regarded as a "gold standard", especially since the disadvantages of requiring contact or coupling and dependence on technique far outweigh the benefits. Today, ultrasound biometry is mostly restricted to cases where optical biometry cannot be performed due to opaque optical media. More theoretical formulae derived in the 1980s and 1990s (e.g. Hoffer Q, Holladay 1 and Haigis) involving several input parameters (e.g. White-to-White or age used in Holladay 2 formula) are now used to improve IOL calculation.

Until Prof. Adolf Fercher published his groundbreaking results on optical non-contact measurement of the eye by partial coherence interferometry in the early 1980s, the measurement of the eye by ultrasound as an acoustic biometry procedure was considered without question as "state of the art". This was changed by the use of partially coherent light as described by Fercher. For the first time a non-contact optical A-scan was made possible—and this represented the first interferometric measurement of the length of the eye. In 1982, Fercher filed his invention for a patent: "*Fercher AF. Verfahren und Anordnung zur Messung der Teilstrecken des lebenden Auges. Offenlegungsschrift DE 3201801 A1; priority date 21.01.1982, Offenlegungstag 08.09.1983*". Based on this patent, Carl Zeiss Meditec developed the first biometric device using this novel technology, the "IOLMaster". With this device, optical biometry made successful debut. For the first time, a technique was available that allowed for distance-independent biometry, providing fast, non-contact and reproducible biometric data of the eye with a significantly higher resolution. Furthermore, the reduced operator dependence of the procedure meant that it could be carried out by less experienced staff. This device provided all of the parameters needed for IOL calculation. For the first time it was possible to determine both the length of the eye and keratometry data in one measurement with one device. This means that the corresponding IOL calculation can be carried out directly, without needing data from external sources, cutting down on transmission errors. The short coherence length light source emits in the visible spectrum, enabling axial length measurement along the fixation axis. In addition, optical biometry is much less susceptible to disturbances such as the medium (vitreous, silicone, gas) filling the posterior chamber of the eye, or the artificial lens when measuring pseudophakic eyes.

With optical biometry, optical distances are measured directly (as opposed to the geometrical measurements in ultrasound biometry). These optical distances are converted into dioptres using the refractive index. Here the variations are significantly smaller compared to ultrasound biometry. Therefore optical biometry is much less dependent on the medium (e.g. native vitreous, silicone oil, dense cataracts or the artificial IOL in pseudophakic eyes).

The proportion of eyes not measurable by optical biometry (and thus requiring ultrasound measurement), has been steadily reduced through optimisation of the measurement strategies and is now well below 5% in industrialised nations. After Zeiss, Haag-Streit brought the "Lenstar" to the market, which provided partial distance measurement for the first time. Today, most modern biometers work non-invasively using optical coherence tomography (OCT), and a variety of devices are available offering eye measurement by means of optical biometry.

Along with this technical evolution numerous formulae have been developed for calculating the optical power of each respective IOL. Intraocular lenses can be calculated using different strategies: with empirical formulae the IOL power is derived from a series of biometric data without any anatomical or physiological background. With the theoretical-optical formulae, which are most commonly used today, the IOL power is extracted from a paraxial optical model which approximates the eye using linear Gaussian optics. With modern raytracing, Snell's law is applied at each refracting surface within the eye and the lens design and power that provide the best focus at the retina are selected (if a plano refraction is favoured for the pseudophakic eye).

Parameters Needed for IOL Calculation

For the main application, several measurements of the eye are taken to calculate the correct lens power before implantation of the intraocular lens. One of the major challenges in IOL calculation is estimating the position where the artificial IOL will finally be located in the eye after surgery. Modelling the cornea and IOL using the thin lens approximation, the distance from the cornea to the IOL is defined as the "Effective Lens Position" (ELP).

1. Ultrasonic axial length

As shown in Fig. 1, acoustical biometry (A-scan) measures the distance between the anterior corneal apex up to the inner limiting membrane (ILM).

2. Axial length measurement with optical biometry

By contrast, optical biometry measures the axial length between the anterior corneal apex and the retinal pigment epithelium (RPE) (distance 2 in Fig. 1). As a

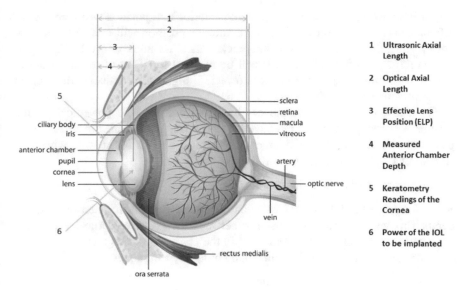

Fig. 1 Important parameters for IOL power calculation

result of these different length measurements, differences can be expected between the results of ultrasound and optical measurements. In most optical biometers, the axial length measurement is calibrated to the immersion ultrasound axial length measurement as this was the gold standard in early times of optical biometry. This calibration is typically performed by subtracting a *standard retinal thickness* of around 200 μm. Therefore, ultrasound and optical axial length measurement may yield different results in individual cases. Today, optical biometry is regarded as the gold standard.

3. Effective Lens Position (ELP)

In theoretical optical calculations the effective lens position is defined as the axial position of a thin intraocular lens implant relative to the corneal anterior vertex of the eye. This ELP is mostly determined from biometric measurements of the eye as well as depending on the design and material of the lens and the placement of the lens in the eye (e.g. capsular bag), and adapts the generally defined formula to an individual eye and IOL type.

The ELP also reduces the model errors and inaccuracies which are inherent in the design of the vergence formulae, which means that the ELP does in general not really reflect the real IOL position in the eye. The improvements in intraocular lens power calculations over the past 30 years are the result of the improved predictability of the variable ELP.

It is important to note that, in an optical system consisting of two thin lenses the ELP will affect the IOL power.

For IOLs with a positive power a more posterior IOL position will increase the refractive power, and conversely a more anterior position will reduce the optical power. Thus, the IOL constants in theoretical optical formulae affect the ELP.

The refractive effect of the ELP will be reduced for IOLs of lower refractive power. With minus lenses the effect is reversed: higher ELP values will result in lesser refractive power of the IOL.

For a given IOL, the lens power obtained from the IOL power calculation scheme will change with the effective lens position. In general, for an IOL with positive power a prediction of a larger ELP implies a larger IOL power, whereas a smaller ELP value implies a lower IOL power.

4. Measurement of the anterior chamber depth

Some formulae for IOL power calculation require the phakic anterior chamber depth. This value refers to the distance between the posterior corneal vertex and the anterior vertex of the crystalline lens in the phakic eye. This measurement can be made using optical as well as ultrasound biometry techniques.

5. Keratometry readings of the cornea

Keratometry generally measures the curvature of the anterior surface of the cornea and reports a radius of curvature in millimetres. Most keratometers offer dioptric powers in dpt in addition to curvature values in mm, but the user should be aware that dioptric powers cannot be measured in general. Conversion from mm radius of curvature of the corneal anterior surface to dioptric power of the entire cornea (the meniscus lens!) requires modelling assumptions about the cornea which may or may not be appropriate in any individual eye. Different keratometer indices which are normally used in different devices on the market refer to different model assumptions, and therefore in an individual patient's cornea the reported dioptric power may vary from device to device even if the base measurement of the radius of curvature of the anterior surface is the same. In order to avoid the potentially erroneous effect of an incorrect keratometer index it is strictly recommended to use radius of curvature measurements (the mm value) instead of dioptric powers for IOL power calculation. To convert between mm and dioptres, it is necessary to know the keratometer index (for example, the conversion from K to radii at a keratometer index of 1.332 would be: $R = 332/K$). Different keratometers use different indices, e.g. 1.3375 (American Optical, the so-called Javal index), 1.336 (Haag-Streit), 1.332 (Zeiss, Gambs, Topcon, the so-called Zeiss index), 1.338 (Hoya).

Importantly, for a given patient the reported radii should be the same on all of the instruments discussed, but the Ks will differ significantly (up to 0.8 D). The default keratometer setting of the IOLMaster is 1.3375 in the USA and 1.332 in all other countries. Also, it is important to consider that each keratometer measures the radius of the corneal anterior surface at a different position, e.g. at distances of 1.25 mm, 1.5 mm or indeed other values.

6. Lens thickness

Furthermore, some IOL-calculation formulae use biometrical values for the thickness of the crystalline lens in calculating the IOL power, e.g. the Olsen formula, Holladay 2 formula and Barrett Universal II formula.

7. Horizontal corneal diameter measurement

The horizontal "white-to-white" distance (horizontal corneal diameter, WTW) is an optional additional measurement. It can be used in the Holladay 2 and some other formulae.

Devices

Ultrasound

Sonic altimeter instruments use echo impulses to measure distances. The A-Scan is used to determine the axial length of the eye. Acoustical biometry can be carried out as applanation contact ultrasound biometry (10 MHz) or immersion ultrasound biometry. Both techniques measure the axial length, anterior chamber depth and thickness of the lens and optionally the thickness of the cornea. In addition, the keratometry must be measured with an external device to determine the refractive power of the cornea.

Applanation scan

In this type of scan the ultrasound probe is placed directly on the cornea. This results in merging of the signal from the ultrasound probe with the echo of the cornea, meaning that the anterior surface cannot be determined by applying this technique. Furthermore, applanation ultrasound biometry produces an unavoidable error, i.e. the corneal applanation or indentation from the probe tip. This compression can induce a shortening of the anterior chamber of anywhere between 100 and 300 microns. As a result, the true axial length is underestimated, leading to an overestimation of the IOL power. Today, patients expect cataract surgery not only to restore visual clarity, but to provide excellent vision in refractive terms as well. Contact biometry is far below the expectations and requirements in terms of accuracy in modern cataract surgery and should be avoided (Fig. 2).

Many examiners consider the contact technique easier and faster than the immersion technique. The disadvantages are clear, as an unavoidable error is produced by compressing the cornea. As a result, the true axial length is underestimated, leading to an overestimation of the IOL power. Even if the axial length is corrected based on the examiner's experience by an offset (rule of thumb) the individual error in a patient measurement cannot be eliminated.

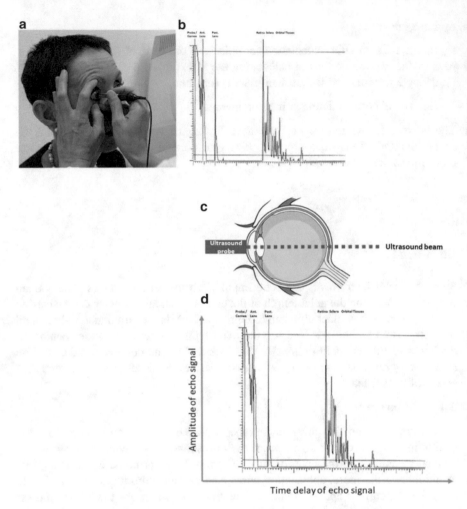

Fig. 2 a–d Applanation scan

Immersion scan

With the immersion technique, there is contact between the cornea and the scleral shell but not with the ultrasound probe. The technician places a small scleral shell on the anesthetised limbus, the probe is either hand-held within the fluid or locked into position in an infusion shell. The fluid is infused into the shell through tubing that connects the shell to either a bottle of BSS or a 5 cm^3 syringe of contact lens saline solution (infusion scleral shells can be used with the patient sitting upright, but it is easier for both patient and technician if the patient is reclined). When the probe is aligned properly, five tall spikes are clearly visible (ideal case) in the scan (representing echoes from the tip of probe, cornea, anterior lens capsule, posterior lens capsule and retina) with the retinal spike rising steeply from baseline then followed by echoes from sclera and orbital fat. The corneal spike is separate from the probe spike and has a double peak representing the epithelial and endothelial layers of the cornea (Fig. 3).

It is important to note that it is not self-evident that measurements are aligned along the visual axis in either applanation or immersion ultrasound biometry. In most cases, measurement is carried out by using applicable ultrasound echoes, which means that the sound signal hits the cornea and the retina perpendicularly, but not necessarily at the fovea. Especially with very long eyes a staphyloma located close to the fovea might lead to overestimation of the axial length, resulting in a calculated IOL power that is too low.

When using immersion ultrasound biometry there is less variation and measurements will be more reproducible, meaning that this technique delivers more

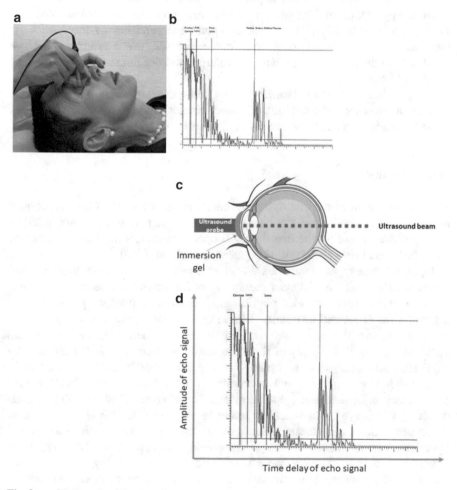

Fig. 3 a–d Immersion Ultrasound

accurate and reproducible results than applanation A-scans. The immersion technique can also be used in dense media, e.g. mature cataract or in eyes with corneal scars. The immersion method also has some disadvantages: the accuracy is lower (120 μm at 10 MHz), the contact between the scleral shell and the eye can induce a change in the eyeball's shape, the accuracy is limited by changes in sound velocity in difficult cases, e.g. pseudophakic eyes or silicone-filled eyes post vitrectomy (settings have to be adjusted appropriately), anaesthesia is required, and experienced operators are needed for application and reading the results. Furthermore, measurements take longer than with optical biometry and have to be carried out in a non-physiological position (reclined). Fixation will be an issue as well: ultrasound probes with an integrated fixation light might offer better fixation but can show an inhomogeneous radiation pattern, whereas probes without an integrated fixation light offer a more homogeneous pattern but might miss conditions such as posterior staphyloma which will require an additional B-Scan.

Both applanation and immersion ultrasound biometry are contact measurements, which always carries the risk of operator dependency of the results. As these techniques are likely to be less frequently used, fewer examiners will be familiar with the procedure and with the interpretation of the results, again raising the risk of errors.

Nevertheless, ultrasound biometry is an indispensable technique for cataract surgery in rare cases where optical biometry cannot be used, for instance in very dense cataracts, vitreous hemorrhages or eyes suffering from corneal scars.

Optical Biometry

With the invention of the first optical biometer in 1999 an option for non-contact measurement of the human eye using the concept of partial coherence interferometry was available for the first time. All optical biometers measure the distance from the corneal apex to the retinal pigment epithelium (RPE).

Optical biometry has numerous advantages over ultrasound methods. Optical biometers allow for a non-contact measurement (no anaesthesia required, no compression of the cornea) under physiological conditions (upright position) with a fixation target located at infinity. Measurements are carried out along the fixation axis of the biometer under fixation (which in general will be close to the visual axis), and the accuracy of the axial length measurement is not affected by pupil size. All settings are adjustable for accurate axial length measurement in silicone-filled eyes, aphakic and pseudophakic eyes. Optical biometers are easy to use, they offer automated operation and are more resistant to failures, even detecting which eye (right or left) is under investigation. As this is a non-contact procedure without anaesthesia measurements can be carried out by less skilled operators. Measurements can be made quickly, in approximately 0.4 s. Most importantly, optical biometry has a significantly higher accuracy, with the resolution of 10 μm being 5–10 times better than ultrasound methods. An optical biometer is almost an all-in-one instrument, scanning simultaneously for axial length, corneal radii and thickness, anterior chamber depth, lens thickness and

White-to-White (WTW) (Figs. 4 and 5). Also, optical biometers calculate the power of the required IOL, eliminating errors caused by transferring or transcribing data. Furthermore such optical biometers typically have an integrated database of optimised IOL constants for several lens types, and modern optical biometers have a direct link to IOL data platforms where lens data and optimised constants can be directly downloaded or updated.

Modern optical biometers are able to measure more than 95% of eyes, with cases involving opaque lenses or significant corneal scars making up the remaining 5%.

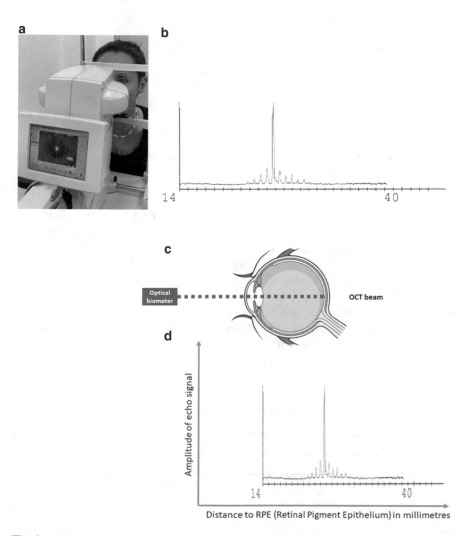

Fig. 4 a–d Non contact optical biometry. The peak refers to the signal of retinal pigment epithelium

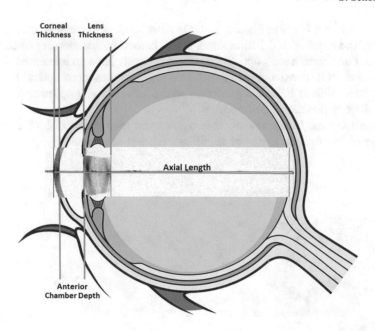

Fig. 5 Hybrid diagram showing OCT image of the cornea and crystalline lens superimposed on a diagrammatic representation of the human eye

Even when considering all striking benefits of optical biometry, ultrasound biometry still has an application in the minority of eyes with significant opacities of the ocular media that make them not amenable to optical measurement.

Both ultrasound and optical measurements are dependent to a certain extent on the modelling of the medium within the eye. With ultrasound, the time delay is converted into a depth in millimetres using an average speed of sound. In optical biometry, the optical path length is converted into a depth in millimetres using an average value for the refractive index. In both methods there can be errors because the conversions are based on estimates of average properties, respectively speed of sound and refractive index. As mentioned in 2.1 however, the variations in optical measurements are significantly smaller compared to ultrasound biometry.

Comparison between ultrasound and optical biometry

Ultrasound	Optical
Contact or immersion	Non-contact
Specially trained personnel needed	Delegable/operator independent results
Measurement is time-consuming	Faster measurement and calculation
Main source of measurement errors today	Higher precision in measurement output
Two procedures (Axial Length/Anterior Chamber Depth—Corneal Radii)	Single procedure (all measurements and IOL calculation)

Influence of Biometric Data for IOL Calculation

Size matters applies in the biometry of the eye. The length of the eye is one of the crucial factors in calculation of the appropriate IOL.

The model calculation for an IOL to achieve emmetropia in an eye with standard axial length of 23.39 mm is based on the appropriate Effective Lens Position (ELP) of 5.2 mm (as shown below). Variations in the axial length, corneal radius of curvature/dioptric power of the cornea or ELP will lead to differences in the IOL power required for emmetropisation of the eye as shown below:

	Short eye	"Normal" eye	Long eye
AL	21 mm	23.39 mm	25 mm
ACD	3,1 mm	3.37 mm	3,6 mm
P (emm.)	31.61 D	21.63 D	16,02 D
$\Delta P/\Delta AL$	−4.80 D/mm	−3.83 D/mm	−3.35 D/mm
$\Delta P/\Delta ACD$	1.27 D/mm	0.81 D/mm	0.57 D/mm
$\Delta P/\Delta R$	7.86 D/mm	8.07 D/mm	8.23 D/mm
$\Delta P/\Delta K$	−1.41 D/D	−1.44 D/D	−1.47 D/D
$\Delta P/\Delta ELP$	3.17 D/mm	2.02 D/mm	1.45 D/mm

Abbreviations used:

AL   Axial Length
ACD Anterior Chamber Depth
P   Lens Power
R   Radius
K   Keratometer
ELP Effective Lens Position.

Potential Sources of IOL Calculation Errors

Incorrect biometric measurements of axial length, anterior chamber depth or lens thickness, resulting from inappropriate instrument settings, outdated instrument calibration or incorrect documentation will unavoidably lead to an incorrect calculation of the IOL's power.

Erroneous interpretation of values, for example the conversion of millimetre (mm) into dioptre (dpt) using an inappropriate keratometer index or not fulfilling the model assumptions for the use of a keratometer index will cause errors in IOL power calculation.

Furthermore, not all formulae fit all eyes, especially in situations after refractive corneal surgery. The use of inappropriate IOL calculation formulae (for instance standard formulae after refractive surgery) or raytracing may lead to incorrect calculation results.

Also, using incorrect formula constants for the respective IOLs (e.g. non-optimised constants or optimised for different environmental conditions) will cause miscalculations in IOL power.

It is important to be aware that when using optical biometry the axial length is measured from the corneal anterior apex to the retinal pigment epithelium, and with ultrasound biometry the measurement is from the corneal apex to the inner limiting membrane, whereas the actual image in the eye is created in between, in the photoreceptor layer. Furthermore, the results displayed by the biometer are not direct measurements since the data for the axial length are calibrated against a precision ultrasound biometer.

Inadequate measurement conditions can also lead to miscalculated IOLs. IOL calculation formulae refer to the best distance vision without correction, plano target refraction. Ophthalmologists understand emmetropia as the best uncorrected vision at 4–6 m distance, based on guidance by the respective ISO standard which specifies that vision tests should be performed at 4–6 m distance (ISO 11979-1:2018). In reality this is not a sufficient distance to qualify as infinity, meaning that such "emmetropic" patients are myopic with a refraction of −0.25 dpt to −0.167 dpt.

Also defined by an ISO standard are the labeling tolerances allowed for IOL manufacturers (ISO 11979-1:2018). Depending on the IOL dioptre range, certain variances in power are considered acceptable (in general, the higher the IOL power, the higher the accepted tolerance in power will be).

Practical Advice on Biometry Measurements

In general

When starting with a new IOL model, the standard process is to perform optical and immersion ultrasound biometry and compare the results. If you have no personal experience with the new lens, it is recommended to check the IOL Con website (www.iolcon.org) to determine if optimised data are available. If not, try to find a lens on this website with the same material and similar geometry and try to work with these constants. If you have personal experience with this lens from contact ultrasound biometry, try to find out how much your A-scan readings and keratometry results typically differ from the optical biometrical results. Refer to the IOL Con website. As a rule of thumb, the A constant selected for applanation ultrasonography should be 0.3–0.4 lower than the value selected for the optical biometry or immersion ultrasonography. If you have personal experience with this lens from immersion ultrasound biometry, you can use your immersion US constants in the optical biometer. Differences between the keratometry readings of both systems may be present; if so, please refer to the above website. It should be possible to use the optimised IOL constants from the IOL Con website for immersion ultrasound biometry. Take your time for the correct positioning of the patient!

Axial length measurement

If the refractive error of the patient is 6 D or higher and there are problems seeing the fixation light, the patient should wear their glasses (for optical biometry). If the pupil is very small or if the patient accommodates too much, mydriasis is recommended. Look out for unexpected results, e.g. an axial length of 27 mm in a patient with a +4 D refractive error. Double-check both eyes if the reported axial length is less than 22 mm or more than 25 mm, if there is a difference in AL greater than 0.33 mm in both eyes which does not correlate with the patient's refraction, or if the measurements do not correlate with the patient's refractive error. In general, myopes would be expected to have eyes longer than 24 mm and hyperopes shorter than 23.5 mm

Keratometry

Keratometry should be performed prior to any contact or immersion measurement of the eye (axial length or anterior chamber depth measurement if US measurement is applied or Goldmann applanation tonometry). Contact or immersion measurements may change the keratometry and the effect persists for a considerable time (as is the case for contact lens use). Ensure, that the patient blinks before measurement, and if needed apply rewetting eye drops and wait for some minutes. Ensure as well that the patient has not worn contact lenses prior to the examination (rigid contact lenses two weeks before examination, soft contact lenses one week).

Confirm the measurement if the average corneal power difference between the two eyes is greater than 1 dioptre. Ask the patient to blink several times to improve reflectivity of the cornea. Ask the patient to open his eye widely. Ensure that keratometry data is always stated in millimetres (not in dioptre!) as millimetre data is retrieved by keratometry.

Double-check both eyes if the corneal power is less than 40 D or more than 47 D, if there is a difference in corneal power greater than 1 D between both eyes, and in case of prior keratorefractive surgery.

Anterior chamber depth measurement

With an optical biometer, ask the patient to look at the fixation light. Modern optical biometers are capable of measuring both phakic and pseudophakic eyes. Modern optical biometers are able to measure eyes with a pupil diameter as small as 3 mm, whereas older optical biometers required ACD measurement under mydriasis to eliminate fluctuations caused by accommodation and to facilitate measurements in cases with small anterior chamber and small pupil size.

IOL calculation

It is recommended to print results from all formulae for a specific lens on one page (4-in-1 function). Choose the appropriate formula in relation to axial length.

Especially for critical eyes, use a formula which considers the measured anterior chamber depth. IOL constants can be optimised using the optimisation feature of the optical biometer or with modern WEB based platforms (e.g. IOL Con) which cover technical data of the lenses as well as formula constants. Double-check the measurements and re-run the IOL calculation if there is a difference in IOL power of more than 1 D between both eyes, if the IOL power correlates poorly with the patient's refractive error (myopes will require <20 D IOLs and hyperopes >23 D IOLs to reach emmetropia), or if the patient has had prior keratorefractive surgery and the calculated power is less than +20 D or more than +23 D. If the lens is to be placed in the sulcus or anterior chamber, use appropriate formula constants for sulcus fixation of the lens, which are typically lower compared to bag fixation of the lens.

Calculation of IOLs

During cataract surgery, the surgeon removes the cataracteous natural lens and replaces it with an artificial intraocular lens (IOL) to compensate for the loss of refractive power. To avoid over- or undercorrection, the IOL has to be chosen according to the patient's needs and the biometry of his/her eye. The IOL-constant links the biometric measurements to the effective axial lens position in the eye. An accurate estimation of the effective lens position is required to decide which IOL power suits your patient best.

Today, all parameters needed for an IOL calculation can be obtained by modern biometry devices: anterior/posterior surface curvature and central thickness of the cornea, axial length, and the respective refractive indices (cornea, aqueous humour, vitreous) can be entered manually and used for calculation.

For the correct calculation of the IOL the biometry data of the pseudophakic eye would be needed, but this is not available before surgery. Therefore, the phakic eye is used as the basis for IOL calculation. Usually the axial length (preferably derived using optical biometry) and the anterior curvature of the cornea are obligatory measurements, and for some formulae additional parameters such as phakic ACD, LT or W2W are also helpful. All other factors involved in IOL calculation are simplifications, assumptions and predictions. The cornea and the IOL are both approximated as infinite thin lenses. The effective lens position (ELP) is estimated from biometric data of the phakic eye. Refractive indices of the aqueous and vitreous humour are taken from schematic eye models, and refractive indices for the cornea and the IOL are not necessary as both are regarded as infinite thin lenses.

Target refraction?

What will be the correct target refraction? The objective should always be to optimise visual quality for a specific cataract patient. Therefore, the lifestyle and major activities of the patient should be taken into account. Emmetropia will probably be the target refraction in most of the cases, however in some cases myopia of −1 to −4 dioptres might be useful for monovision or for reduction of anisometropia.

Especially with multifocal lens implantations, care must diligently be taken to reach emmetropia so that the patient gets the most benefit from multifocality and reaches the highest possible level of spectacle independence. Success factors in achieving emmetropia are: use of optimised IOL constants, choice of proper IOL formula for biometry, use of optical biometry and consistent optical biometry readings.

However, even after considering all of these factors, the IOL recommended by biometry might not be available exactly in the requested dioptre or the IOL formulae might generate different results. These obstacles can be overcome only through experience with the respective IOL and with biometry. Some general guidelines might be: first of all, each printout of the optical biometer should contain the results of all IOL formulae (too often the printout shows the results with one formula but for different lenses, which is of limited value) and the results with the different IOL formulae should be compared to each other.

Evolution of Formulae

Many published and unpublished IOL formulae are available today. Over time different approaches for IOL calculation have evolved:

The simplest 'theoretical-optical' formula was devoloped by Swjatoslaw Nikolajewitsch Fjodorow around 1970 with Vo′ being the target refraction at the spectacle plane (d0 in front of corneal vertex), d1 refers to the IOL position, and d1 + d2 to the retinal position, both relative to the corneal anterior vertex (Fig. 6).

$$P_{IOL} = \frac{n_{Vitreous}}{Axial\,Length - ELP} - \frac{1}{\cfrac{1}{\cfrac{1}{\frac{1}{P_{Glasses}} - d_{Corneal\,Vertex}} + P_{Cornea}} - \frac{d_{Anterior\,Chamber}}{n_{Aqueous\,Humor}}}$$

P = Power
n = Refractive Index
d = Distance
ELP = Effective Lens Position

Fig. 6 The Fjodorow formula

$$IOLP = A - 0.9 \cdot K - 2.5 \cdot AL$$
$$IOLP = A_{mod} - 0.9 \cdot K - 2.5 \cdot AL$$

Fig. 7 SRK and SRK2 formula

The **empirical approach**, which is independent of any anatomical or physiological eye model, relies on a "big data" approach. Here you'll find simple formulae like SRK, SRK2, which should not be used anymore due to their limited accuracy (Fig. 7).

Where "A" is the A constant of the IOL, "K" for keratometry data, "AL" for axial length and "A_{mod}" as A + offset as function of AL.

But also modern approaches, like Hill RBF use a "big data" approach.

Theoretical-optical formulae are those formulae generally in use today (including the use of the thin lens approximation and Gaussian optics) as well as those with a significant empirical element (estimation of ELP, fudge factors or assumptions about architecture of the 'corneal dome').

The most modern option for calculating IOL power, **Ray Tracing**, works with or without simplifications of the thin lens approximation or the cornea and/or the IOL and relies as well on a significant empirical component (estimation of ELP).

Current IOL Formulae

There are numerous suitable IOL calculation formulae available today, some of which have been published, and others that are proprietary and available for purchase in dedicated software tools or together with an optical biometer. Some are more suitable for long eyes and others for eyes with a history of corneo-refractive surgery (Figs. 8 and 9).

The formulae marked in *red* in Fig. 8 are those most frequently used in Europe. Since these are published formulae, they are available free of charge. The *grey* ones are the basic formulae. These were the first formulae, published around 1970. With the *blue* ones we will find formulae which are suitable after refractive surgery (these have been published and may be used without charge). The *violet* ones are commercial formulae which have not been published and for which a fee is charged.

A remark on SRK/SRK 2 (Sanders Retzlaff Kraff) and the Hill RBF formula, as these have something in common even though SRK/SRK 2 are outdated and Hill RBF a modern formula: both of these rely on the "big data"-approach—and use empirical strategies without consideration of any anatomical model eye (Fig. 9).

None of these formulae reflect the situation after refractive surgery—yet these patients present more and more for cataract surgery these days. SRK/SRK2 are outdated, SRK/T is a classic formula still frequently used, the Haigis formula might show some effect on patient age as the crystalline lens is growing over time

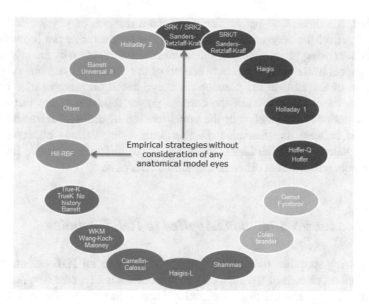

Fig. 8 Selection of IOL calculation formulae (this list is not intended to be exhaustive)

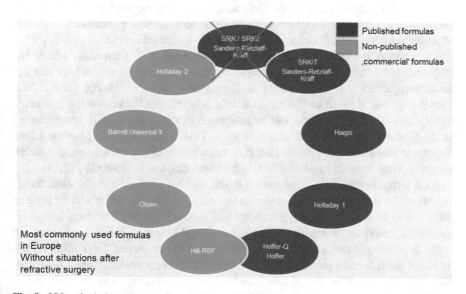

Fig. 9 IOL calculation schemes commonly used in Europe

decreasing the ACD and increasing LT, Hill-RBF uses artificial intelligence (AI) for selecting an appropriate IOL out of a huge amount of biometrical data. The Olsen formula determines the ELP from the anterior and posterior vertex of the crystalline lens by considering the ACD as well as LT.

In fact, the theoretical-optical formulae are a mixture of physics and empiricism and reflect the respective philosophy of the originator of the formula which includes also using various factors, values and constants set up by the originator.

One aspect of the differences between all of the formulae available today is the estimation of the ELP in the pseudophakic eye based on pre-operative biometry data. Also, the interpretation of the corneal power resulting of the values of the corneal anterior surface radius or the consideration of different refractive indices may differ between the formulae. Furthermore, using various offset values for biometric values or "fudge factors" and the use of different refractive indices for ocular media will result in different calculated IOL powers.

Simplifications/Assumptions Applied to IOL Formulae

The following simplifications and assumptions apply to **all IOL calculation formulae**: that no change of the geometry of the cornea is expected (the anterior and posterior surface, corneal thickness and refractive index stay the same), or that such changes can be predicted from the preoperative situation. The axial length remains unchanged.

Only in formulae using a simplified model regarding the cornea and the IOL as thin lenses will the ELP be relevant. The ELP is an estimated parameter which can be predicted from pre-OP biometry results (axial length and corneal power).

The following simplifications apply to **traditional IOL formulae**, which are frequently used today. Both the cornea as a convex-concave meniscus lens and the IOL are regarded as a **thin lenses** (i.e. lenses with no volume). For the IOL the refractive power is given by the manufacturer, whereas for the cornea the geometry of the corneal anterior surface will be measured in millimetres. With keratometers the radii of the cornea are measured in mm. This value has to be converted into dioptres as this is the value needed for IOL calculation. Using the keratometer index the appropriate formula to convert mm values into dioptres is shown in Fig. 10.

As a simplification the keratometer index will be used as a calibration factor instead of the model of the cornea which includes the anterior and posterior surface curvature as well as the central thickness and refractive index. The focal length of the cornea could be defined with respect to the principal plane as is common in optics or relative to the anterior or posterior vertex of the cornea. Depending on the choice of the reference plane we will obtain different keratometer indices: for a cornea according to the Gullstrand schematic model eye we obtain a keratometer index of 1.3315 for the principal plane as reference, for the anterior vertex we obtain 1.332 (Zeiss Index) and for the posterior vertex we obtain 1.3375 (Javal index).

$$\text{Corneal power} = (1 - n_K)/Ra$$

Fig. 10 Calculating the corneal power (with n_K as keratometer index and R_a as radius)

Ray Tracing

The theory of Ray Tracing has been known for a long time, but has only been applied to calculating IOLs for a few years with increasing interest today. Many surgeons are still using third generations formulae for calculating the IOL power. Such formulae use Gaussian optics with well known simplifications of paraxial optics. Furthermore, such formulae implement more simplification regarding the cornea and IOL as both are approximated as thin lenses. These principles have been used for decades to provide IOL power calculation formulae.

Especially for eyes post refractive surgery or very long eyes such classic IOL calculation formulae may fail. Instead of an analytical solution the calculation can now be solved by numerical methods requiring a computer. Before computers were common for IOL calculation, formulae with a set of assumptions and simplification were needed in IOL calculation.

The optics of the pseudophakic eye can be described by using Ray Tracing and modern biometry techniques, and this new method offers a reliable prediction of the actual IOL postion. Ray Tracing is a very modern technique which calculates the path (trace) of a single ray of light through an optical system. The ray of light is refracted at each optical surface of the system and changes its direction depending on the refractive power of the respective surface and according to Snell's law. For a single ray passing multiple surfaces the calculation is mathematically too complex to be carried out using classic analytical formulae.

For Ray Tracing, data of acoustic axial lengths are needed and will be entered into the Ray Tracing calculation or directly transferred from the biometry device. The Ray Tracing program also includes all relevant data for the major IOLs on the market. Ray Tracing uses a pseudophakic eye model. The parameters of the anterior and posterior corneal surfaces should be measured using tomography.

IOL Calculation in Special Cases

"Long" and "Short" Eyes

A general source of error is the simplification and model assumptions in biometry when optical lengths are converted into geometric lengths. The axial length of "short" and "long" eyes has to be adjusted when the axial length has been obtained by optical biometry as optical biometers may show a systematic error in reporting higher values with increasing length. Calculating IOL power based on optical biometry data and using classic formulae (which are based on using the average refractive index, without taking the real axial length into account) will lead to miscalculation of IOL power in both extremes: in long eyes the corneal and lens power will be underestimated in relation to the vitreous humour, which will be overestimated and which would result in IOL power leaving the patient with hyperopia. In short eyes the corneal and lens power will be overestimated, the vitreous humour underestimated which would result in an IOL power leaving the patient with myopia.

The Haigis formula and newer generation formulae, e.g. Holladay 2, Olsen and Barrett will provide good results. If Holladay 1, SRK/T, Haigis and Holladay 2 are used, an adjustment is required with high myopes. When using the Barrett Universal II formula, no axial length adjustment is required. It is worth bearing in mind that, depending on the patient population, the anatomy of the anterior segment and the errors involved, it might be questionable if such an adjustment will make sense or if better results are only provided statistically on average.

Recommendation: Use all your previous surgical data from eyes with axial length >25 mm and derive your own IOL constants accordingly. Adapt the axial length as appropriate to reflect the longer depth of the vitreous humour. Avoid using this in eyes post refractive sugery.

Also, the labelling tolerance of the IOL manufacturers has to be taken into account as the IOL power for hyperopic patients might be e.g. +35 dpt which allows ±1 dpt tolerance in IOL production.

Eyes After Refractive Surgery

After refractive surgery the relation between anterior and posterior corneal curvature is impaired. In myopic LASIK/PRK the corneal anterior surface is flattened in the center, whereas in hyperopic corrections the center is steepened. This leads to an overestimation of corneal power after myopic corrections and to an undercorrection after hyperopic corrections. The consequence of this is that after myopic corrections the IOL power is underestimated and the patient will end up with hyperopia after LASIK, whereas the initially hyperopic patient will end up with myopia after refractive surgery and subsequent cataract surgery.

Another problem which may arise after refractive surgery performed in childhood by PRK/LASIK is the transition zone around the small optical zone of around 5.5 or 6 mm in diameter. If a keratometer measures curvature (especially in decentered refractive procedures) at the transition zone, this will cause again an overestimation of corneal power/underestimation of IOL power after myopic correction and vice versa after hyperopic correction.

The estimation of the ELP will be incorrect if IOL calculation schemes are used where the ELP calculation is based on keratometry. Especially in these cases the approximation of the cornea as a "thin lens" will result in miscalculations for IOL power as such a lens can not be calculated from the anterior radius and classical keratometer indices.

With myopic LASIK the curvature of the anterior cornea is reduced selectively, meaning that such a cornea can not be described by a classic eye model any more. After myopic LASIK or PRK the eye length is longer comparable to normal eyes. Using appropriate formulae for "long" eyes is strongly recommended. After myopic LASIK the refractive index will be overestimated and consequently the

IOL underestimated, making such patients hyperopic after cataract surgery. When performing hyperopic LASIK/PRK the central corneal curvature is increased and becomes steeper due to circular ablation in the periphery. As eyes post hyperopic LASIK/PRK are shorter, classic formulae for calculating IOLs will also fail in these cases, and formulae appropriate for short eyes should be used.

Classic US-American IOL formulae assess the IOL position from the corneal curvature (SRK/T, Holladay, Hoffer-Q). After PRK/LASIK the IOL will be placed at a different (incorrect) position by such formulae: with myopic LASIK the cornea becomes more flat, leading to a more anterior placement of the IOL, which results in IOLs with less power and leaves the patient with a hyperopic refractive outcome. In patients having undergone hyperopic LASIK, the cornea has become steeper, the IOL placement will be more posterior leading to a higher IOL power resulting in a myopic refractive outcome.

Our recommendation: Either consider IOL calculation formulae which do not use k-values for assessing the ELP or make use of strategies which incorporate a "thick" cornea initially.

Recommendations for biometry in eyes post refractive Laser surgery:

Never use standard formulae for eyes post-LASIK/PRK. The corneal power measurements will be incorrect because the approximation of the cornea as a thin lens is longer valid. In such cases assessing the radii might lead to incorrect data because of the changes in asphericity. The Haigis or Olsen formulae will give better results if the estimate of the ELP is based on the corneal refractive power (as with Hoffer-Q, Holladay and SRK/T).

In general, when calculating IOLs for post-LASIK eyes it has to be differentiated if the patietnt´s pre-LASIK refractive data of the cornea will be available (eyes "with history") or not (eyes "without history"). In patients having data prior to refractive surgery it is possible to calculate the IOL based on the situation before the refractive intervention. In such cases the latest measurement of the cornea is needed as well as refraction before and after LASIK or the corneal refractive data before LASIK. Usually, it will be difficult to obtain such data many years after LASIK surgery. Even if a "LASIK Passport" had been provided to the patient after sugery it might have got lost in between the LASIK and the cataract surgery.

In patients without such data, one option is to use the estimation of the correction when performing LASIK and compare it to standard corneal data. Another option might be to use corneal tomography as it is essential for assessing the real refractive power of the complete cornea without the simplifying approximation of the cornea as a thin lens. In these cases no pre-LASIK data will be needed. With OCT- and/or Scheimpflug technology now available, this should be the standard method for post-LASIK eyes.

Furthermore, ensure that the ELP is not estimated based on the corneal radii after PRK/LASIK (Fig. 11).

The ASCRS website offers helpful tools when calculating IOL power, also post refractive surgery (https://ascrs.org/online-tools).

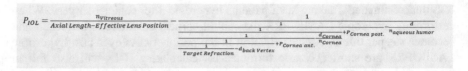

$$P_{IOL} = \cfrac{n_{vitreous}}{Axial\,Length - Effective\,Lens\,Position} - \cfrac{1}{\cfrac{1}{\cfrac{1}{\cfrac{1}{Target\,Refraction} - d_{back\,Vertex}} + P_{Cornea\,ant.}} + P_{Cornea\,post.}} + \cfrac{d_{Cornea}}{n_{Cornea}} + \cfrac{d}{n_{aqueous\,humor}}$$

Fig. 11 IOL calculation formula including all corneal data

Eyes Post Cross-linking

Caution must be exercised in this case, since everything discussed so far refers to a standard eye. After Cross-linking the relation of the radii will change and the refractive index of the cornea will be higher, therefore the refractive power of the eye will be lower and accordingly the dioptre of the IOL has to be lower.

Children

The exact estimation of the IOL power required in congenital cataract is very difficult as the axial length and the corneal curvature changes constantly as a result of the growth of the eyeball in the first 5 years of life. Most surgical strategies involve selecting IOLs which leave the child hyperopic initially, with the expectation of achieving emmetropia in the following years as a result of the eyeball's further growth. Alternatively the IOL power could be specified for emmetropia anticipating the implantation of an add-on IOL at a later date as soon as the child becomes myopic. Another option would be simultaneously or subsequently implanting two IOLs (one in the capsular bag, the other one in the sulcus (=add-on lens) to adjust the IOL power according to the growth of the eyeball. The add-on lens can be easily replaced at any time if necessary.

Aphakic Eyes

Here the question is whether the capsular bag will still be available for secondary IOL implantation or whether sulcus implantation, anterior chamber or iris fixated IOL are possible options. In such cases different constants are needed which will be significantly lower as a result of the higher distance to the retina for IOLs implanted in these ways. Optical biometers should be used with settings adjusted appropriately for aphakic eyes. Ultrasound biometry would produce an image missing the two signals for the crystalline lens and with one signal for the anterior surface of the vitreous humour. In these eyes Ultrasound biometry will only provide valid data if the aphakic measurement mode is used—this is based on a more appropriate average sound velocity for an aphakic eye.

Pseudophakic Eyes

Using ultrasound biometry in such eyes a very strong signal can be seen representing the IOL mostly followed by Ultrasound echoes which might overlay the retinal signals. Especially in ultrasound biometry it is extremely important to know the material of the implanted IOL, e.g. silicone IOLs show a significantly lower speed of sound.

In general, optical biometry with settings adjusted to pseudophakic eyes is highly favourable in such eyes as these biometers offer correct measurements and appropriate correction factors for different IOLs. As with aphakic eyes the central question in pseudophakic eyes concerns the condition of the capsular bag. If the capsular bag is unstable or absent then sulcus or iris fixated IOLs together with anterior chamber IOLs are the method of choice taking account of the different, lower constants in such eyes.

Posterior Segment Surgery

Due to the differences in speed of sound depending on the different ocular media (vitreous, silicone, gas) Ultrasound biometry is not the diagnostic technique of choice in such eyes. Optical biometry using the specific settings appropriate to native vitreous, silicone or gas will do far better.

Need for (Optimised) IOL Constants

The choice of correct IOL-power can be improved by continuous optimisation of IOL constants. Reliable IOL-constants require a high number of pre-surgical biometry measurements together with the respective refractive outcomes and information on which lens has been implanted. With a continuously growing database of refractive success, IOL-calculation can become more and more reliable.

One parameter that appears to be essential in calculating the individual IOL power for the respective patient is the correct value of the IOL constant provided by the manufacturer. Such constants have to be updated on an ongoing basis with the accumulation of more and more surgical data. Usually an IOL calculation has only one constant, although some have more (e.g. the Haigis formula uses three). All constants characterise material properties (e.g. the refractive index of the IOL material), the shape of the optic of the IOL (e.g. the ratio of anterior to posterior radii), the center thickness of the IOL, and the angulation and properties of the haptics.

It is assumed that constants are the same for all IOLs within one product range, which may not always be the case as the characteristics (e.g. the relation of anterior and posterior radii of an IOL) will most probably vary when referring to the complete dioptre range of a respective IOL.

The IOL constant is furthermore responsible for compensating for systematic errors such as inaccurate conversion from corneal radius of curvature to dioptric power, conversion of the reference plane (principal plane of the cornea to apex plane), incorrect calibration of the biometer (calibration for targeting the RPE instead of photo receptor layer), incorrect measurement of post-OP refraction, the individual technique of the examiner/surgeon and the variation of the IOL geometry covering the whole IOL model range (e.g. central thickness, relationship of radii).

Today, IOL constants are personalised/individualised to compensate for systematic errors of the specific IOL. In the near future IOL constants will additionally be optimised with regard to factors such as the biometer, keratometer, topographer, tomographer, the refraction technique used to capture postoperative refraction, the technique of the surgeon and the ethnicity of the patients.

Standard optimisation procedures include evaluating the outcome of post cataract surgery data (keratometry, axial length, phakic anterior chamber depth, stable refractive results (e.g. 6 months post surgery), IOL model and IOL refractive power).

In optimizing the constants used in Haigis' formula for each eye, firstly the ELP is calculated and then a regression regarding Axial Length and pACD using all data sets is carried out to calculate a_0, a_1 and a_2.

For other IOL calculation formulae the idea of inverse calculation using the ideal constant for each eye is extremely helpful. This involves deriving a "perfect" formula constant for each eye, matching the preop biometry, postop refraction and the power of the implanted IOL. Statistics (ideally the median as this is robust for outliers) are needed for all eyes with SRK/2´s A_{SKRK2}, $A_{SKR/T}$, $pACD_{Hoffer}$, $SF_{Hollday}$, $C_{Olsen,}$ a_0 (for standard values for a_1 and a_2).

Tools

IOL Con

After 20 years of optical biometry and the need for optimised IOL constants, and given that the ULIB database has not been updated for more than three years now, a new encyclopedic database, the IOL Con database, has been established. This database containing IOL specifications has been established to fulfill the increased needs of modern cataract surgery and IOL calculation. IOL Con holds an ongoing agreement to incorporate the ULIB data within the IOL Con database.

The concept of IOL Con is evolving on an ongoing basis, in cooperation with manufacturers of IOLs and biometry devices as well as with cataract surgeons from all around the world. Optimisation algorithms for published IOL formulae (SRK/T, Haigis, HofferQ, Holladay 1) have been implemented. With the dedicated collaboration of cataract surgeons, IOL manufacturers, manufacturers of biometry devices and scientists, a company-independent database for optimal IOL selection which takes all important factors into account has recently been created. IOL Con is an open online database for continuous and automated optimisation and compilation of (IOL) constants for cataract surgery.

This globally available and active database, which has been set up as an "Alliance for Better Vision" is an internet platform which, on the one hand enables all IOL manufacturers to provide all the relevant technical data and specifications of their lens models, while on the other hand IOL Con offers a platform for characteristics of intraocular lenses and the optimisation of lens constants for all ophthalmic surgeons worldwide. By collecting many datasets (consisting of pre-OP biometry data, implanted IOLs and post-OP refraction) IOL Con is able to offer reliably optimised IOL constants for formula-based IOL calculation. The volume and the quality of the data is the crucial factor here: the more reliable data that ophthalmic surgeons upload to the platform, the more reliable the optimised constants are. In establishing IOL Con a new and modern web-based, publicly accessible database for continuous archiving and automatic, manufacturer-independent optimisation of IOL constants for common IOL calculation formulae (e.g. calculation according to SRK/T, Hoffer Q, Holladay 1, Haigis) has been made available.

The data regarding IOLs is provided internationally by both IOL manufacturers and ophthalmic surgeons. It is continually adapted, expanded and updated which allows a timely and standardised publication and distribution of optimised IOL constants for the benefit of physicians and patients. This database offers physicians a comprehensive overview of lens models and their technical specifications, easy IOL selection of models based on criteria and/or manual selection as well as the option of individual optimisation of lens constants. Biometry device manufacturers are implementing IOL Con´s open XML interface to integrate IOL Con with their devices.

Surgeons can register at IOL Con for free at https://www.IOLCon.org and can use the various search functions of the platform and check their parameters with the most up-to-date-constants by IOL Con. Additionally, surgeons can upload their pre- and postoperative results to obtain globally and personally optimised IOL-constants.

Summary and Advice

Today, optical biometry is regarded as a standard diagnostic tool and essential basis for IOL calculation prior to cataract surgery. It is an indispensable part of ophthalmology, and has fundamentally revolutionised cataract surgery. Some aspects should be kept in mind:

Biometers cannot be used interchangeably at the moment, there is a high need for optimised constants applicable to different biometers.

Be careful with keratometer values. Corneal power cannot be measured directly by any instrument—a conversion from millimetres into dioptres is always needed. Even in normal corneas the conversion from mm to dpt is not valid in all cases, and the refractive power is quite often overestimated. In some cases this conversion is even more incorrect, e.g. after refractive surgery, with intracorneal rings, after CXL etc.

Set up your own quality system. If you have collected a sufficient quantity of surgical data with one IOL type, set up your own quality control. Tune your IOL constants according to your own individual technique, biometer, keratometer or Topo-/Tomographer, and technique of refractometry.

Issues with extremely long and short eyes are problems resulting from the use of an average refractive index, and it is recommended not to use this any more.

The problem of cataract surgery following refractive surgery will be solved when using tomography to measure the anterior and posterior surface curvature and corneal thickness rather than evaluating/comparing the results of many different strategies with and without clinical history. In most clinical cases the measurement of corneal power and refraction BEFORE refractive surgery and/or refraction before myopisation due to cataract may be missing.

The best IOL calculation and optimised constant cannot compensate for errors in the biometry. Take your time and take an overall view of all measurements in order to ensure consistency.

However, the ongoing improvement of optical biometry over the past two decades has led to patients with higher expectations regarding the refractive outcome after cataract surgery. Additionally post-LASIK patients are now presenting for their cataract surgery or refractive lens exchange wishing for a life without glasses. Such demanding patients put special pressure on ophthalmic surgeons requesting an optimal post-operative refractive outcome. Thanks to the more precise measurement results of modern optical biometry, patients' expectations can be met far better than with ultrasonic measurements as the IOL calculation is much more accurate. By implication, modern IOL concepts such as EDOF lenses have become possible only as a consequence of the immense accuracy of IOL calculation using optical biometry.

Teaching Phacoemulsification Cataract Surgery

John Desmond Ferris

Introduction

Across the globe there are pressures on surgical training in all specialties. Long training programmes, virtually unlimited access to surgical cases and a 'see one, do one, teach one' approach are all a thing of the past. Training programmes are getting shorter, there are fewer surgical opportunities on operating lists which are filled to capacity and, not before time, a greater emphasis is being placed on improving the safety of surgical training. All of these factors contribute to reduced surgical opportunities for our current trainees.

There are also concerns that despite the adoption of competency based surgical training programmes we are still producing ophthalmologists who are struggling surgically. A survey of 58 US programme directors revealed that 9% of residents had trouble mastering surgical skills, a quarter of these had poor hand eye coordination, one in five had poor intraoperative judgement and a third had still not overcome these difficulties by graduation [1].

The aim of this chapter is to provide a practical, evidence based, guide of how to teach phacoemulsification cataract surgery safely and efficiently using a combination of virtual reality and model eye simulation techniques and modern assessment tools.

There is nowadays no doubt that increased time spent in practising surgical technique will speed up the learning curve. There is also, however, no doubt that being taught the correct thing to practise is as important. No single technique is uniquely better than another and for the trainee it is very important to learn a range of techniques so that surgical adaptability is built up.

So what are the core surgical skills we are trying to teach for any type of surgery and how can simulation help develop these skills? Surgery is not just about

J. D. Ferris (✉)
Gloucestershire Eye Unit, Gloucestershire, UK
e-mail: johndferris@me.com; john.ferris2@nhs.net

© Springer Nature Switzerland AG 2021   115
C. Liu and A. Shalaby Bardan (eds.), *Cataract Surgery*,
https://doi.org/10.1007/978-3-030-38234-6_8

learning isolated technical skills, developing manual dexterity, the basics of instrument handling, dissection and suturing skills are important building blocks for any surgeon and simulation can certainly help to hone these skills, but surgery is much more complex than this. A good surgeon will have the ability to deal with evolving and unexpected situations, be able to give, listen to and act upon instructions, as well as have the ability to make good decisions in pressurised situations. If all simulation training does is to teach technical skills then we have missed an opportunity to fine tune the attributes that set surgeons apart from technicians.

So how do we go about designing a surgical training program that will produce competent, confident and adaptable surgeons? I would suggest that the first step is to have some understanding of the educational theories, which are the bedrock of successful surgical training programs.

Educational Theory

Learning can be defined as the process of acquisition, assimilation and consolidation of attitudes, skills, and knowledge. Learning is about how we perceive the world, our understanding, about making meaning. As trainers and educators, we preferably strive for learners to engage in deep, rather than surface learning. Teaching can be seen as the process of transmitting, transferring, facilitating, or intrinsically motivating someone's development.

Adult Learning

Andragogy refers to adult learning, in contrast to pedagogy or childhood learning. The American educator Malcolm Knowles defined andragogy in the 1980s as the "art and science of helping adults learn" [2].

As an adult matures, they develop from being a dependent individual and become more self-directed. Mature adults have accumulated a reservoir of experiences that become a rich resource for learning. Adults develop readiness to learn when they experience a need to know or understand something. Children tend to be more subject-centred with an outlook of postponed application of knowledge, contrasting with adults who are more problem-centred and who display a greater immediacy of application of knowledge. Finally, as individuals mature, their most powerful motivators to learn are internal. Self-directedness and personal motivation are crucial for surgical training, and especially simulation-based surgical education. An eye surgeon who has not grasped self-directed learning and not fostered their own motivation will struggle, and the achievement of mastery and expertise will be almost impossible.

Personal motivation in surgical training is critical. This can however be internal or external. Internal motivators may be the desire to accomplish a task, to succeed, or to be able to serve patients. External motivators are varied and many faceted, including career progression, financial reward, respect from colleagues, certification or more simply required assessment and examinations.

Constructivism

In contemporary psychology, constructivist theories are used to describe how people learn: they propose that we learn by fitting new knowledge and understanding in, and together with what we already know and understand; expanding or even replacing old with new. There are a number of types of constructivist theory, but their central notion is that of continuous building and amending of structures, or schemata, in the mind that hold knowledge [3].

Constructivism describes knowledge being derived from processes where the learner is an active participant rather than a passive bystander or passive recipient of knowledge. Furthermore, knowledge and meaning are changeable over time, depending on the individual's prior experience or knowledge. A practical example of this is encouraging trainees to be proactive with their training and seek out training opportunities, rather than relying on their trainers to "spoon-feed" them.

Experiential Learning

Surgical training has traditionally relied on an apprentice model. However, this apprentice model, with its 'see one, do one, teach one' approach to surgical training, is being replaced by methods which have adopted a more nuanced form of experiential learning.

Experiential learning describes the process of gaining knowledge continuously through personal and environmental experiences. This constructivist perspective on learning is based on the idea that understanding is not unchangeable or fixed, but can be formed or reformed by experiences. The learner must be able to reflect on the experience, use analytical skills to conceptualise the experience, and actively use the ideas gained by the experience to make decisions and solve problems.

Reflection

Reflection and reflective practice can be seen as a critical aspect of experiential learning as it transforms experience into learning. Donald Schön described two different types of reflection within educational development: reflection in action, and reflection on action [4]. Reflection in action might be a trainee commenting on their surgical performance during surgery, and reflection on action relating to a commentary of a video recording of their performance.

Reflection and reflective practice are a cornerstone of surgical education, including ophthalmic surgical training. Encouraging a trainee to reflect on their cataract surgical performance is an important learning exercise. Once this becomes embedded in the education and training process, it can develop into a life-long learning tool for surgeons as they constantly strive for improvement of their skills.

Zone of Proximal Development

Lev Vygotsky's suggested that trainees' learning is best when activities are focussed within their zone of proximal development (ZPD) [5]. Trainee novices (or advanced beginners) may already possess a few skills, which they have mastered and can perform solo; however there are other tasks or skills, which are too distant or hard for them to perform alone. The space in between these two poles of learning is the ZPD. An experienced trainer will know where the ZPD is for a particular trainee and structure the training to constantly take them just beyond their previous level of competence, without asking them to attempt a new manoeuvre that is several increments above their current level of competence.

Communities of Practice

Communities of practice and situated learning describe groups of people who share a concern or a passion for something they do and learn how to do it better as they interact regularly. This certainly applies to surgical trainees who work together as peers, and with their more senior surgeon trainers.

Ophthalmologists operate within a variety of communities of practice, these may include peers and seniors in an institution, country or international region; within multi-disciplinary teams of ophthalmic nurses, orthoptists, optometrists, and technicians; as well as health-care professionals throughout many departments of a hospital. The overarching ethos of these communities of practice and their attitudes towards teaching and learning is perhaps one of the most important factors in establishing a successful surgical training program.

Sustained Deliberate Practice

Psychologist K. Anders Ericsson has published widely on theories of expertise. He challenged the view that merely engaging in a sufficient amount of practice, regardless of the structure of the practice, automatically leads to maximal performance. In other words how an individual becomes expert at a particular skill has more to do with the how of practice, rather than merely performing that skill a great number of times [6].

There are a number of important facets to deliberate practice. It is facilitated by feedback. It encompasses the continual practicing of a skill at progressively more challenging levels with the intent of mastering the skill. One of the challenges of providing feedback of simulation-based deliberate practice is that a trainer or assessor may not be available to observe performance. One potential solution is the use of video recording of surgical simulation procedures, and subsequent assessment of the recorded performance.

Simulation provides a great platform for gaining of expertise and mastery of specific skills, as it provides the opportunity for extensive sustained deliberate practice.

These key concepts proposed by the various educational theorists, should be used to underpin curriculum development and the delivery of training which aims to;

- Offer a personal motivation to students.
- Be active and collaborative.
- Consist of concrete observations, abstract conceptualisation and active experimentation, to benefit the student through experiential learning.
- Allow for re-examination and reflections of experience.
- Be focused on the zone of proximal development, i.e. the area of knowledge between novice and competency or expertise.
- Offer a community of practice where learning can be shared.
- And finally offer the opportunity for sustained deliberate practice of the learned skill.

Preparation Before Commencing Surgery

The following topics are essential components of any cataract surgery training programme and are covered in some depth in other chapters of this book. Needless to say it is essential that all trainees have a sound grasp of these before undertaking surgical training;

- Ocular anatomy and pathophysiology of cataracts.
- Preoperative assessment of a patient for cataract surgery—history taking and examination skills.
- Knowledge of biometry, intraocular lenses and refractive aims of surgery.
- How to consent a patient for cataract surgery.
- Anaesthetic techniques.
- Principles of sterile technique—hand washing, donning gowns and gloves.
- How to operate the surgical microscope.
- Phaco-dynamics and how to set up phacoemulsification equipment in preparation for surgery.

- Knowledge of the surgical instruments and blades.
- An understanding of each step of phacoemulsification surgery and some of the different options for performing each of these steps.
- Knowledge of the intraoperative and post-operative complications of cataract surgery and how to manage them.

Simulation Based Training

In ophthalmology, as with other medical specialties, there has been a focus on highly sophisticated technology models of simulation training. However, not all simulation needs to be high-tech nor expensive, in fact there is an argument to be made that high-tech does not always imply high-fidelity simulation. There is also a danger that "surgical simulations are often accepted uncritically, with undue emphasis being placed on technological sophistication at the expense of educational theory-based design" [7].

When considering the fidelity, reliability and validity of a training approach and implementation it is important to bear in mind the four criteria for validating simulation-based training. In the domain of medical and surgical education, validity refers to the degree to which an instrument measures what it sets out to measure. *Face validity* describes whether the chosen tasks resemble those that are performed during a surgical procedure in a real-life situation. *Content validity* is whether the test actually resembles a specific skill, for example does the capsule of a model eye behave in the same way as the human lens capsule during capsulorrhexis? The reliability, or *construct validity*, pertains to the ability of a tool or simulator to differentiate between the performances of a procedure of novice and expert surgeons. In other words, construct validity is the degree to which the test actually captures the skill level it was designed to measure, for example does it discriminate between experts and novices. *Predictive validity* is often the most difficult to assess, and it relates to future performance and transfer of skills acquired during simulation to the operating theatre. Simulation modalities that meet these four criteria are highly likely to enhance surgical training.

Virtual-Reality Simulators

Three computerised simulators have been used for cataract surgical training in ophthalmology: the Eyesi (VRMagic Holding AG, Mannheim, Germany), MicroVisTouch (ImmersiveTouch, Chicago, USA), and PhacoVision (Melerit Medical, Linkoping, Sweden).

The Eyesi is the most widely used of these virtual-reality simulators (Fig. 1).

It consists of a mannequin head, instruments, foot pedals and a virtual-reality interface, which is seen through the operating microscope. The cataract interface

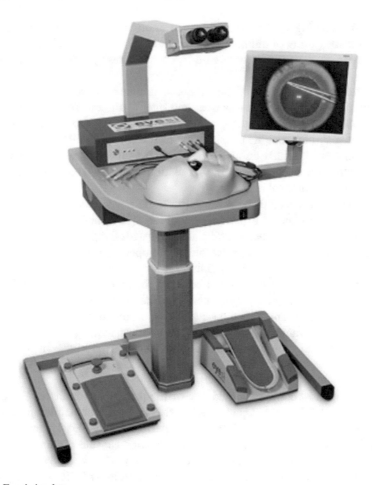

Fig. 1 Eyesi simulator

consists of all the major steps of the cataract procedure apart from creating an incision, in addition to abstract modules, which train basic skills, such as navigation within the anterior chamber, anti-tremor training and bimanual training. All modules can be used on different difficulty levels.

The automated assessment provided by the simulator consists of 21–33 different outcomes categorized into five main outcomes:

– Target achievement
– Efficiency, which is based on the total time that instruments are inserted in the eye
– Instrument utilization
– Tissue damage e.g. corneal, iris, lens or posterior capsule trauma
– Microscope usage.

Parts of the scoring system are based on motion-tracking technology, which involves the measuring of millimeter movement of instrument tips and the number of instrument closings (i.e. how often a forceps is closed), whilst others are time based.

One of the great strengths of the simulator is the ability to carry out sustained deliberate practice, repeating tasks over and over again and seeing improvement. Some of its features like focussing and zooming with the foot pedal controls are just like the real thing, but the physical feel of the simulation is somewhat lacking and it is very much reliant on visual rather than tactile feedback. There is also a facility to playback a recording of the simulation undertaken and the software will highlight errors in surgical technique.

Construct validity studies have proven that the EyeSi can distinguish between novice and intermediate or experienced surgeons [8, 9] and a number of studies have demonstrated that technical skills acquired with EyeSi training, such as capsulorrhexis performance, are transferable to the operating theatre [10], so proving that there is a degree of predictive validity.

A high correlation has been found between the automated EyeSi performance scores and real-life cataract surgery performance, as measured by motion tracking metrics [11]. The same group have also demonstrated that a proficiency-based EyeSi training programme improved surgical performance by 32% in novice cataract surgeons (had only performed steps of surgery) and 38% in intermediate surgeons (1–75 cases) as measured by an Objective Structured Assessment of Cataract Surgical Skill rating scale [12].

Perhaps the most convincing evidence of the predictive validity of Eyesi training is the Royal College of Ophthalmologists National Ophthalmology Database study [13]. In this series of 17,831 cases performed by 265 1st and 2nd year UK residents between 2010 and 2016, the posterior capsule rupture (PCR) rates for trainees who had access to an Eyesi fell from 4.2 to 2.6%, a 38% reduction. In those hospitals where there was no access to Eyesi training PCR rates only fell by 3% during the study period.

In light of this study it could be argued that Eyesi training should be mandatory for all trainees prior to commencing live phacoemulsification surgery.

Model Eyes

Artificial eyes made with plastic and other synthetic materials have been used and developed over the past decade for ophthalmic simulated training.

In the UK, Phillips Studio have developed a wide range of artificial eyes for use in training for cataract, glaucoma, corneal, strabismus and vitreo-retinal surgery (Phillips Ophthalmic Simulated Surgery: Phillips Eye Studio). The Simulated Ocular Surgery website (*simulatedocularsurgery.com*) demonstrates how these eyes can be used to simulate a wide variety of surgical procedures.

There are two types of cataract eyes, a basic and an advanced model. The basic eyes are hemispherical The cornea has a similar feel to a real cornea, allowing trainees to practice wound construction and their corneal suturing skills. The lens has an anterior capsule, which has very similar properties to the human capsule and enables trainees to practice capsulorrhexis techniques (Fig. 2).

The lens itself is made from a gel-like material of varying consistencies, to mimic different types of cataracts. These lenses behave in a similar way to the human lens during phacoemulsification surgery, enabling the trainee to practice their sculpting, cracking and segment removal techniques, but they do not have a lens cortex. Once the lens has been removed an IOL can be inserted.

The advanced phaco eyes are spherical and have an anterior and a posterior chamber (Fig. 3). The lens is encased within a capsule and the lens comes in a number of different densities, to simulate different types of cataract. The posterior chamber can be filled with egg white as a vitreous substitute. These eyes can be

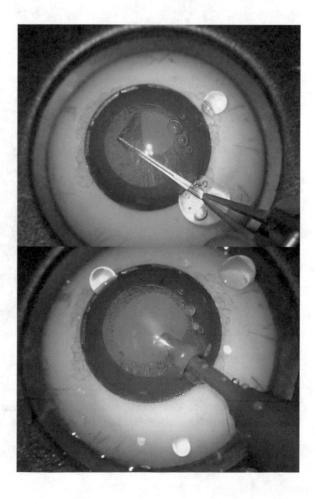

Fig. 2 Phillips Studio—capsulorrhexis and nucleus sculpting with basic cataract eye

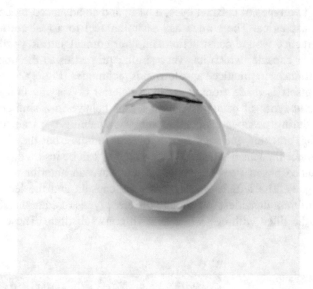

Fig. 3 Phillips Studio—advanced cataract eye

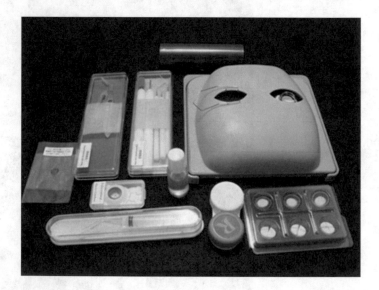

Fig. 4 Kitaro Dry-lab

used to simulate either routine or complicated surgery such as posterior capsule rupture with vitreous loss, a dropped nucleus, a zonular dialysis +/− vitreous loss and even an expulsive haemorrhage. Videos of these types of simulation can be found on the Simulation Gallery website (gallery.simulatedocularsurgery.com)

'Kitaro DryLab' is a tool to teach and learn some steps of cataract surgery (Fig. 4). It is mobile, and can be used on a desktop, and without the use of an

Table 1 Comparison of simulation tools for each step of phacoemulsification surgery

	Eyesi	Phillips eyes	Kitaro eyes	Bioniko eyes	Porcine eyes
Wound construction	NA	++	++	+	+++
Capsulorrhexis	+++	++	++	++	+
Hydrodissection	++	+	+	+	++
Nucleus sculpting	+	+++	++	++	+
Nucleus cracking and segment removal	+	++	++	++	+
Aspiration of lens cortex	+++	NA	NA	NA	+
Implanting IOL	++	+++	++	++	+

+++ Excellent, ++ Good, + Fair, NA not applicable

operating microscope (Frontier Vision Co. Ltd., Hyogo, Japan). The Kitaro models are particularly useful for practicing capsulorrhexis techniques and for nucleus cracking.

The Bioniko system uses 3D printed model eyes which can be used to simulate a wide variety of surgical procedures, including phacoemulsification surgery (Bioniko Models, Florida USA). The OKULO Brown 8 is the model used for phacoemulsification surgery and can be used to practice all of the steps of surgery except aspiration of the lens cortex.

Guilden Ophthalmics have developed 'phaco practice patient replacement eyes'. A number of steps of phacoemulsification cataract surgery can be practiced, including the capsulorrhexis (Guilden Ophthalmics, Elkins Park, PA, USA).

Although animal eyes such as goats eyes soaked in formalin, cows eyes and most commonly porcine eyes, have been used for decades for practicing wound construction, capsulorrhexis and sculpting of the nucleus, they all need to have a dedicated wet-lab, as the use of these eyes in a normal operating theatre would have serious health and safety, and ethical barriers. It is also important to recognise that in certain countries, cultural and ethical sensitivities preclude the use of certain animal models.

With the advent of relatively low cost, high fidelity model eyes, which have no issues with storage or disposal and can be used in an operating theatre or a wet-lab, the use of animal eyes is being phased out of most training programs.

Table 1 Summarises the strengths and weakness for the Eyesi, Phillips Eyes, Kitaro eyes and porcine eyes for simulating the 7 steps of phacoemulsification surgery.

Assessment Tools in Ophthalmic Surgical Training

As post-graduate surgical education has changed over the past decade to a competency-based model, surgical training programmes have been directed by the Royal Colleges and General Medical Council (GMC) in the UK and the Accreditation

Council for Graduate Medical Education (ACGME) in the US, to provide evidence of the attainment of competence by trainees.

In 1997, the ACGME endorsed the use of educational outcomes measures as a tool in assessing residency programmes' accreditation status. They specifically identified six areas of competence for residency education in ophthalmology including medical knowledge, patient care practice-based learning, interpersonal and communication skills, professionalism, and finally systems-based practice. The seventh area of competence, surgery, was subsequently included by the American Board of Ophthalmology.

The long-term goal of implementing the ACGME guidelines is to improve resident medical and surgical education by using outcomes measures to improve feedback and teaching techniques. In ophthalmic surgery, the goal is also specifically to assess surgical skill, improve the surgical learning curve.

For this, training institutions and programmes need valid assessment tools. A number of assessment tools, for both live and simulated surgery, have been developed for surgical training in the field of ophthalmology.

OSACSS (Objective Structured Assessment of Cataract Surgical Skill)
The OSACSS was developed as an objective performance-rating tool. The grading system contained global as well as phacoemulsification cataract surgery task-specific elements [14]. The global rating system was adapted from the previously validated objective structured assessment of technical skill (OSATS) tool previously validated for assessment of technical skills in simulated and live surgeries. The OSACSS system records the trainee's performance, and has advantages over direct observation as it is free of direct observational bias as the grading can be anonymised. OSACSS has construct validity for phacoemulsification cataract surgery.

OASIS (Objective Assessment of Skills in Intra-ocular Surgery)
The OASIS was developed in Harvard, Boston in 2005 [15]. The aim was to develop an objective ophthalmic surgical evaluation protocol to assess surgical competency and improve outcomes—developed specifically for phacoemulsification cataract. A unique database of all resident cataract cases over a one-year period at a tertiary hospital, and constructive feedback by experts in resident teaching assisted in creating a single page evaluation form. This provides an in-depth record of pre-operative, intra-operative, and post-operative data. OASIS has face and content validity and can be used to assess, objectively, surgical events and surgical skill. The main purpose of OASIS is the direct observation of live surgery, and surgical assessment.

GRASIS (Global Rating Assessment of Skills in Intraocular Surgery)
Complementary to OASIS, the GRASIS is a more subjective measurement [16]. It can be used to assess an ophthalmic surgical trainees' surgical care as well as their surgical knowledge, preparedness, and inter-personal skills. It has face and content validity.

SPESA (Subjective Phacoemulsification Skills Assessment)
The Subjective Phacoemulsification Skills Assessment (SPESA) [17] assesses trainee performance in cataract surgery by combining a global approach, very similar to GRASIS and ESSAT, with detailed stage-specific criteria of the critical components of cataract surgery.

OSCAR (Ophthalmic Surgical Competency Assessment Rubric) Origins
An assessment matrix (Ophthalmic surgical competency assessment rubric—OSCAR) for live ocular surgery has been developed and validated by the International Council of Ophthalmology [18]. These OSCARs were originally based on the OSACSS described by Saleh, however they have been expanded by creating a set of behaviourally-anchored scoring matrices that precisely and explicitly define what is expected for each step (Table 2). The rubric was based on a modified Dreyfus model [19], however the final 'expert' category was omitted, as trainees were not expected to become experts during training.

OSSCAR (Ophthalmic Simulated Surgical Competency Assessment Rubric)
OSSCARs are modifications of the ICO OSCAR matrices to be used with model eyes (Table 3). The principal modification is that OSSCARS only have three stages of competence, Novice, Advanced Beginner and Competent and surgical steps that cannot be simulated with the model eyes have been removed.

The learning outcome would be that a trainee is able to perform all the stages of the technique to a level of clearly defined 'competence', and thus be able to progress to live, supervised surgery in the operating theatre.

Although the OSCAR/OSSCARs at first glance look like rather wordy matrices, trainers very quickly learn to gauge which column a trainee falls into without having to slavishly read each descriptor.

Preparation for Live Surgery

As there is now clear cut evidence that Eyesi training improves performance in live surgery and significantly reduces PCR rates it should be viewed as the "Gold Standard" for training prior to commencing live phacoemulsification surgery. However, as has been discussed in section 'Model Eyes' of this chapter, model eye simulation should also play an important and complementary role alongside Eyesi training, on the journey towards live surgery.

How to Get the Most Out of Eyesi Training

The Eyesi has a pre-installed Surgical Courseware which is a structured ready-to-use training curriculum. The courseware has ascending degrees of difficulty and to

Table 2 ICO-Ophthalmology Surgical Competency Assessment Rubric: phacoemulsification (ICO-OSCAR: Phaco)

International Council of Ophthalmology's Ophthalmology Surgical Competency Assessment Rubric (ICO-OSCAR)

The International Council of Ophthalmology's "Ophthalmology Surgical Competency Assessment Rubrics" (ICO-OSCARs) are designed to facilitate assessment and teaching of surgical skill. Surgical procedures are broken down to individual steps and each step is graded on a scale of novice, beginner, advanced beginner and competent. A description of the performance necessary to achieve each grade in each step is given. The assessor simply circles the observed performance description at each step of the procedure. The ICO-OSCAR should be completed at the end of the case and immediately discussed with the student to provide timely, structured, specific performance feedback. These tools were developed by panels of international experts and are valid assessments of surgical skill.

ICO-OSCAR Instructor Directions

1. Observe resident phacoemulsification surgery.
2. Ideally, immediately after the case, circle each rubric description box that you observed. Some people like to let the resident circle the box on their own first. If the case is videotaped, it can be reviewed and scored later but this delays more effective prompt feedback.
3. Record any relevant comments not covered by the rubric.
4. Review the results with the resident.
5. Develop a plan for improvement (e.g. wet lab practice/tips for immediate next case).

Suggestions:

- If previous cases have been done, review ICO-OSCAR data to note areas needing improvement.
- If different instructors will be grading the same residents, it would be good that before starting using the tool they grade together several surgeries from recordings, so they make sure they are all grading in the same way.

Table 2 (continued)

Date ___ Resident ___ Evaluator ___	Novice (score = 2)	Beginner (score = 3)	Advanced Beginner (score = 4)	Competent (score = 5)	Not applicable. Done by preceptor (score= 0)
	ICO-Ophthalmology Surgical Competency Assessment Rubric: Phacoemulsification (ICO-OSCAR: Phaco)				
1 Draping:	Unable to start draping without help.	Drapes with minimal verbal instruction. Incomplete lash coverage.	Lashes mostly covered, drape at most minimally obstructing view.	Lashes completely covered and clear of incision site, drape not obstructing view.	
2 Incision & Paracentesis: Formation & Technique	Inappropriate incision architecture, location, and size.	Leakage and/or iris prolapse with local pressure, provides poor surgical access to and visibility of capsule and bag.	Incision either well-placed or non-leaking but not both.	Incision parallel to iris, self sealing, adequate size, provides good access for surgical maneuvering.	
3 Viscoelastic: Appropriate Use and Safe Insertion	Unsure of when, what type and how much viscoelastic to use. Has difficulty accessing anterior chamber through paracentesis.	Requires minimal instruction. Knows when to use but administers incorrect amount or type.	Requires no instruction. Uses at appropriate time. Administers adequate amount and type. Cannula tip in good position. Unsure of correct viscoelastic if multiple types available.	Viscoelastics are administered in appropriate amount and at the appropriate time with cannula tip clear of lens capsule and endothelium. Appropriate viscoelastic is used if multiple types of viscoelastics are available.	
4 Capsulorrhexis: Commencement of Flap & follow-through.	Instruction required, tentative, chases rather than controls rhexis, cortex disruption may occur.	Minimal instruction, predominantly in control with occasional loss of control of rhexis, cortex disruption may occur.	In control, few awkward or repositioning movements, no cortex disruption.	Delicate approach and confident control of the rhexis, no cortex disruption.	
5 Capsulorrhexis: Formation and Circular Completion	Size and position are inadequate for nucleus density & type of implant, tear may occur.	Size and position are barely adequate for nucleus density and implant type, difficulty achieving circular rhexis, tear may occur.	Size and position are almost exact for nucleus density and implant type, shows control, requires only minimal instruction.	Adequate size and position for nucleus density & type of implant, no tears, rapid, unaided control of radialization, maintains control of the flap and AC depth throughout the capsulorrhexis.	
6 Hydrodissection: Visible Fluid Wave and Free Nuclear Rotation	Hydrodissection fluid not injected in quantity nor place to achieve nucleus rotation.	Multiple attempts required, able to rotate nucleus somewhat but not completely. Tries to manually force rotation before adequate hydrodissection.	Fluid injected in appropriate location, able to rotate nucleus but encounters more than minimal resistance.	Ideally see free fluid wave but adequate if free nuclear rotation with minimal resistance is achieved. Aware of contraindications to hydrodissection.	

Table 2 (continued)

#	Skill					
7	Phacoemulsification Probe and Second Instrument: Insertion Into Eye	Has great difficulty inserting the probe or second instrument, AC collapses, may damage wound, capsule or Descemet's membrane	Inserts the probe or second instrument after some failed attempts, may damage wound, capsule or Descemet's membrane.	Inserts probe and second instrument on first attempt with mild difficulty, no damage to wound, capsule or Descemet's membrane.	Smoothly inserts instruments into the eye without damaging the wound or Descemet's membrane.	
8	Phacoemulsification Probe and Second Instrument: Effective Use and Stability	Tip frequently not visible, has much difficulty keeping the eye in primary position and uses excessive force to do so.	Tip often not visible, often requires manipulation to keep eye in primary position.	Maintains visibility of tip at most times, eye is generally kept in primary position with mild depression or pulling on the globe.	Maintains visibility of instrument tips at all times, keeps the eye in primary position without depressing or pulling up the globe.	
9	Nucleus: Sculpting or Primary Chop	Frequently incorrect power used during sculpting, applies power at inappropriate times, excessive phaco probe movement causes constant eye/nucleus movement, unable to engage nucleus (chop method) or the groove is of inadequate depth or width (divide and conquer). Unable to correctly work foot pedals.	Moderate error in power used while sculpting, tentative, frequent eye/nucleus movement produced by phaco tip, difficult to engage nucleus (chop technique) or groove adequately after many attempts (divide and conquer), poor control of phacodynamics with frequent anterior chamber depth fluctuations. Has difficulty working foot pedals.	Uses correct power with minimal error when sculpting, occasional eye/nucleus movement caused by phaco tip, some difficulty in engaging or holding nucleus (chop method) or groove adequate with minimal repeat attempts, fairly good control of phacodynamics with occasional anterior chamber depth change. Minimal mistakes using foot pedals.	Sculpting is performed using adequate ultrasound power regulated by the pedal, with forward movements that do not change the eye position or push the nucleus, the nucleus is safely engaged (with chop method) or the groove is appropriate in depth and width (divide and conquer technique), phacodynamics are controlled as evidenced by the internal anterior chamber environment. Adept at foot pedal control.	
10	Nucleus: Rotation and Manipulation	Unable to rotate nucleus.	Able to rotate nucleus partially and with zonular stress.	Able to rotate nucleus fully but with zonular stress.	Nucleus is safely and efficiently manipulated producing minimal stress on zonules and globe.	

Table 2 (continued)

Nucleus: Cracking or Chopping With Safe Phacoemulsification of Segments 11	**CRACKING**: Grooves are not centered or deep enough and go into epinucleus, nucleus is constantly displaced from central position, unable to crack nucleus at all, eye constantly moving. **CHOPPING**: Always endangers or engages adjacent tissue, unable to accomplish chop of any piece. **SEGMENT PHACOEMULSIFICATION**: produces significant wound burn, great difficulty pursuing fragments around the anterior chamber and into the bag, poor awareness of second instrument tip and difficulty keeping the second hand instrument under the phaco tip.	**CRACKING**: Some grooves are centered and deep enough and some go into epinucleus, displaces nucleus in most grooves, attempts to split nucleus with instruments too shallow in groove, able to crack portion of nucleus, eye often moving. **CHOPPING**: endangers or engages adjacent tissue in most chops, able to accomplish chop of some pieces. **SEGMENT PHACOEMULSIFICATION**: produces light wound burn, pursues most fragments around the AC and into the bag, the second hand instrument is sometimes under the phaco tip	**CRACKING**: Most grooves are centered and deep enough, rarely goes into epinucleus, rarely displaces nucleus, sometimes attempts to split in mid-nucleus but succeeds, eye usually in primary position. **CHOPPING**: endangers or engages adjacent tissue in some chops, able to accomplish chop of most pieces. **SEGMENT PHACOEMULSIFICATION**: produces minimal wound burn, pursues some fragments around the AC and into the bag, the second hand instrument is usually under the phaco tip	**CRACKING**: Grooves are centered, deep enough to ensure cracking, length does not reach epinucleus, nucleus is not displaced from central position, places instruments deep enough to easily and successfully crack nucleus, eye stays in primary position. **CHOPPING**: Nucleus engaged and vertical or horizontal chop technique undertaken with no inadvertent engagement of adjacent tissue (especially capsule). Full thickness nuclear chop of all pieces in a controlled and fluid manner. **SEGMENT PHACOEMULSIFICATION**: No wound burns, Pieces are "floated" to the tip without "pursuing" the fragments around the anterior chamber and the bag, The second hand instrument is kept under the phaco tip to prevent posterior capsule contact if surge arises.
Irrigation and Aspiration Technique With Adequate Removal of Cortex 12	Great difficulty introducing the aspiration tip under the capsulorrhexis border, aspiration hole position not controlled, cannot regulate aspiration flow as needed, cannot peel cortical material adequately, engages capsule or iris with aspiration port.	Moderate difficulty introducing aspiration tip under capsulorrhexis and maintaining hole up position, attempts to aspirate without occluding tip, shows poor comprehension of aspiration dynamics, cortical peeling is not well controlled, jerky and slow, capsule potentially compromised. prolonged attempts result in minimal residual cortical material.	Minimal difficulty introducing the aspiration tip under the capsulorrhexis, aspiration hole usually up, cortex will engaged for 360 degrees, cortical peeling slow, few technical errors, minimal residual cortical material.	Aspiration tip is introduced under the free border of the capsulorrhexis in irrigation mode with the aspiration hole up, Aspiration is activated in just enough flow as to occlude the tip, efficiently removes all cortex, The cortical material is peeled gently towards the center of the pupil, tangentially in cases of zonular weakness.

Table 2 (continued)

13	Lens Insertion, Rotation, and Final Position of Intraocular Lens	Unable to insert IOL, unable to produce adequate incision for implant type NON-FOLDABLE: unable to place the lower haptic in the capsular bag, unable to rotate the upper haptic into place FOLDABLE: unable to load IOL into injector or forceps, no control of lens injection, doesn't control tip placement, lens is not in the capsular bag or is injected upside down.	Insertion and manipulation of IOL is difficult, eye handled roughly, anterior chamber not stable, repeated attempts result in borderline incision for implant type NON-FOLDABLE: repeated hesitant attempts result in lower haptic in the capsular bag, upper haptic is rotated into place but with excessive force on capsulorrhexis and zonules and repeated attempts are necessary FOLDABLE: difficulty loading IOL into injector or forceps, hesitant, poor control of lens injection, difficulty controlling tip placement, excessive manipulation required to get both haptics into capsular bag.	Insertion and manipulation of IOL is accomplished with minimal anterior chamber instability, incision just adequate for implant type NON-FOLDABLE: the lower haptic is placed inside the capsular bag with some difficulty, upper haptic is rotated into place with some stress on the capsulorrhexis and zonule fibers FOLDABLE: ; minimal difficulty loading IOL into injector of forceps, hesitant but good control of lens injection, minimal difficulty controlling tip placement, both haptics are in the capsular bag.	Insertion and manipulation of IOL is performed in a deep and stable anterior chamber and capsular bag, with incision appropriate for implant type. NON-FOLDABLE: The lower haptic is smoothly placed inside the capsular bag; the upper haptic is rotated into place without exerting excessive stress to the capsulorrhexis or the zonule fibers. FOLDABLE: Able to load IOL into injector or forceps, lens is injected in a controlled fashion, fixation of IOL is symmetric; the optic and both haptics are inside the capsular bag.
14	Wound Closure (Including Suturing, Hydration, and Checking Security as Required)	If suturing is needed, instruction is required and stitches are placed in an awkward, slow fashion with much difficulty, astigmatism, bent needles, incomplete suture rotation and wound leakage may result, unable to make incision water tight or does not check wound for seal. Improper final IOP.	If suturing is needed, stitches are placed with some difficulty, resuturing may be needed, questionable wound closure with probable astigmatism, instruction may be needed, questionable whether all viscoelastics are thoroughly removed, Extra maneuvers are required to make the incision water tight at the end of the surgery. May have improper IOP.	If suturing is needed, stitches are placed with minimal difficulty tight enough to maintain the wound closed, may have slight astigmatism, viscoelastics are adequately removed after this step with some difficulty, The incision is checked and is water tight or needs minimal adjustment at the end of the surgery. May have improper IOP.	If suturing is needed, stitches are placed tight enough to maintain the wound closed, but not too tight as to induce astigmatism, viscoelastics are thoroughly removed after this step, the incision is checked and is water tight at the end of the surgery. Proper final IOP.

Table 2 (continued)

Global Indices				
15	Wound Neutrality and Minimizing Eye Rolling and Corneal Distortion	Nearly constant eye movement and corneal distortion.	Eye often not in primary position, frequent distortion folds.	Eye usually in primary position, mild corneal distortion folds occur.	The eye is kept in primary position during the surgery. No distortion folds are produced. The length and location of incisions prevents distortion of the cornea.
16	Eye Positioned Centrally Within Microscope View	Constantly requires repositioning.	Occasional repositioning required.	Mild fluctuation in pupil position.	The pupil is kept centered during the surgery.
17	Conjunctival and Corneal Tissue Handling	Tissue handling is rough and damage occurs.	Tissue handling borderline, minimal damage occurs.	Tissue handling decent but potential for damage exists.	Tissue is not damaged nor at risk by handling.
18	Intraocular Spatial Awareness	instruments often in contact with capsule, iris and corneal endothelium'; blunt second hand instrument not kept in appropriate position.	Occasional accidental contact with capsule, iris and corneal endothelium, sometimes has blunt second hand instrument between the posterior capsule and the activated phaco tip.	Rare accidental contact with capsule, iris and corneal endothelium. Often has blunt second hand instrument between the posterior capsule and the activated phaco tip.	No accidental contact with capsule, iris and corneal endothelium, when appropriate, a blunt, second hand instrument, is always kept between the posterior capsule and the tip of the phaco when the phaco is activated.
19	Iris Protection	Iris constantly at risk, handled roughly.	Iris occasionally at risk. Needs help in deciding when and how to use hooks, ring or other methods of iris protection.	Iris generally well protected. Slight difficulty with iris hooks, ring, or other methods of iris protection.	Iris is uninjured. Iris hooks, ring, or other methods are used as needed to protect the iris.
20	Overall Speed and Fluidity of Procedure	Hesitant, frequent starts and stops, not at all fluid.	Occasional starts and stops, inefficient and unnecessary manipulations common, case duration about 60 minutes.	Occasional inefficient and/or unnecessary manipulations occur, case duration about 45 minutes.	Inefficient and/or unnecessary manipulations are avoided, case duration is appropriate for case difficulty. In general, 30 minutes should be adequate.

Comments:

Golnik KC, Beaver H, Gauba V, Lee AG, Mayorga E, Palis G, Saleh GM. Cataract surgical skill assessment. Ophthalmology. 2011 Feb;118(2):427.e1-5.

Adapt and translate this document for your non-commercial needs, but please include ICO attribution. Access and download ICO-OSCARs at icoph.org/ico-oscar

Table 3 Ophthalmic Simulated Surgical Competency Assessment Rubric: phacoemulsification (OSSCAR: Phaco)

Trainee: _____ Evaluator: _____ Date: _____

Ophthalmic Simulated Surgical Competency Assessment Rubric – Phacoemulsification (OSSCAR:Phaco)

		Novice (score = 0)	Advanced Beginner (score = 1)	Competent (score = 2)	Score (Not done score = 0)
1	Incision and paracentesis formation technique	Poor wound construction and paracentesis placement. Traumatises conjunctiva	Correct positioning of incision and paracentesis but incision architecture is not yet correct	Well constructed incision and paracentesis with careful tissue handling	
2	Viscoelastic: appropriate use and safe insertion	Incomplete fill +/- damage to capsule	Appropriate fill but still hesitant	Safe and smooth insertion of viscoelastic	
3	Capsulorrhexis: Commencement of flap	Poor positioning of initial flap with disruption of underlying cortex	Good positioning of flap but slightly hesitant in raising the flap	Neat creation of a flap of an appropriate size in the correct position.	
4	Capsulorrhexis: Formation and circular completion	Unable to create a complete capsulorrhexis with poor understanding of tearing vectors	capsulorrhexis is completed but is either too small, too large or eccentric	Smooth creation of an appropriately sized and circular capsulorrhexis	
5	Hydrodissection: visible fluid wave and free nuclear rotation	Cannot insert cannula in the correct tissue plane / excessive or insufficient force used / incomplete freeing of the nucleus	Cannula inserted correctly under the anterior capsule but more than one attempt is needed to achieve free nucleus rotation	Efficient and safe hydrodissection with free nuclear rotation	
6	Phaco probe and second instrument: effective use and stability within the eye	Unsure of the positioning of the instruments within the eye / phaco probe is frequently close to the capsulorrhexis / inefficient use of the second instrument	Phaco probe and second instrument generally positioned correctly / no iris trauma / capsulorrhexis not endangered	Confident instrument handling with phaco probe always kept in a safe position	
7	Nucleus: sculpting or primary chop	Hesitant use of the phaco probe / tendency to push the lens / timid sculpting with poor use of full range of phaco power	More efficient use of phaco power and appropriate vacuum settings to create a groove or perform a primary chop / still some stress placed on zonules	Fast and efficient sculpting or chopping technique	
8	Nucleus: Rotation and manipulation	Incorrect positioning of the instruments / excessive posterior pressure on the lens / rounds off the edges of the quadrants leaving a bowl	Good positioning of instruments but still some hesitancy using the second instrument / some posterior pressure whilst rotating the nucleus	Confident use of both phaco probe and second instrument to rotate the lens with no posterior pressure on the zonules	
9	Nucleus: cracking or chopping	Attempts to crack the lens before groove is deep enough / places instruments too superficially in the groove / excessive posterior pressure	Forms a grove of the correct depth and width before cracking / still requires several attempts to crack the nucleus	Good groove construction and cracks / chops nucleus at first attempt	

Table 3 (continued)

		during cracking		
10	Nucleus: segment removal	Chases segments with phaco probe / poor use of the second instrument / endangers capsule / phaco probe positioned too close to posterior capsule or endothelium	Appropriate use of vacuum to engage segments / second instrument being used more efficiently / less of a tendency to phaco too deep in capsular bag or too close to the endothelium	Safe enagement of nuclear segments and efficient removal with good use of the second instrument
11	Irrigation and aspiration technique with adequate removal of cortex	Aspiration port not safely positioned in the capsular bag / inappropriate vacuum used / hesitant engagement of cortex	Better positioning of aspiration port / still not using vacuum efficiently / occasionally engages the anterior capsule	Efficient removal of the cortex with no danger to the capsular bag or capsulorrhexis
12	Lens insertion, rotation and final position of IOL	IOL not placed in the capsular bag / unable to rotate the lens into the correct position	IOL placed in the capsular bag but haptics still require manipulation	IOL completely placed within the capsular bag at the first attempt
13	Wound closure: hydration, suturing if required and checking security	Ineffective hydration technique / does not check would security / poor placement and tying of 10/0 suture	Wound hydration performed correctly / suture tying hesitant / suture slightly too tight or too loose	Wound hydration performed correctly / good suturing technique with correct tension
	Global Indices			
14	Tissue handling:	Tissue handling is often unsafe with inadvertent damage to the conjunctiva, cornea, iris or capsule / excessively aggressive or timid.	Tissue handling is safe but sometimes requires multiple attempts to achieve desired manipulation of tissue.	Tissue handling is efficient, fluid and almost always achieves desired tissue manipulation on first attempt.
15	Eye positioning and use of the microscope	Eye is frequently in an eccentric position. Focusing and X-Y movement of the microscope is erratic.	Eye is mainly kept in a central position and focusing of the microscope is becoming smoother.	Eye is maintained in a central position throughout the procedure and the point of interest is always in focus.
16	Overall speed and fluidity of the procedure	Hesitant and lacks fluidity with multiple pauses between manouevres	Beginning to string the different steps together with minimal guidance from trainer	All steps completed in a timely manner with minimal input from trainer

Overall Difficulty of Procedure: Simple   Intermediate   Difficult

Good Points: _____

Suggestions for development: _____

Agreed action: _____

Signature of assessor _____   Signature of trainee _____ advance through a course trainees must meet a required performance level on each task.

The following are tips to get the maximum benefit from Eyesi training.

– Induction session with trainee to introduce them to the instrumentation, and Courseware.
– Supervision by a trainer (this can be a more senior trainee) at least for the first hour of Eyesi training and then periodic observed sessions to make sure the correct techniques are being adopted.
– Monitoring of training data. This can be done individually with trainees by viewing their scores on the local Eyesi or by using VRmNet, VR Magic's web-based training portal through which supervisors can view their trainee's training history online and compare their results to peer group training data.
– Practicing in pairs. Many trainees find it helpful to work through the Courseware in pairs, giving each other tips about how to pass the trickier modules.
– Revisiting Eyesi training if a trainee is consistently finding a particular manoeuvre difficult during live surgery, or to help rebuild confidence after a surgical complication.
– Creating bespoke courses for more advanced trainees who are moving towards independent live surgery. Although there are pre-set courses with variable degrees of difficulty for different stages of surgery such as capsulorrhexis and nucleus sculpting, it is possible to create courses designed to practice a specific task. This is helpful when a trainee wants to practice a new capsulorrhexis technique, or change from a "divide and conquer" technique to a "stop and chop" technique.

As trainees progress through the Eyesi Courseware levels they can be introduced to simulation using model eyes. Although this training traditionally takes place in a wet-lab, if there is access to such a facility, the model eyes should also be used in the operating theatre where a trainee will be performing live surgery. This form of immersive simulation gives the trainee the opportunity to get comfortable with the operating microscope and phacoemulsification equipment they will be using in live surgery and enables them to practice the more tactile elements of surgery, such as wound construction, nucleus sculpting and manipulating nuclear fragments.

Once a trainee has completed the Eyesi Courseware A and B and has demonstrated their competence on the model eyes with the phacoemulsification OSSCAR, they are ready to be introduced to live surgery.

Live Surgery

Prior to commencing live surgery it is important to set some ground rules about how the trainee and trainer will communicate with each other and with the patient during surgery. Trainees need to be reminded that patients will be able to hear exactly what is being said during surgery and may pick up on certain phrases and perhaps, more importantly, the tone of voice being used. It is essential that a calm reassuring tone is used throughout and that words such as "sorry" should be avoided. Having some coded phrases which indicate when a trainee should stop what they are doing and listen for further instruction, or hand over to the attending surgeon, are also helpful.

Ideally the first exposure to live surgery should be on dedicated training lists, with reduced numbers of patients, who have no ocular or systemic comorbidities. Patients should be informed during the consent process that part of their surgery will be performed by a trainee surgeon under close supervision and that the trainee has demonstrated their competence to perform these parts of the operation on a simulator.

Trainees should have spent a number of lists assisting their trainer so they can observe how he/she communicates with the scrub team and patients and how they perform each step of the operation.

The Steep Part of the Learning Curve—Cases 1–20

A number of models of training have been used for teaching cataract surgery, the most commonly used of which are repeating the same part of the procedure several times on a list and so-called "reverse chaining" or "backing in", wherein the steps of the procedure are learned from the end of the procedure forwards, so in theory at least the trainee is operating in good conditions all the time.

Most trainers use a combination of these two teaching methods and will have a personal preference for the order they teach the different stages, for example;

- Correct draping procedure.
- Removing viscoelastic at the end of a case.
- Inserting the IOL and then removing the viscoelastic.
- Corneal and side port incisions and filling anterior chamber with viscoelastic.
- Aspiration of cortical lens material.
- Removal of nuclear fragments and using the second instrument to manipulate lens fragments.
- Sculpting of the nucleus, rotating and cracking nucleus.
- Capsulorrhexis—trainees who have trained on the Eyesi often find capsulorrhexis relatively straightforward and so this stage can be introduced after a trainee has mastered wound construction.

As a trainee gains confidence and competence with each of these stages the next step is to start stringing these stages together, whilst being mindful of the length of time being taken for each procedure. The concept of the Zone of Proximal Development is worth bearing in mind, as trainees progress through these stages.

The following are common stumbling blocks trainees may encounter in the early part of their training and the remedies for addressing them.

– Pressing on the main incision or side port incisions causing the anterior chamber to shallow. This is something that trainees are not penalised for during Eyesi training, in fact they may actually consciously press posteriorly on the mannequin eye to stabilise it and so improve their score. Using the Phillips or Kitaro model eyes helps to correct this fault.
– Tentative capsulorrhexis technique. The best way to address this is more supervised Eyesi training.
– Not grooving deeply enough before trying to crack the nucleus and/or not placing the phaco tip and second instrument deeply enough into the groove before attempting to crack the nucleus.
– Rounding off the edges with a divide and conquer technique leading to the creation of a nuclear bowl.
– Poor nuclear rotation technique with too much posterior pressure being applied.
– Poor use of the second hand instrument, because they are concentrating so much on the phaco tip.
  All of these problems dealing with the nucleus are best addressed using the Phillips or Kitaro eyes, as they require tactile feedback.
– Problems with cortex aspiration such as failing to occlude the aspiration tip with the cortex before applying vacuum, or being in the incorrect plane relative to the capsulorrhexis. Further supervised Eyesi training will correct these faults.

Feedback should be given immediately after each case, pointing out what aspects of the surgery went well and making suggestions for improvements, with the aid of sketched diagrams. Reviewing recordings of the surgery is incredibly valuable as it enables the trainer to point out aspects of a trainee's technique, which could be modified and practiced on the Eyesi and/or model eyes before the next theatre list.

Getting in the Groove—Cases 20–100

Once a trainee can consistently perform all of the steps of phacoemulsification and is starting to perform operations from start to finish, the next step is to consolidate what they have learnt and concentrate on improving the flow and efficiency of their surgery. If trainees have access to two or more operating lists of suitable cases per week, the majority will progress rapidly during this phase of training. Reviewing recordings of their surgery is also invaluable at this stage as trainees can often identify when they are carrying out unnecessary manoeuvres or are being inefficient.

A wider variety of cataract morphologies can be selected, but it would still be prudent to avoid mature cataracts, pseudoexfoliation cases, smaller pupils and very hypermetropic or myopic eyes. Once a trainee is consistently performing complete procedures in less than 20 min, with minimal intervention from their trainer, they are ready to learn different surgical techniques using a combination of Eyesi (Intermediate Courseware C) and model eye training. For example, using forceps instead of a cystatome needle to perform a capsulorrhexis, or performing a "stop and chop" instead of a "divide and conquer" technique for nuclear fracture.

It should be emphasised that no one technique is better than another and that mastering a range of techniques will help them become more adept and adaptable surgeons.

Increasing Case Complexity—Cases 100+

It is at this stage that trainees are, in general, ready to take on more complicated cases with ocular and systemic comorbidities which will make surgery more challenging. There are Eyesi modules to simulate more difficult capsulorrhexis scenarios, mature cataracts and weak zonules, which trainees should undertake before tackling more complex cases. Closer supervision is required during these cases, as a trainer can often pick up subtle signs of an imminent problem, such as a deepening of the anterior chamber, and intervene before a complication occurs.

It is almost inevitable that complication rates will rise during this phase of training and it is imperative that trainees are offered support and encouragement if they encounter complications.

Management of Posterior Capsule Rupture and Vitreous Loss

One of the unintended consequences of improved phacoemulsification training is that even trainees who have performed 300 or more surgeries may have had very few opportunities to manage cases where there has been a PCR and vitreous loss. Although PCR is associated with an increased risk of endophthalmitis and retinal detachment, if managed correctly the visual prognosis can still be excellent, with preservation of the anterior capsule support and placement of an IOL in the sulcus.

Once again a mixture of Eyesi and model eye simulation techniques can be used to simulate PCR and vitreous loss. The latest Eyesi software includes a PCR and vitreous loss module, which enables trainees to familiarise themselves with the anterior vitrectomy instrumentation and the use of triamcinolone to stain the

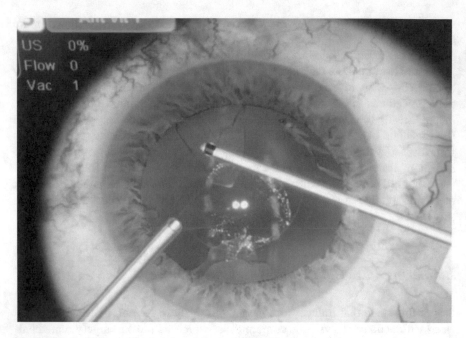

Fig. 5 Eyesi—PCR module showing vitreous stained with triamcinolone

vitreous (Fig. 5). The foot pedal controls can be used to switch from vitrectomy to aspiration mode and the simulation of removing the vitreous from the capsular bag and anterior chamber is very realistic.

Phillips advanced cataract eyes have been designed to be used for simulating complicated cataract surgery. The posterior chamber of these eyes can be filled with egg white, to simulate vitreous and the posterior capsule and/or the "zonules" can be tampered with to induce a posterior capsule rupture or zonular dialysis. Videos of how to set up these eyes for this type of simulation and of the Eyesi PCR modules can be found on the Simulation Gallery website (gallery.simulate-docularsurgery.com)

The following is an example of modular PCR training:

– Didactic teaching about how to prevent PCR and how to manage patients who have had complicated surgery post-operatively.
– The principles behind anterior vitrectomy for PCR and IOL implantation options.
– Videos of correct and incorrect management of PCR with vitreous loss
– Eyesi PCR modules—this training should be under the supervision of a trainer and not undertaken solo.
– How to set up for the phaco for an anterior vitrectomy.
– Practice anterior vitrectomy techniques with Phillips advanced cataract eyes by intentionally piercing the posterior capsule once the cataract has been removed

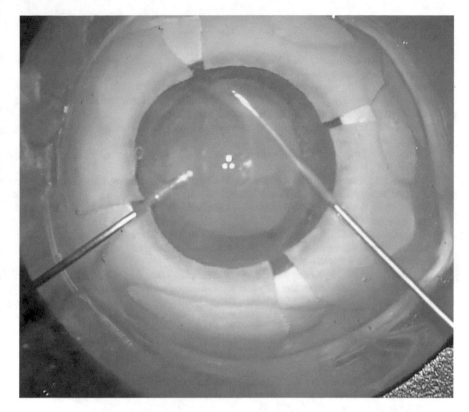

Fig. 6 Anterior vitrectomy simulation with Phillips Studio eye and triamcinolone substitute

by phacoemulsification (Fig. 6) This enables trainees to transfer skills acquired with the Eyesi to the theatre environment.
- Simulate complicated cataract surgery without trainees or scrub team being aware of what complications might ensue. This truly immersive simulation is akin to the simulation undertaken by pilots and aircrew, who are not aware of what problem they are going to encounter before the simulation commences. This vitreous loss "fire drill" training is an excellent way of making sure all members of the theatre team know what is required of them in the event of a PCR [20].

At the conclusion of this chapter it is appropriate to mention that the simulation is not just for trainees and that even experienced surgeons can benefit from time spent on the Eyesi or using the model eyes. This is especially true when it comes to practicing the management of surgical complications or when trying a new surgical technique. The desire to continually improve one's surgical skills should be a lifelong quest and we are fortunate to have the tools to achieve this, without compromising the safety of our patients.

Acknowledgements I would like to thank my friend and colleague Will Dean, for his assistance with the Educational Theory section of this chapter.

References

1. Binenbaum GM, Nicholas MD, Volpe J. Ophthalmology resident surgical competency: a national survey. Ophthalmology. 2006;2006(113):1237–44.
2. Knowles M. Andragogy in action. Houston: TX, Gulf Publishing; 1984.
3. Fry H, Ketteridge S, Marshall S. A handbook for teaching and learning in higher education: enhancing academic practice. New York: Routledge; 2009.
4. Schön DA. The reflective practitioner: how professionals think in action. London: Temple Smith; 1993.
5. Vygotsky L. Interaction between learning and development. Harvard University Press; 1979.
6. Ericsson KA, Krampe RT, Tesch-Romer C. The role of deliberate practice in the aquisition of expert performance. Psychol Rev. 1993;100:363–406.
7. Kneebone R. Evaluating clinical simulations for learning procedural skills: a theory-based approach. Acad Med. 2005;80:549–53.
8. Mahr MA, Hodge DO. Construct validity of anterior segment anti-tremor and forceps surgical simulator training modules: attending versus resident surgeon performance. J Cataract Refract Surg. 2008;34:980–5.
9. Spiteri AV, Aggarwal R, Kersey TL, Sira M, Benjamin L, Darzi AW, et al. Development of a virtual reality training curriculum for phacoemulsification surgery. Eye. 2014;28:78–84.
10. McCannel CA, Reed DC, Goldman DR. Ophthalmic surgery simulator training improves resident performance of capsulorhexis in the operating room. Ophthalmology. 2013;120:2456–61.
11. Thomsen ASS, Smith P, Subhi Y, Cour M, Tang L, Saleh GM, et al. High correlation between performance on a virtual-reality simulator and real-life cataract surgery. Acta Ophthalmol. 2017;95:307–11.
12. Thomsen ASS, Bach-Holm D, Kjaerbo H, Hojgaard-Olsen K, Subhi Y, Park YS, et al. Operating room performance improves after proficiency based virtual reality cataract training. Ophthalmology. 2017;124:524–31.
13. Ferris JD, Donachie PHJ, Johnston RL, Barnes B, Olaitan M, Sparrow JM. Royal College of Ophthalmologists' National Ophthalmology Database study of cataract surgery: report 6. The impact of EyeSi virtual reality training on complication rates of cataract surgery performed by first and second year trainees. BJO. 2020;104:324–29.
14. Saleh GM, Gauba V, Mitra A, Litwin AS, Chung AK, Benjamin L. Objective structured assessment of cataract surgical skill. Arch Ophthalmol. 2007;125:363–6.
15. Cremers SL, Ciolino JB, Ferrufino-Ponce ZK, Henderson BA. Objective assessment of skills in intraocular surgery (OASIS). Ophthalmology. 2005;112:1236–41.
16. Cremers SL, Lora AN, Ferrufino-Ponce ZK. Global rating assessment of skills in intraocular surgery (GRASIS). Ophthalmology. 2005;112:1655–60.
17. Feldman BH, Geist CE. Assessing residents in phacoemulsification. Ophthalmology. 2007;114:1586.
18. Golnik KC, Beaver H, Gauba V, Lee AG, Mayorga E, Palis G, Saleh GM. Cataract surgical skill assessment. Ophthalmology. 2011;118(427):e421–5.
19. Dreyfus SE, Dreyfus HL. A five-stage model of the mental activities involved in directed skill acquisition; 1980.
20. Lockington D, Belin M, McGhee CNJ. The need for all cataract surgeons to run a regular vitreous loss fire drill. Eye. 2017;31:1120–1.

Challenging Cases

**Ahmed Shalaby Bardan, Riddhi Thaker, Rawya Abdelhadi Diab,
Vincenzo Maurino and Christopher Liu**

Objectives of This Chapter

1. To recognise the degree of complexity in each and every case,
2. To describe and formulate the detailed planning required for complex cases,
3. To illustrate surgical approach and techniques in a whole range of challenging situations,
4. To introduce the concept that complexity is just simplicity multiplied, a mind trick to enable surgical calm, taking one step at a time,
5. To ensure patient satisfaction and safety through adequate counselling, discussing risk–benefit ratios to achieve proper informed consent, and referral to an appropriate cataract sub-specialist when necessary.

A. S. Bardan (✉)
Faculty of Medicine, Alexandria University, Alexandria, Egypt
e-mail: Ahmedbardan@gmail.com

A. S. Bardan · R. A. Diab · C. Liu
Sussex Eye Hospital, Brighton and Sussex University Hospitals NHS Trust, Brighton, UK

R. Thaker
Northampton General Hospital, Northampton, UK

R. A. Diab
Sudan Eye Centre, Khartoum, Sudan

V. Maurino
Moorfields Eye Hospital NHS Foundation Trust, London, UK

C. Liu
Brighton and Sussex Medical School, Brighton, UK

Tongdean Eye Clinic, London, UK

© Springer Nature Switzerland AG 2021
C. Liu and A. Shalaby Bardan (eds.), *Cataract Surgery*,
https://doi.org/10.1007/978-3-030-38234-6_9

Introduction

There are numerous circumstances and/or conditions that combine to make cataract surgery more challenging. These can be related to previous surgical treatment (e.g. laser refractive surgery, corneal surgery or vitrectomy) or can be associated with ocular co-morbidity (e.g. uveitis or corneal diseases such as Fuchs' endothelial dystrophy) or patient's general condition (such as extreme kyphoscoliosis and related posturing difficulties).

Surgeons and patients should be aware of factors that might make cataract surgery more difficult, or that may adversely affect the outcome. This awareness will inform decisions about the surgical technique, and grade and experience of the operating surgeon required as well as the pre- and post-operative care. Most importantly, it will influence the counselling and advice given to patients about their surgery and enable patients to make an informed decision on whether or not and when to proceed with surgery. (See chapter "Risk Stratification" for more details).

Mastering cataract surgery is a matter of becoming a specialised cataract surgeon who can deal with complex cataract situations consistently and reliably. The learning curve is steep for the most difficult cases because such cases are uncommon and in small centres might be very exceptional. In this chapter, we will provide a guide for the cataract surgeon and their team to identify, counsel, prepare for, and manage difficult cataract cases.

Pre-Operative Challenges

Immunosuppressed

Immunosuppressed patients are more vulnerable to infections and inflammation post-cataract surgery. Patients may be immunosuppressed due to different causes or patients may be taking immunosuppressant medication for autoimmune diseases (for example post-organ transplant treatment and cancer). Taking a careful history including an extensive past medical and medication history is vital to identifying patients' systemic morbidities that may affect cataract surgery outcomes.

It is important to ensure that a multidisciplinary approach is followed for such patients and that counselling involves in detail the specific higher risks of infection/inflammation and this is balanced against the benefit of seeing better after cataract surgery. Patients on immunosuppressant therapy must be informed of the increased risks of sight threatening infection compared to the general population [1]. Full blood count may be helpful for checking level of risk. Perfect wound construction for watertightness is mandatory. Where there is doubt, place a suture to ensure watertightness. A scleral tunnel incision could also be considered.

Hypertension

A blood pressure of below 180 mmHg systolic (SBP) and 110 mmHg diastolic (DBP) is generally considered acceptable to proceed with phacoemulsification. However, uncontrolled blood pressures can increase the risk of adverse medical events (e.g. cardiovascular and neurological). Furthermore, it is linked to increased risk of ocular haemorrhage which can be sight threating [2].

Patients with SBP ≥ 180 mm Hg and/or DBP ≥ 110 mm Hg are believed to have an increased risk of major adverse perioperative cardiovascular and neurological events. However, this evidence is mostly derived from patients undergoing major cardiac or vascular surgery and may not be applicable to cataract surgery. A UK series of 734 hypertensive cataract patients, including 87 patients (12%) with SBP ≥ 180 mm Hg or DBP ≥ 110 mm Hg, had no systemic adverse events, including cardiac arrest, myocardial infarction or stroke. This study concluded that since the risks are usually low, delaying cataract surgery in patients undergoing local anaesthesia just for isolated increased in blood pressure is not reasonable. However, all 734 patients did have previously well controlled hypertension [3].

Studies show that rather than pre-operative hypertension, fluctuations in blood pressure is more associated with cardiovascular risk factors. Therefore, it is recommended that during the perioperative period the mean blood pressure should remain within 20% of baseline [2, 4].

Diabetes and Hyperglycaemia

As patients may be required to fast for cataract surgery, fluctuations in glucose levels may result. It is therefore advisable to put patients with diabetes especially those who are insulin dependent earlier on the surgical list especially if planned for sedation.

Surgical stress can lead to peri-operative hyperglycaemia. Pre-operative hyperglycaemia is linked to adverse events including delayed wound healing, infection, diabetic ketoacidosis and non-ketotic hyperosmolar state. There can be an increased risk of cystoid macular oedema (CMO) and worsening of retinopathy. Furthermore, patients with high glucose levels may need insulin infusion.

HbA1c of <8.5% (69 mmol/mol) should be considered as acceptable for surgery according to the UK guidelines [5]. HbA1c may be used as an indicator of overall glycaemia control.

It is advisable in patients with active diabetic retinopathy to get advice on concurrent management of the retinopathy from a medical retina colleague prior to proceeding with surgery. There is significant interplay between diabetic retinopathy (DR) and cataract. The cataract can cause difficulty examining, diagnosing and treating DR and inversely cataract removal can exacerbate untreated DR/maculopathy.

Pre-operative optical coherence tomography (OCT) of the macula is a must to identify cases of clinically significant macular oedema (CSMO) so that it can be treated accordingly. An injection of anti-VEGF can be done at the end of cataract surgery to prevent worsening of macular oedema. Where there is inadequate view, early follow up within days is mandatory as cataract surgery can set off acute progression of maculopathy.

A combined pars plana vitrectomy with phacoemulsification and intraocular lens (IOL) insertion should be considered for patients with advanced diabetic eye disease—these are usually younger patients with Type 1 DM. These cases should be handled by surgeons trained in vitreo-retinal surgery.

There is a higher risk among the diabetic patients of developing post cataract surgery cystoid macular oedema (CMO). This has created a debate on whether to give prophylactic non-steroidal anti-inflammatory drops (please see chapter "Pseudophakic Cystoid Macular Oedema" for more details). The evidence is to add prophylactic non-steroidal anti-inflammatory drops to the steroids for all diabetics and we should add this.

It is also important to consider those patients who have a dense cataract with a poor fundus view for cataract surgery. Cataract extraction would allow visualisation of the macula and retina, facilitating management for diabetic retinopathy. Therefore, cataract surgery is recommended sooner rather than later in these cases, as their DR can be assessed, and subsequent follow-up can be established.

Finally, to aid good fundal view for diabetic retinopathy screening, fundoscopy in clinic and potential pan-retinal photocoagulation (PRP), a good sized anterior capsulorrhexis is recommended to reduce the risk of anterior capsular fibrosis and phimosis. Special design IOLs (e.g. square edge) and biomaterials which reduce the risk of capsular contraction syndrome (CCS) and opacification should be used.

Anticoagulants

Anticoagulants such as warfarin, direct oral anticoagulants (DOACs) and novel oral anticoagulants (NOACs) are life-saving medications. The more recent DOACs and NOACs should be stopped 48–72 h in advance to reduce risk of bleeding in local anaesthesia surgery. These anticoagulants cannot be reversed readily [6]. The cataract surgeon should weigh-up the risks and benefits of stopping anticoagulation, balancing general health risks with minimising bleeding during cataract surgery. It is useful to liaise with the original prescribing physician to ensure the safest course of action. CHA_2DS_2-VASc and HAS-BLED calculator scores can be used to assess the patient's risk of clotting and bleeding, respectively [6]. Most cataract surgeons tend not to stop anticoagulation if there is a high general health risk for the patient's general health and proceed with cataract surgery having properly counselled the patients on the bleeding risk and possible but unlikely consequences such as blindness.

When patients are using anticoagulants like warfarin it is important to check the INR as close as possible to the day of surgery and make sure it is within the range where risk of bleeding during cataract surgery is thought to be minimal. The authors are happy to perform cataract surgery with no sharp block local anaesthesia when INR is below 3.5. The cataract national dataset electronic multicentre audit [7] showed significant increase in minor complications of sharp needle and sub-Tenon's cannula but no increased risk of vision-threatening local anaesthetic or operative haemorrhagic complications in patients using warfarin and clopidogrel.

In these patients, it is best to always perform cataract surgery under topical anaesthesia or when indicated under sub-Tenon's block, whilst sharp needle local anaesthesia (peribulbar and retrobulbar) should be always avoided as recommended by the Royal College of Ophthalmologists [8] to help significantly reduce the risk of bleeding related vision-threatening complications of sharp needle anaesthesia. Anticoagulants are usually restarted the same day as normal if surgery has been uneventful.

Periocular Disease

All patients undergoing cataract surgery must have a full eye examination including the adnexa. For example, an ectropion/entropion can increase the risk of endophthalmitis post-operatively. Severe blepharitis and acne rosacea can also increase the risk of endophthalmitis. Such conditions need to be treated prior to cataract surgery. Furthermore, the ocular surface and the tear film must be evaluated. Any adnexal and ocular surface problems must be addressed prior to surgery. An oculoplastic referral will be needed promptly to correct ectropion/entropion [8].

Orthoptic Challenges/Orthoptic Imbalance

Motility and binocularity examination are essential parts of a cataract assessment. Being aware of ocular motility problems will enable the surgeon to better counsel the patient. A good history must include previous strabismus of any type and particularly patients with cranial nerve palsies, and thyroid eye disease. Cataract surgery can be used also to treat patients with intractable diplopia, photophobia or other complex neurological symptoms where an opaque IOL can be used as last resort to eliminate the troublesome symptoms (placement in the sulcus will facilitate removal if circumstances change) (Fig. 1) [9, 10]. Liu et al. described a black-on-clear piggyback technique of implanting both a black occlusive device

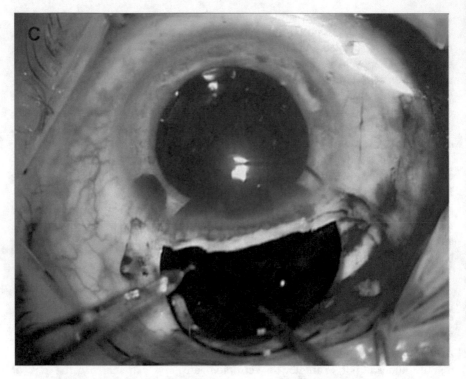

Fig. 1 Custom-made black implant of 10 mm "optic" diameter being inserted into the eye. Credit Christopher Liu

and a clear polymethyl methacrylate IOL in the capsular bag to allow safer and easier explantation of the black occlusive device should the need arise at a later date, avoiding the need for IOL exchange [11].

Patients with pre-existing ocular motility issues that put them at risk of post-operative diplopia should be counselled properly and this risk amply explained, discussed and documented. If there is any history of double vision a formal pre-operative orthoptic assessment would be required.

Surgeons must be aware that local anaesthetic injection can also cause extraocular muscle damage and induce diplopia after cataract surgery. To reduce the risk of post local anaesthetic diplopia, topical anaesthesia should be the default choice [12].

Management of post cataract surgery diplopia requires orthoptic and strabismic assessment in most cases. Temporary extraocular muscles paresis causing diplopia can be treated with prismatic correction. Orthoptic exercises can also be offered to patients with convergence insufficiency or temporary fusion disruption [12].

Challenging Situations in Cataract Surgery

Patients with Difficult Positioning and Back Problems

Adequate positioning of the patient is of paramount importance for patient and surgeon comfort and to ensure surgical safety by reducing the risk of operative complications. Positioning may be difficult to achieve in patients with ankylosing spondylitis, and patients with severe forms of kyphosis and or scoliosis. An adequate past medical history is required to reveal the potential difficulties for the patient to allow proper steps to be taken prior to the operation. Surgical positioning should be tested prior to planned surgery in severe cases. Most patients with physical disability can be operated on with little disruption to them or to the normal surgical regimen. Positioning of patients with spinal mobility restriction is facilitated if surgical trolleys specifically adapted for ophthalmic surgery are used. Position adjustment adds to theatre time (both perioperative and actual surgical) so allocation of extra time is important to avoid unexpected delay of the flow of the operating theatre.

Positioning options for challenging cases include:
For patients who have bent spine/neck, otherwise well consider using Trendelenburg position; Patients can be positioned in a chair which is then tipped backward, so that the patient's feet are above their head. It only works for patients who can tolerate this position therefore it is not suitable for older patients who may have coexisting orthopnoea. This position may increase the vitreous pressure during cataract surgery because the head is lower than the rest of the body.

    For patients who cannot lie flat but have flexible neck, the patient can be seated upright and the surgeon standing. This position helps in patients with orthopnoea (e.g. heart failure or severe COPD) who have a flexible spine so they can extend their neck. The headrest is adjusted so that the patient can extend the neck and look up to the overhead microscope.

    For patients who cannot lie flat and cannot extend their neck, consider face-to-face upright seated position. The patient sits upright and comfortable on the surgical chair. The microscope is rotated forwards to face the eye, and the surgeon sits (or stands) facing the patient. Cataract surgery is done through an incision in the lower half of the cornea: right-handed surgeons may find it easier to use a temporal incision (0 degrees) for a left eye and inferior incision (270 degrees) for a right eye. Because the eye is higher above the floor than normal, the infusion bottle height should be raised accordingly. It's worth spending time to ensure that patient and surgeon should remain comfortable for what may be a longer operation [13, 14].

Patients with Severe Anxiety and Special Needs (E.g. Learning Difficulties, Cognitive Impairment)

Preparation for this category of patients should start from the pre-assessment visit. The cataract team should identify those who will find it difficult to cope with the surgical theatre setting as this can exaggerate their responses and cause undue fear. If general anaesthesia (GA) is preferred, one may also consider immediately sequential bilateral cataract surgery to save the patient having a GA twice.

Claustrophobia and severe anxiety can affect the patient's ability to keep still and co-operate during surgery. These patients need special counselling as well as anaesthetic review to consider the best anaesthetic approach such as the type of local anaesthesia that must include sedation to allow relaxation during surgery. Appropriate draping (trial of draping at assessment, transparent drape, cutting a hole over the patient's nose and mouth) are possible further measures.

Some patients may not have the capacity to give consent; one should consider thorough assessment of capacity and presume adequate capacity unless otherwise proven. Depending on the country/institution using the correct type of procedure and consent form is vital if a patient is deemed to have no capacity. Involving other professionals if communication is difficult with the patient (for example interpreter to prevent language barriers and support workers for patients with special needs) and encouraging the patients to express themselves is important to deal with these issues. This all takes time and organisation.

Enophthalmos, Deep Set Eyes and Highbrow

It is vital to recognise challenging socket anatomy preoperatively and how to plan cataract surgery so that variations of orbital anatomy do not become an impediment. Causes of abnormal orbital anatomy that can make surgery difficult are age and prostaglandin analogue which can cause deep-set eyes secondary to orbital fat atrophy [15, 16]. Previous orbital trauma, developmental craniofacial abnormalities like sagittal synostosis or highbrow can cause structural enophthalmos. Other causes include silent sinus syndrome, sphenoid wing dysplasia in neurofibromatosis and Paget disease of bone.

Cataract surgery in the presence of abnormal orbital dimension and very deep-set eyes is challenging especially for a beginning surgeon. Deep set eyes and enophthalmos cause pooling of fluid, which makes visualisation difficult. Furthermore, access of the instruments through the superior limbus is more difficult.

Using the temporal approach is always advised, proper head positioning (slight face turn towards the temporal side) and a draining speculum to avoid pooling of fluid can also be helpful. Extension of the neck is also advised for improved access if positioning allows [17]. In addition, a sub-Tenon's anaesthetic can help push the eye forwards. Vertical recti bridle sutures can be needed in extreme enophthalmos cases to pull the eyeball upwards and improve surgical access.

Head Tremor

Head tremor if present will require special planning. Head tremor is most common in patients with Parkinson's disease, heart problems or can be idiopathic. Patients with involuntary limb movements especially leg movements can also have those movements transmitted to the head. Theatre staff as well as the anaesthetist, if present, should be briefed at the commencement of the operating list. Pre-operatively the extent of head tremor needs to be evaluated and the operating surgeon needs to decide if surgery under local anaesthesia is possible based on his/her expertise/experience. Good head support is important to reduce the tremor. In cases with significant tremor that can make surgery difficult, general anaesthesia should be considered. It is imperative to explain the extra surgical risks due to significant head tremor at the counselling stage and these should be reflected in the consenting process.

Dense (Brunescent) Cataract

One of the challenges during cataract surgery arises when the cataract is very dense, so patients should be counselled on the higher risks of surgery in such cases. This adds to the difficulty of most of the steps starting from the continuous curvilinear capsulorrhexis (CCC). Visualisation can be difficult in brunescent cataract surgery and hence trypan blue assisted CCC can be useful to improve visualisation. Emulsification of dense cataract requires more ultrasound energy and time, which can lead to prolonged postoperative corneal oedema and may permanently damage corneal endothelial cells. Corneal wound burn with its sequelae of increased postoperative astigmatism and even inability to close the wound although rare is more common in brunescent cataract surgery. Likewise, the risks of posterior capsular rupture and vitreous loss are higher in such cases.

We consider using soft shell technique to protect the corneal endothelium, avoid very tight wounds to prevent wound burn and adjust phacoemulsification parameters i.e. avoid continuous phaco and preferably use torsional phaco with or without simultaneous longitudinal phaco and bevel down phaco to achieve the maximum ultrasound power concentration on the hard lens [18].

Although less likely with modern phaco machine technology, potential conversion to extracapsular cataract extraction (ECCE) has to be considered whilst operating on a brunescent/black cataract.

In summary the steps to minimise risks in brunescent cataract surgery aim to perfect the cataract surgical steps with special attention to:

CCC visualisation and size → Using vision blue to see better and aiming for a large CCC size to prevent CCC tears when removing large lens fragments.

High power phacoemulsification settings to deal with the excessive cataract density → torsional, longitudinal power simultaneously as well as bevel down phaco and making sure the phaco metal tip is well exposed.

Nucleofractis → deep and central nucleus grooving is a must to enable lens cracking which can be difficult due to the leathery brunescent lens density.

Chopping techniques; either horizontal or vertical chopping can be useful in brunescent cataract.

White (Mature Cortical) Cataract (Fig. 2)

Pre-operative examination is important to differentiate between white cataract (without high intra-lenticular pressure) and white intumescent cataract (with high intra-lenticular pressure) since the surgical approach will differ. In any case visualisation can be helped by using vision blue assisted CCC.

If the lens is intumescent, the intra-lenticular pressure will be high and opening the anterior capsule can cause a rapid extension of the opening with anterior capsular tear that can extend beyond the equator causing the dreaded Argentinian flag sign. To prevent that, tamponade with heavy ophthalmic viscosurgical device (OVD) like Healon GV® or similar during the CCC is useful. The authors use vision blue with heavy OVD and a capsulotomy needle to make a small incision of the anterior capsule, then suck with a lacrimal cannula the plume of milky lens matter inside the capsular bag (the lacrimal cannula is inserted inside the capsular

Fig. 2 Showing white cataract. (Photo credit professor Christopher Liu)

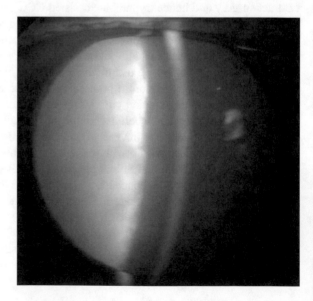

opening by 1 mm) and release the intra-lenticular pressure to enable safe CCC completion. Forceps are preferred in these cases due to the shearing force achieved that can bring the CCC back in if there is tendency to extend outwards.

In case of anterior capsular tear, intraocular micro scissors such as Ong capsular micro scissors or vitreoretinal micro scissors can be used to change the linear capsular opening into a more curvilinear one. A dispersive OVD is recommended to express the nucleus into the anterior chamber. It is advised to reduce the irrigation and pressure of the phaco machine and commence cautious aspiration of the nucleus. If the tear is noticed to extend to the posterior lens capsule, follow the steps of managing posterior capsule rupture discussed later in section "Management of Vitreous Loss" of this chapter.

Cataract in Presence of Corneal Pathology

Corneal assessment in patients is important prior to cataract surgery. Careful slit lamp examination is key in determining the expected intraoperative visualisation during surgery and different techniques that may need to be adopted to improve visualisation. Using the diffuse filter during the slit-lamp examination will enable surgeons to appreciate and estimate a more similar view of the operating microscope. This is vital because, abnormal cornea geometry, scars and neovascularisation make intraoperative view worse compared to what is seen through a slit lamp view. In situations where the view is extremely poor, it may be better to opt for other techniques such as Small Incision Cataract Surgery (SICS) or ECCE or else use assisted visualisation with retinal pipe light.

For the purposes of assessing risk versus benefit, prognosis and obtaining consent, coexisting corneal opacity and cataract need careful attention. One must identify which is the main cause of reduced vision, and whether it is possible to do cataract surgery with poor view.

- **Corneal Opacity**

If a corneal scar is longstanding, discrete, and has not changed recently, and it is the cataract which has become visually significant, then cataract surgery should restore vision. The reverse is also true, and the surgeon can perform corneal surgery and reserve the cataract for later refractive including astigmatic correction. Remember the time after penetrating keratoplasty (PKP) or deep anterior lamellar keratoplasty (DALK) it takes to achieve refractive stability though and the risk of endothelial cell loss with cataract surgery.

Various techniques can be used to improve visualisation through opaque corneas during surgery. It is important to obtain favourable contrast in the surgical field by adjusting the illumination [19]. Red reflex can be increased by switching off the paraxial peripheral light while increasing the central coaxial light. Moving the eye around to look through clear cornea to do surgery, the use of capsular stain, increased magnification, and dimming room lights all help. Using 2% hydroxypropyl methycellulose (HPMC)-OcuCoat®, Bausch and Lomb) to coat the cornea can also help improve visualisation. Consider using glycerol to achieve deturgescence of the cornea in cases of corneal oedema and removing the epithelium if there is epithelial oedema. Chandelier endo-illumination system can be used at the limbus or in the anterior chamber to improve visualisation in poor view cases [19].

While doing capsulorrhexis, avoid the area under the corneal opacity and look for a transparent window to initiate continuous curvilinear capsulorrhexis, then perform "continuous" capsulorrhexis with a constant tethered force under the opaque area. Non-continuous capsulorrhexis is likely to cause radial tearing and intraoperative complications are hard to manage in eyes with poor corneal clarity. Therefore, patients must be aware of alternative surgical options and second procedures during preoperative consultation. Ocular surface diseases such as mucous membrane pemphigoid (MMP) and viral keratitis can be exacerbated by uneventful cataract surgery and limit surgical outcomes. Prophylactic oral antiviral regimes are recommended in cases of corneal opacities due to Herpes simplex keratitis. In cases of MMP, cataract surgery is not supposed to cause flare up of the condition if a clear corneal incision is used [20].

- **Peripheral Ulcerative keratitis (PUK) and Mooren's ulcer (MU) Fig.** 3

Cataract surgery should be planned after achieving corneal quiescence. Immunosuppression is key to control corneal inflammation and melting. Topical, oral or intravenous immunosuppression can be used as per a stepladder approach [21, 22]. Keratoconjunctivitis sicca is common in PUK and MU and needs addressing before cataract surgery [23] Biometry can be difficult due to the corneal disease. Preoperative cataract counselling should aim to explain the generic and specific risks of the cataract procedure and the sight improvement that can be achieved.

Fig. 3 Mooren's ulcer.
(Photo credit Mr. Vincenzo
Maurino)

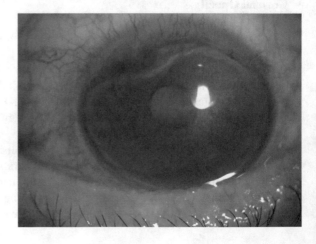

To improve visualization, the surgeon should follow the steps mentioned above (See corneal opacity section above). Phacoemulsification surgical incisions in patients with PUK and MU are another challenge due to a very thin and abnormal cornea in the affected areas which must be avoided. Incisions in thin abnormal cornea are difficult to seal and can cause post-operative complications such as wound leak. Thinning, vascularization and stromal opacities can extend for one quadrant or more. MU usually affects 6–7 clock hours [24] with inferior and nasal quadrants more often involved. Clear cornea incisions for phacoemulsification can be placed in the healthy cornea while areas of previous ulceration or thinning should be avoided and, in those cases, incisions must be into sclera (under a conjunctival flap if necessary). When planning scleral incisions, it is important to remember that scleral involvement is rare in MU but frequent in PUK specially when associated to systemic vasculitis and Wegener's granulomatosis [25]. Having clear preoperative drawings of cornea/scleral involvement will help in planning the incisions.

For post-operative treatment, preservative free (PF) drops are preferred. An intense regime of preservative free steroid drops to taper down slowly is recommended. Additional immunosuppression to avoid corneal disease relapse triggered by the cataract surgery might be needed [24].

- **Corneal endothelial disease (Fuchs' endothelial corneal dystrophy)**

Any corneal endothelial condition, including Fuchs' endothelial dystrophy (FED), can impair visualisation during cataract surgery. The use of dispersive OVD to coat the corneal surface together with the aforementioned techniques can help with the visualisation. It can also be used to coat and protect the endothelium during the cataract procedure.

Limbal incision can help reduce endothelial cell loss, being further away from the central cornea. To avoid damage to the endothelial cells, fluidics should be controlled, and the surgeon should be careful to avoid fluid currents that move lens particles within the eye which by hitting the endothelium can cause mechanical trauma to the corneal endothelial cells.

Pre-operative assessment will involve decision making in terms of corneal endothelial keratoplasty and if it can be deferred or needs to be performed at the time of the cataract surgery. If corneal endothelial transplant is expected in the future, it is good practice implanting hydrophobic IOLs to reduce the possibility of IOL opacification after endothelial keratoplasty with air/gas injection. If the endothelial cell density (ECD) is <600/mm^2, central corneal thickness (CCT) is >640 microns, or if there is significant diurnal visual variation (morning blur on awakening), or dense central pigmented endothelial guttata, a combined cataract extraction and Descemet's membrane endothelial keratoplasty should be considered.

Prolonged post-operative corneal oedema and pseudophakic bullous keratopathy can occur more commonly in pre-existent cornea guttata/ FED and adequate pre-operative counselling as always is important. If corneal oedema after cataract surgery persists for over 3 months, endothelial keratoplasty is recommended.

- **Prior Penetrating Keratoplasty (PKP)**

Prior PKP increases the risk of complications during cataract surgery as well as long-term effects on the survival of the corneal graft. Some key areas of difficulty for these patients to consider are pre-operative astigmatism, visualisation, fragility of the graft-host interface, damage to endothelium, damage to suture (if still present, especially a single running suture), as well as inducing graft rejection. Ideally these cases should be allocated to an experienced surgeon or a cornea consultant.

Visualization can be severely compromised, and the epithelium can slough. The frequent use of topical balanced salt solution (BSS) and or the use of small amount of dispersive OVD such as Viscoat (Alcon) with some BSS can help. Anaesthetic drops like Tetracaine should be avoided as it can compromise the cornea. Trypan blue should be used to stain the anterior capsule as capsulorrhexis edges can be lost, particularly if the tear is anywhere near the graft-host junction or hidden by peripheral corneal pathology.

During cataract surgery, the endothelium can be affected by ultrasound power. The corneal graft can fail readily, with even a small amount of marginal endothelial cell loss. The management is similar to that of cataract surgery in patients with FED. Therefore, inject and regularly reinject dispersive OVD to the corneal dome. This is important to prevent endothelial loss. Additionally, it is essential to minimize the ultrasound time during nucleus removal. Lowering the bottle height during the procedure will reduce the intraocular pressure (IOP) and reduce stress on the graft host junction. Removal of cataract should be at an earlier stage rather than leaving it until the cataract becomes harder.

To prevent corneal rejection, steroids eyedrops frequency and concentration may be increased a few weeks prior to cataract surgery and may need to be maintained for a longer period.

Graft related astigmatism and refractive error are other issues to be considered. Cataract surgery can be considered after full suture removal and achieving refractive stability [26]. Toric IOL can be used to correct residual astigmatism when the corneal astigmatism is not irregular.

- **Previous Kerato-Refractive Surgery**

Previous refractive surgery is one of the major risk factors for poor refractive outcomes after cataract surgery. There are two types of corneal refractive surgery; laser vision correction (LVC) and radial keratotomy (RK). LVC procedures includes laser-assisted in situ keratomileusis (LASIK), photorefractive keratectomy (PRK), small incision lenticular extraction (SMILE) and laser subepithelial keratomileusis (LASEK). These procedures involve changes to the anterior surface of the cornea mainly. Radial keratotomy (RK) on the other hand, involves flattening of the anterior and posterior surface of the central cornea.

A standard keratometry measures only the anterior corneal curvature, (the posterior curvature is extrapolated based on the normal anterior/posterior curvature ratio). Since the anterior surface has been changed during refractive surgery, the extrapolation is no longer valid [27]. Therefore, cataract surgery on a patient who has previously undergone refractive surgery can be challenging in terms of achieving the desired refractive outcome and patients should be counselled about the higher refractive unpredictability. Even in eyes without previous refractive surgery there is a 20–25% of cases which can suffer from a prediction error in refraction higher than 0.5 dioptres (D) [28]. Other sources of error include incorrect estimation of effective lens position (ELP), difficulty with measuring K, and alterations in refractive index. It is essential to counsel patients about these methods and request them to bring in the pre-refractive surgery notes so that all the relevant data is available for the special calculations [28].

One of the Following Formulae Can Be Used:

Haigis-L Formula; This formula is part of the built-in software of the IOLMaster. It is based on LASIK data and only suitable for post-LVC cases, not post-RK cases.

The newer formulae including the Barrett True-K and OCT-based IOL power calculation (OCT formulae) have been included in the American Society of Cataract and Refractive Surgery (ASCRS) calculator in eyes with previous myopic LASIK/ PRK after showing promising results [29].

Barrett True-K formula; A study involving 88 eyes concluded that this formula was either equal to or better than alternative methods available on the ASCRS online calculator for predicting IOL power in eyes with previous myopic LASIK or photorefractive keratectomy [30].

For post RK patients the Barrett true K and Haigis formulae both perform well [28].

The surgeon is faced with many options for IOL calculation and usually the median/ average IOL or combinations of these are used, especially the more myopic target is recommended to prevent hyperopic shift.

Despite all the choices of formulae and several methods of computing the average of recommended lens, the predictability of refractive outcome of cataract surgery after previous refractive surgery is still not as good as the results obtained from a virgin eye. The patients who have undergone previous refractive surgery should be warned about the potential need for refractive correction after their cataract surgery.

- **Abnormal Corneal Thinning**

Areas of abnormally thin cornea and sclera should be identified and drawn correctly as adjustments may need to be made for intraoperative incisions and planning to these damaged areas. This will help to reduce the risk of wound leakage, risk of infection and flat anterior chamber post-operatively. The normal central corneal thickness ranges between 503–565 μm [31].

It is vital to look out for pathology causing thinning of the cornea—these include a range of conditions such as keratoconus (KC), Ehlers–Danlos syndrome

(EDS) (types I, II, and VI), osteogenesis imperfecta, Marfan syndrome and brittle cornea syndrome (BCS). The latter is an autosomal recessive disease and is characterised by the presence of extreme, limbus-to-limbus corneal thinning and structurally abnormal corneal biomechanics causing corneal rupture after minor/trivial trauma during childhood. Clinically characterised by blue sclera and high myopia. Extraocular features may be seen like deafness, joint hypermobility, congenital hip dysplasia, juvenile hypotonia and soft, doughy skin [31].

Such cases need to be counselled regarding the high risk of corneal perforation during cataract surgery and surgical approach should not be considered until the sight is so badly affected that there are no other options. During surgery, the IOP should be controlled below 20 mmHg with the Alcon centurion phacoemulsification system to avoid spontaneous extension of corneal incisions. Glue, 11-0 nylon, and bandage contact lens should be available in theatre in case of wound enlargement or rupture. Fluorescein 2% should be used to check for any wound leak. Since wound sutures are challenging in the abnormal cornea, cyanoacrylate glue and bandage contact lens or even corneal tissue should be available [31].

Glaucoma

Lens extraction is an important intervention in the armamentarium of management of angle closure glaucoma as proven by the EAGLE study [32]. Cataract surgery in angle closure disease poses unique difficulties due to the shallowness of the anterior chamber, possible presence of laser peripheral iridotomy and zonular weakness. The use of capsular hooks/pupil devices and or capsule tension rings should be considered in cases of zonulopathy. Due to the increased risk of iris trauma and iris prolapse in patients with shallow anterior chamber angle, proper wound construction is particularly important and the use of intracameral phenylephrine may also help.

Those patients with axial length below 19 mm carry higher risk of suprachoroidal and expulsive haemorrhage and use of intraoperative Acetazolamide/Mannitol has been recommended. Prophylactic sclerostomy is no longer recommended.

Counselling as always is key and should include the surgery aims: improve vision if cataract and/or reduce risk of glaucoma sight loss if no cataract but surgery performed mainly to avoid acute or chronic angle closure attacks and therefore cure the glaucoma. Counselling must include the extra risks typical of small eyes.

Patients with open angle glaucoma especially those who had previous filtering surgery are another challenge. Making sure the IOP does not go too high during the procedure is vital as this can cause damage to their vulnerable optic nerve or cause a thin walled bleb to burst. A clear temporal corneal wound is advocated, well away from the filtration bleb. Dispersive OVD is preferable to cohesive, and all OVD should be removed even more carefully than usual with attention to behind the IOL, reducing the risk of postoperative pressure spikes. Topical anaesthesia when possible would be preferable to sub-Tenon's or peribulbar anaesthesia, to avoid high intra-orbital pressure which can cause irreversible sight loss by choking an already damaged optic nerve head. It is important to ensure the IOP does not rise in the immediate post-operative period by giving prophylactic IOP lowering medications for the first few days after the operation. Post-operative follow up visits should be planned more frequently to allow for IOP evaluation.

Increasing filtration through the bleb during the cataract procedure and the possibility of post-operative hypotony may occur. Furthermore, in cases where there is an existing filtering bleb, its function can be reduced by fibrosis and healing. To prevent this, consider temporal clear corneal incision to avoid the bleb area. We also advocate more prolonged use of post-operative topical steroid eye drops and also intraoperative bleb injection of 5 FU and Avastin can be used to prevent bleb scarring caused by the cataract surgery induced inflammation.

Extremes of Axial Length

A. High Myopia

In highly myopic eyes IOL power calculations may be less reliable although with modern fourth generation formula refractive outcomes are ever improving. The use of the recommended IOL formulae for each axial length can help reduce the possibility of an error (Barrett true K is a new formula which is good for all and has substituted the need for different formulae). The use of ultrasound B scan should be considered to exclude the presence of posterior staphyloma. Optical biometry ensures foveal fixation even if it lies within a staphyloma.

Highly myopic eyes are more prone to peripheral retinal tears, holes and lattice degeneration and have a higher risk of retinal detachment after cataract surgery than normal axial length eyes especially in the younger population; screening for any such lesions is important and counselling the patients about symptoms of possible retinal detachment postoperatively can help.

Anterior chamber depth fluctuation during the cataract procedure is also common in high myopic eyes; adjusting the infusion pressure (bottle height) can help. Avoidance of AC fluctuations and trampolining of iris lens diaphragm may theoretically help reduce the risk of forcible posterior vitreous detachment and subsequent retinal tear. A single iris hook, or tenting of the iris with a second instrument, will break the reverse pupil block by equalizing the pressure between anterior and posterior chambers when the irrigation enters the eye. With that in place, it no longer causes severe deepening of the anterior chamber.

B. High Hyperopia

Please see section "Glaucoma". Difficulty calculating IOL power can cause postoperative refractive surprises, which can be reduced by using the most advanced 4th generation biometry formula.

Prior Pars Plana Vitrectomy

Cataract formation occurs in 80% of eyes after pars plana vitrectomy. Usually after vitrectomy procedure patient will need cataract surgery within 2 years [33]. Problems encountered during post vitrectomy cataract surgery such as capsular instability, possible previous posterior capsule damage and fluctuating anterior chamber depth make cataract surgery more challenging. Anterior chamber depth fluctuation can be managed the same way as in highly myopic eyes using techniques to break reverse pupil block. It is very important to take care during phacoemulsification as a posterior capsular tear can easily occur. Keeping the phacoemulsification probe above the lens segment and always keeping the tip, bevel up, in view is important. Removing the second instrument while aspirating the final nuclear quadrant may reduce leak and stabilise the anterior chamber depth.

Intraoperative miosis is often encountered and can be managed with intracameral phenylephrine, iris hooks, or pupil expanders (please see section "Small Pupil" for management). A weakened lens capsule and zonules can also be common (see section "Zonulopathy" for management). Increased nuclear sclerosis and lens hardness may also be encountered (see section "Dense (Brunescent) Cataract" for management). Presence of posterior capsular plaques is a common finding so primary posterior CCC or early postoperative YAG laser capsulotomy need to be considered [34].

Reported post-cataract re-detachment rates can be up to approximately 6%, therefore patients need to be informed about the increased risk during consenting [5].

Patients Who May Require Subsequent Vitreo-Retinal Surgery

Patients who may require vitreo-retinal surgery after cataract surgery should be identified, as adequate counselling and intraoperative precautions are necessary. For example, patients with advanced diabetic eye disease, who do not yet need vitrectomy at the time of cataract surgery but may need it later.

The use of Acrylic rather than silicone IOLs is recommended as the use of silicone IOLs will limit the visibility if silicone oil will be used for vitreo-retinal surgery. A wide CCC is recommended and the use of large diameter IOL optic >6 mm when possible is advised for better visualization to enable surgical access to the peripheral vitreous and retina if necessary, later.

Patients Who Have or at Risk of Developing Age-Related Macular Degeneration (AMD)

This group of patients carry specific problems related to the nature of their macular disease. Since for most the visual prognosis would be guarded, managing the patient expectation and the implementation of proper counselling and informed consent are essential. Inadequate preoperative counselling can cause misunderstanding and potential dissatisfaction of the patients after cataract surgery.

Pre-operative macular OCT is a must in these patients to classify the condition, identify the prognosis and manage the wet type of AMD with anti-VEGF injections when needed.

Multifocal IOLs are generally contraindicated in AMD as they decrease contrast sensitivity, can increase the risk of dysphotopsia and reduce optical quality. Multifocal IOL are best used in patients with otherwise healthy eyes and not in the presence of macular pathology.

Small Pupil

Causes of small pupil are summarised in Table 1. Small pupil (<6 mm) should be identified prior to cataract surgery as it can reduce surgeon's view, causing increased difficulty in manoeuvring within the capsular bag. Subsequently this can lead to posterior capsular rupture, higher risk of extended post-operative inflammation, iris damage, CMO and retinal detachment (please see chapter "Risk Stratification"). Furthermore, an adequate pupil size is required for a decent sized capsulorrhexis because an inadequate diameter of anterior capsulorrhexis increases the risk of retention of OVD and capsular distension syndrome. It also raises risks of capsular fibrosis and phimosis.

To prevent these, an experienced surgeon may use several techniques to improve intraoperative view. Preoperative Mydriasert® and phenylephrine (2.5% or 10%) can help dilate the pupil to an optimal size. Intracameral phenylephrine 1.5% or Mydrane® can also be used.

Intraoperative techniques to dilate the pupil include; viscodilatation by injecting OVD at the pupillary plane. Another technique involves bimanual stretch with iris repositors. It is vital to augment anaesthesia using topical, intracameral or sub-Tenon's method as iris manoeuvres can cause pain. Other methods include creating radial sphincterotomies measuring approximately 0.50 mm, limited to the iris sphincter which is cut at equal intervals around the iris border using 23G Prasad scissors. This snips the pupillary sphincter muscle and causes paralysis. It has now become almost redundant as new devices involving iris rings and pupil

Table 1 Causes of small pupil during cataract surgery

Intraoperative floppy iris pupil syndrome (IFIS)
Diabetic patients
Pseudoexfoliation (PXF)
After long-term miotic treatment for glaucoma
Trauma
Previous eye surgery
Old age
Opioid use

expanders have developed. Generally speaking, avoiding mechanical iris dilatation is preferable as it can tear the sphincter muscle, cause an irregular and non-constricting pupil, and lead to post-operative fibrinous uveitis. Pupil expanders like Malyugin ring and Morcher pupil expander can also be used with ease. Using iris hooks to dilate the pupil is another alternative with an added benefit in cases of zonular weakness due to pseudoexfoliation syndrome (PXF) as the hooks can be used to stabilise the capsular bag (by transferring the hook to the anterior capsulorrhexis rim, provided it is intact) to prevent zonular dehiscence.

Intraoperative floppy iris syndrome (IFIS) is one of the causes of small pupil during cataract surgery in patients using α1-adrenergic antagonist (especially tamsulosin) characterised by iris billowing, iris prolapse, and progressive intraoperative miosis. Wound architecture is of paramount importance in such cases; a longer wound with the internal wound further away from the angle can reduce the risk of iris prolapse. If iris prolapse occurs intraoperatively, the surgeon should follow steps to minimise the difficulty and avoid complications. Initially, direct reposition of the iris and injection of OVD through the port should be avoided as this can exacerbate the prolapse. It is advised to start reducing the pressure in the eye through one of the side ports and encourage the iris to get back in by gentle massage around the wound. If the iris goes back in, consider the above-mentioned methods to reduce the risk of further prolapse. If it does not, continue reducing the pressure by expressing the OVD out through one of the side ports and use an iris repositor to reposition the iris using another port. A new port may need to be created to access the one that has the iris prolapse.

Zonulopathy

Zonular weakness and dehiscence can be caused by PXF syndrome, Marfan syndrome, spherophakia, trauma, iris colobomata, previous angle closure (See Table 2 for the list of causes).

Thorough slit-lamp evaluation is very important in such cases to look for signs of zonular weakness by asking the patient to look side to side to check for zonular fibres damage and abnormal lens mobility (phacodonesis).

Zonular laxity or instability can have significant implications during and after cataract surgery. Vitreous loss, IOL tilt and decentration and late dislocation of IOL can occur. These may need further surgery to rectify. Therefore, ensuring that these issues are dealt with in the correct way is vital. If zonular laxity was noticed during cataract surgery, it is advised to insert a capsular tension ring (CTR) into the capsular bag, which may help reduce the risk of future dislocation (Fig. 4) [35].

Accelerated posterior capsule opacification can occur in these patients. This risk can be reduced by thorough aspiration of the lens epithelial cells. It is also important to consider early YAG capsulotomy before capsule contraction and IOL decentration.

Table 2 Causes of zonulopathy

Ocular causes
Pseudoexfoliation syndrome
Traumatic zonulysis
Iatrogenic zonulysis (previous eye surgery)
Brunescent cataracts
Retinitis pigmentosa
Aniridia
Axenfeld Rieger syndrome
Advanced age
Systemic causes
Marfan syndrome
Homocystinuria
Weil-Marchesani syndrome
Ehlers Danlos syndrome
Sulfite oxidase deficiency
Hyperlysinemia
Sturge-Weber syndrome

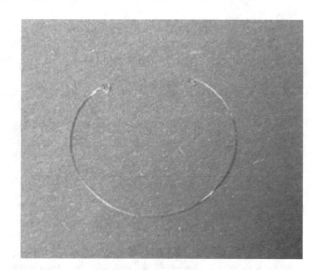

Fig. 4 Showing a capsular tension ring (CTR). *Source* Tribus et al.

Anterior capsular fibrosis and capsular contraction syndrome can result after cataract surgery in PXF due to a combination of a small CCC and contractile forces unopposed by zonular weakness [36, 37]. It is important to create an adequately sized CCC after viscoexpansion or iris hooks insertion and consider insertion of a CTR and using a strong haptic IOL (3-piece IOL) to resist the contraction forces [38].

Uveitis and Pre-existing Posterior Synechiae

Patients who develop cataract after previous episodes of uveitis represent a challenge for any cataract surgeon. The behaviour of the iris, anterior chamber and the lens differs from case to case. Iris adhesions and intraoperative miosis are common amongst this group of patients (please see section "Small Pupil"). The surgeon can also use OVD, pupil stretch techniques to break formed adhesions.

There is higher possibility of iris bleed, for example in patients with known Fuchs uveitis syndrome (so called Amsler-Verrey sign). Visco-tamponade is advised should significant bleeding take place and waiting for a few seconds for the bleeding to stop is essential.

Prolonged postoperative inflammation can occur. To prevent this, the cataract procedure should be planned only after adequate control of the inflammation preoperatively is achieved. Meticulous aspiration of all the lens matter including epi-nucleus and cortex during surgery is key to minimise the risks already higher than normal of post-operative inflammation. A prolonged course of postoperative steroids and non-steroidal anti-inflammatory drugs is usually necessary in those cases.

Other post-operative complications in this group of patients include post-operative CMO and secondary glaucoma, which may require IOP lowering topical medications. Systemic acetazolamide and referral to a glaucoma surgeon may also be necessary.

There is a potential for protein and cellular deposits on the IOL. This can be minimised by using biocompatible substance like Acrylic IOLs rather than silicone IOLs and use of prolonged postoperative steroids course. YAG capsulotomy can help if the deposits are on the posterior capsule and in cases of posterior capsular distension [39].

Posterior Polar Cataract (Fig. 5)

This is one of the big challenges even for an experienced cataract surgeon as there may be a defect in the posterior capsule. It is imperative to identify posterior polar cataract at pre-operative assessment to counsel on the likely need for anterior vitrectomy and the higher surgical risks. These cases will need an experienced cataract surgeon and take longer than standard cataract surgery. Whilst the appearance of posterior polar cataract is typical and almost unique, it is quite difficult to establish if a capsule hole is present or not in the majority of cases. White dots in the anterior vitreous that move with the degenerated vitreous like a fish tail is sometimes obvious, and it confirms a posterior capsule defect.

Pre-operative Anterior segment OCT and ultrasound biomicroscopy (UBM) imaging can be very useful to identify cases of posterior polar cataract with higher risk of posterior capsule tear allowing better surgical planning and pre-operative

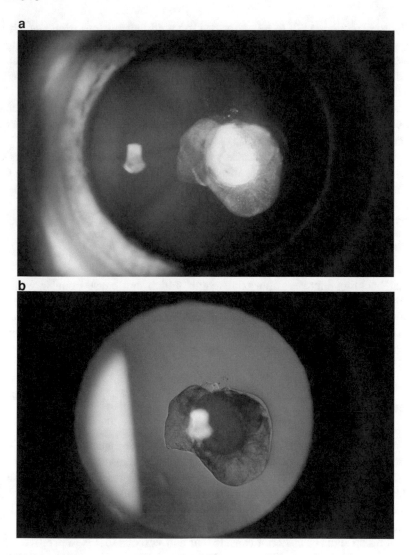

Fig. 5 Posterior polar cataract. (Photo credit Mr. Vincenzo Maurino)

counselling [40, 41]. If in doubt it is always better to treat any suspected polar cataract as such and perform surgery accordingly.

The main steps to modify are:

CCC needs great care and precision. It must be well centred and not smaller than 4.5 mm, not larger than 5.5 to allow IOL optic capture if needed.

Hydrodissection is not to be performed to avoid lens/nucleus drop since it will open up the pre-existing capsular posterior hole at an early stage of the surgery. Hydrodelineation must be achieved instead to allow first removal of the nucleus and then dealing with epi-nucleus and cortex afterwards and separately to eliminate the chances of nucleus drop.

The use of low fluidics and avoiding sudden shallowing of the anterior chamber, especially at the end of the procedure can help minimise vitreous forward movement that can lead to extension of a posterior capsular (PC) tear.

It is important to prepare theatre staff for management of vitreous loss and choose the appropriate IOL e.g. sulcus versus IOL optic capture within the CCC (For more details see section "Management of Vitreous Loss" of this chapter).

Prior Scleral Buckling Surgery

Scleral buckling increases the axial length which can cause zonular weakness and increases risk of lens subluxation. Scleral buckle surgery can also cause conjunctival scarring, and it increases the risk of scleral perforation with injection of sub-Tenon's anaesthetic. Re-detachment rates after post scleral buckle cataract surgery are low unlike post pars plana vitrectomy [42].

Management of Vitreous Loss

Vitreous loss can occur through a tear in the posterior capsule or through weak dehisced zonules. Posterior capsular tear can occur as a result of extension of anterior capsular tear. There are some preoperative characteristics that increase the likelihood of having a posterior capsule tear such as posterior polar cataract and pre-existing posterior capsule damage after intravitreal anti VEGF injections. (See the chapter "Risk Stratification" for more details).

Picking up signs of posterior capsule tear and vitreous loss is imperative. These include deepening of the anterior chamber, pupil widening, lens nucleus no longer centred, particles no longer coming to phaco or irrigation/ aspiration (I/A) probes, and the lens no longer rotating freely.

If phacoemulsification is still in progress, this should stop, and the probe carefully withdrawn from the anterior chamber in a way that minimises traction on the vitreous. OVD may be injected into the anterior chamber at this stage to reduce vitreous prolapse as the phacoemulsification probe is withdrawn and to stabilise any remaining lens fragments. It is most important that the surgeon should then pause for assessment of the state of affairs. While an assessment of the situation takes place, time can be gainfully used for setting up the equipment for vitrectomy and adding a sub-Tenon's anaesthetic, if needed (see Table 3).

Table 3 Tips and pearls for anterior vitrectomy during cataract surgery

Place the dispersive OVD in the area of PC tear prior to removing any instruments
Irrigation cannula should be inserted through a separate paracentesis
Consider suturing the original wound to keep the anterior chamber formed if the AC is unstable due to leaking port (e.g. phaco wound burn)
Settings: For anterior vitrectomy, use low vacuum 150 mmHg range, as high as possible cutting rate (newer machines have high cut rates up to 5000 c/min)
Try to aspirate the residual cortical material using the vacuum on, cutter off setting
Whenever possible, try to convert a PC tear into a posterior CCC to avoid its extension and losing the capsular bag
Place intraocular lens in sulcus if possible (adjust power)
Miochol should be administered to constrict the pupil

The aims of vitreous loss management are removal of any vitreous strands from the anterior chamber and surgical wound, completion of cataract removal, and safe intraocular lens implantation [43]. Management plan depends on size, location of the tear and stage of the procedure.

A small rupture of the posterior capsule during the stage of nuclear emulsification can be managed as follows;

After pushing the vitreous backwards with OVD, use low-flow, low-vacuum settings to remove the remaining nuclear and cortical fragments. Reducing the risk of vitreous aspiration and further damage to the capsule can be achieved by maintaining full occlusion of the phaco probe and minimal phaco power.

A large capsular tear in the early part of nuclear removal when most of the nucleus remains, further attempts at phacoemulsification can lead to nucleus drop in the vitreous cavity and the preferred approach is to enlarge the incision and convert to mechanical removal of the nucleus with a loop. OVD injection behind the nucleus to lift it upwards can help with its delivery. If nuclear fragments are dislocated posteriorly behind the posterior capsule, aggressive efforts to retrieve these without pars plana vitrectomy can result in giant retinal tears and retinal detachment and must be avoided [43].

A small capsular rent in the late part of surgery during aspiration of the cortex and the vitreous face remains intact, the surgeon should attempt to remove the residual cortex without expanding the tear using low flow I/A to avoid disruption of the vitreous face.

If vitreous prolapse is noticed, it is important to remove all vitreous from the anterior chamber initially as this will facilitate removal of residual lens matter and reduce vitreoretinal traction. While doing anterior vitrectomy, it is important to ensure the vitreous cutter and irrigation device are separated at a distance. The vitreous cutter needs to be placed low (at the level of the posterior capsule) while the irrigating cannula needs to be held high (towards the anterior chamber angle). This prevents hydration of the vitreous by the irrigating fluid (see Table 3).

The general rule of thumb is that the infusion should be low. Just enough to keep the AC formed and not so high that the fluid is forced out as this means that the vitreous can be brought up with it. A high cut rate is advisable; the cutting rate should be set at 600–700 cuts/min (or up to 5000 cuts/min on newer machines), with a vacuum of 150–200 mm Hg. The high cut rate minimizes the risk of retinal traction while the vitreous is cut and removed. The cutter is placed through the tear, pointing toward the optic nerve, with the cutting port positioned behind the posterior capsule to minimize the risk of engaging the capsule during the vitrectomy. Most of the anterior vitreous is drawn backward and efficiently removed [44].

Remaining lens matter after anterior vitrectomy can be removed with the cutter, reducing the cut rate to 300 cuts/min and increasing vacuum to draw the firmer lens material into the cutting port and allowing it to engage sufficiently to permit cutting. The cortex can then be engaged, using the vacuum-only setting of the cutter, and stripped off the capsule. The cortex is freed and drawn into the centre, and the cutting action is activated to remove it [44].

In most cases, there will be adequate capsular support enabling the surgeon to implant an IOL either in the capsular bag or in the sulcus. If the PC tear is small and central and can be converted to a posterior circular capsulorrhexis, then in-the-bag IOL implantation can be done safely. If there is large PC tear but the anterior capsulorrhexis is intact and central, the IOL can be placed in the sulcus. For sulcus placement the overall diameter of the IOL should be at least 13 mm, consider optic capture by the anterior capsulorrhexis for a more stable position. If the anterior capsulorrhexis is split or zonular loss resulting in an eccentric rhexis is suspected, implant the lens into the sulcus with no optic capture.

Vitreous Loss Due to Zonular Dehiscence

Previous eye trauma, pseudo-exfoliation, and Marfan's syndrome are common causes of zonular weakness that can lead to zonular laxity and dehiscence. Consider referring those with severe zonular dehiscence and subluxated lens to vitreoretinal colleagues where a pars plana lensectomy might be safer. If an anterior approach is planned; try to support the capsular bag with a CTR [35], a capsular tension segment (CTS), or capsular hooks after performing CCC [45]. If vitreous loss is suspected, triamcinolone can be used to identify the vitreous strands and area of weak zonules and careful anterior vitrectomy should be performed to clear the vitreous. Dispersive OVD should be placed in the area of weak zonules then place cohesive OVD on top forcing dispersive into area of weak zonules sealing it off. Perform CCC if not already done. Place a CTR with lead eyelet of the ring heading out of inserter toward the area of weak zonules to minimize stress of insertion [44, 46].

IOL insertion in cases of zonular weakness can be challenging. It is always useful to place a 3-piece IOL with haptics towards the weak zonular area to minimise the risks of IOL late displacement. CTR can be used to support the bag if less than 4 clock hours of zonular dehiscence. Sutured CTR (Cionni ring) or capsular tension segment (Ahmed CTS) should be considered if more than 4–5 clock hours of zonular dehiscence are present [44].

Staining with Triamcinolone

The transparency of vitreous makes it difficult to visualise, making the surgeon dependant on indirect clues, such as a peaked pupil or a wick presenting through an incision to guide complete removal. Using triamcinolone to visualize vitreous prolapse into the anterior chamber was described in 2003 by Burk et al. [47]. However, it is to be noted that there have been reports of sterile and infectious endophthalmitis with its use in vitreo-retinal surgery. The recommended measure for using triamcinolone in cataract surgery is to dilute the non-preserved triamcinolone 10:1.

References

1. Montan PG, Koranyi G, Setterquist HE, Stridh A, Philipson BT, Wiklund K. Endophthalmitis after cataract surgery: risk factors relating to technique and events of the operation and patient history: a retrospective case-control study. Ophthalmology. 1998;105(12):2171–7. https://doi.org/10.1016/S0161-6420(98)91211-8.

2. Kumar CM, Seet E, Eke T, Joshi GP. Hypertension and cataract surgery under loco-regional anaesthesia: not to be ignored? Br J Anaesth. 2017;119(5):855–9. https://doi.org/10.1093/bja/aex247.

3. Agarwal PK, Mathew M, Virdi M. Is there an effect of perioperative blood pressure on intraoperative complications during phacoemulsification surgery under local anaesthesia. Eye. 2010;24(7):1186–92. https://doi.org/10.1038/eye.2010.4.

4. Hanada S, Kawakami H, Goto T, Morita S. Hypertension and anesthesia. Curr Opin Anaesthesiol. 2006;19(3):315–9. https://doi.org/10.1097/01.aco.0000192811.56161.23.

5. Kumar CM, Seet E, Eke T, Dhatariya K, Joshi GP. Glycaemic control during cataract surgery under loco-regional anaesthesia: a growing problem and we are none the wiser. Br J Anaesth. 2016;117(6):687–91. https://doi.org/10.1093/bja/aew305.

6. Dubois V, Dincq A-S, Douxfils J, et al. Perioperative management of patients on direct oral anticoagulants. Thromb J. 2017;15(1):14. https://doi.org/10.1186/s12959-017-0137-1.

7. Benzimra JD, Johnston RL, Jaycock P, et al. The cataract national dataset electronic multicentre audit of 55 567 operations: antiplatelet and anticoagulant medications. Eye. 2009;23(1):10–6. https://doi.org/10.1038/sj.eye.6703069.

8. Special considerations in cataract surgery: five cornea challenges—American Academy of Ophthalmology. https://www.aao.org/eyenet/article/special-considerations-in-cataract-surgery-five-co. Accessed November 24, 2019.

9. Lee RMH, Dubois VDJP, Mavrikakis I, et al. Opaque intraocular lens implantation: a case series and lessons learnt. Clin Ophthalmol. 2012;6(1):545–9. https://doi.org/10.2147/OPTH.S27972.

10. Dubois VDIP, Mavrikakis I, Vickers SLC. Black opaque intraocular lens implantation in three patients: diagnoses leukocoria; loss of fusion; and alternating hypotropia with image delay. Ophthalmic Res. 2005;376:52.

11. Byard SD, Lee RMH, Lam FC, Simpson ARH, Liu CSC. Black-on-clear piggyback technique for a black occlusive intraocular device in intractable diplopia. J Cataract Refract Surg. 2012;38(1):5–7. https://doi.org/10.1016/j.jcrs.2011.10.020.

12. Gawwcki M, Grzybowski A. Diplopia as the Complication of Cataract Surgery. 2016. https://doi.org/10.1155/2016/2728712.

13. Lee RMH, Jehle T, Eke T. Face-to-face upright seated positioning for cataract surgery in patients who cannot lie flat. J Cataract Refract Surg. 2011;37(5):805–9. https://doi.org/10.1016/j.jcrs.2011.03.023.

14. Sohail T, Pajaujis M, Crawford SE, Chan JW, Eke T. Face-to-face upright seated positioning for cataract surgery in patients unable to lie flat: case series of 240 consecutive phacoemulsifications. J Cataract Refract Surg. 2018;44(9):1116–22. https://doi.org/10.1016/j.jcrs.2018.06.045.

15. Athanasiov PA, Prabhakaran VC, Selva D. Non-traumatic enophthalmos: a review. Acta Ophthalmol. 2008;86(4):356–64. https://doi.org/10.1111/j.1755-3768.2007.01152.x.

16. Filippopoulos T, Paula JS, Torun N, Hatton MP, Pasquale LR, Grosskreutz CL. Periorbital changes associated with topical bimatoprost. Ophthal Plast Reconstr Surg. 2008;24(4):302–7. https://doi.org/10.1097/IOP.0b013e31817d81df.

17. Martz TG, Karlin J, Prum BE, Karcioglu ZA. Cataract surgery and the deep-set eye. JCRS Online Case Reports. 2018;6:62–4. https://doi.org/10.1016/j.jcro.2018.05.003.

18. Allen D, Benjamin L, Chawla JS, Foss A, Kervick GLC. Top ten tips: phacoemulsification of hard cataracts. Refract Eye News. 2004;3(1):16.

19. Srinivasan S, Kiire C, Lyall D. Chandelier anterior chamber endoillumination-assisted phacoemulsification in eyes with corneal opacities. Clin Experiment Ophthalmol. 2013;41(5):515–7. https://doi.org/10.1111/ceo.12037.

20. Ho YJ, Sun CC, Chen HC. Cataract surgery in patients with corneal opacities. BMC Ophthalmol. 2018;18(1). https://doi.org/10.1186/s12886-018-0765-7.

21. Maurino V, Matarazzo F. Cirugía de catarata en la queratitis ulcerativa periférica y la úlcera de Mooren. In: Silva RV, Moore M-S, editors. Madrid: INDUSTRIA GRÁFICA MAE; 2020:180–3.

22. Ashar JN, Mathur A, Sangwan VS. Immunosuppression for Mooren's ulcer: evaluation of the stepladder approach—topical, oral and intravenous immunosuppressive agents. Br J Ophthalmol. 2013;97(11):1391–4. https://doi.org/10.1136/bjophthalmol-2012-302627.

23. Yagci A. Clinical ophthalmology update on peripheral ulcerative keratitis. Clin Ophthalmol. 2012;6–747. https://doi.org/10.2147/OPTH.S24947

24. Das S, Mohamed A SVJCRS 2017 A-1049. Clinical course and outcomes in patients with Mooren ulcer who had cataract surgery. J Cataract Refract Surg. 48(8):1044–9.

25. Garg PSV. Immunosuppression for Mooren's ulcer: evaluation of the stepladder approach—topical, oral and intravenous immunosuppressive agents. Cornea Fundam Diagnostic, Manag. 2011; (3rd ed. St. Louis, MO: Elsevier).

26. Javadi MA, Feizi S, Moein HR. Simultaneous penetrating keratoplasty and cataract surgery. J Ophthalmic Vis Res. 2013;8(1):39–46.

27. Savini G, Hoffer KJ. Intraocular lens power calculation in eyes with previous corneal refractive surgery. https://doi.org/10.1186/s40662-018-0110-5.

28. Turnbull AMJ, Crawford GJ, Barrett GD. Methods for intraocular lens power calculation in cataract surgery after radial keratotomy. Ophthalmology. 2019. https://doi.org/10.1016/j.ophtha.2019.08.019.

29. Wang L, Tang M, Huang D, Weikert MP, Koch DD. Comparison of newer intraocular lens power calculation methods for eyes after corneal refractive surgery. Ophthalmology. 2015;122(12):2443–9. https://doi.org/10.1016/j.ophtha.2015.08.037.

30. Abulafia A, Hill WE, Koch DD, Wang L, Barrett GD. Accuracy of the Barrett True-K formula for intraocular lens power prediction after laser in situ keratomileusis or photorefractive keratectomy for myopia. J Cataract Refract Surg. 2016;42(3):363–9. https://doi.org/10.1016/j.jcrs.2015.11.039.

31. Maurino V, Matarazzo FAF. Cirugía de catarata en el Síndrome de Córnea Frágil. In: Silva, Moore, Martinez-Soroa, editors. Cataracta & Cornea y Superficie Ocular. Madrid: INDUSTRIA GRÁFICA MAE; 2020:183–5.

32. Azuara-Blanco A, Burr J, Ramsay C, et al. Effectiveness of early lens extraction for the treatment of primary angle-closure glaucoma (EAGLE): a randomised controlled trial. Lancet. 2016;388(10052):1389–97. https://doi.org/10.1016/S0140-6736(16)30956-4.

33. Cole CJ, Charteris DG. Cataract extraction after retinal detachment repair by vitrectomy: visual outcome and complications. Eye. 2009;23(6):1377–81. https://doi.org/10.1038/eye.2008.255.
34. Grusha YO, Masket S, Miller KM. Phacoemulsification and lens implantation after pars plana vitrectomy. Ophthalmology. 1998;105(2):287–94. https://doi.org/10.1016/s0161-6420(98)93133-5.
35. Mavrikakis I, Georgiou T, Syam PP, Eleftheriadis H, Liu C. Capsular tension rings, iris retraction hooks, and intraocular prosthetic iris devices: a review. Eye News. 2003;10(1):7–15.
36. Waheed K, Eleftheriadis H, Liu C. Anterior capsular phimosis in eyes with a capsular tension ring. J Cataract Refract Surg. 2001;27(10):1688–90. https://doi.org/10.1016/S0886-3350(01)00766-0.
37. Dubois VDJP, Ainsworth G, Liu CSC. Unilateral capsular phimosis with an acrylic IOL and two capsular tension rings in pseudoexfoliation. Clin Experiment Ophthalmol. 2009;37(6):631–3. https://doi.org/10.1111/j.1442-9071.2009.02051.x.
38. Liu CS, Eleftheriadis H. Multiple capsular tension rings for the prevention of capsular contraction syndrome. J Cataract Refract Surg. 2001;27(3):342–3. https://doi.org/10.1016/S0886-3350(01)00778-7.
39. Gomaa A, Liu C. Nd:YAG laser capsulotomy: a survey of UK practice and recommendations. Eur J Ophthalmol. 2011;21(4):385–90. https://doi.org/10.5301/EJO.2010.6085.
40. Chan TCY, Li EYM, Yau JCY. Application of anterior segment optical coherence tomography to identify eyes with posterior polar cataract at high risk for posterior capsule rupture. J Cataract Refract Surg. 2014;40(12):2076–81. https://doi.org/10.1016/j.jcrs.2014.03.033.
41. Guo Y, Lu C, Wu B, et al. Application of 25MHz B-scan ultrasonography to determine the integrity of the posterior capsule in posterior polar cataract (2018). https://doi.org/10.1155/2018/9635289.
42. Mehdizadeh M, Afarid M, Haghighi MS. Retinal redetachment after cataract surgery in eyes with previous scleral buckling. J Ophthalmic Vis Res. 2011;6(1):73–5. https://www.ncbi.nlm.nih.gov/pubmed/22454712. Accessed November 26, 2019.
43. Jacobs PM. Vitreous loss during cataract surgery: prevention and optimal management. Eye. 2008;22:1286–9. https://doi.org/10.1038/eye.2008.22.
44. Oetting TA. Cataract Surgery for Greenhorns (2012). https://webeye.ophth.uiowa.edu/eyeforum/tutorials/instruments/Phacoemulsification/index.htm. Accessed November 26, 2019.
45. Osher RH. Slow motion phacoemulsification approach. J Cataract Refract Surg. 1993;19(5):667. https://doi.org/10.1016/s0886-3350(13)80025-9.
46. Eleftheriadis H. Capsular tension ring insertion technique tips. J Cataract Refract Surg. 2002;28(7):1091–2. https://doi.org/10.1016/S0886-3350(02)01477-3.
47. Burk SE, Da Mata AP, Snyder ME, Schneider S, Osher RH, Cionni RJ. Visualizing vitreous using Kenalog suspension. J Cataract Refract Surg. 2003;29(4):645–51. https://doi.org/10.1016/S0886-3350(03)00016-6.

Pseudophakic Cystoid Macular Oedema

Marta Ugarte

Introduction

Pseudophakic cystoid macular oedema (PCMO), also known as Irvine-Gass syndrome [1–4], is defined as oedema newly formed after cataract surgery, which is associated with symptomatic vision loss 6/12 or worse.

The presentation can be any time after cataract surgery with the majority presenting within 5 weeks. Those occurring more than 4 months post-operatively are designated as late-onset. The great majority will resolve spontaneously within 6 months but some can be difficult to treat and become chronic. There are very few studies comparing visual morbidity in eyes with and without PCMO but some patients do develop permanent visual loss making it a serious complication. There is evidence published in the USA showing that the cost of cases with PCMO is 41% higher compared to controls [5]. The most common complaint is blurriness, which can be noticed after an initial period of improved vision post cataract surgery. Less common presentations include central scotomas, metamorphopsia, mild photophobia and reduced contrast sensitivity [6]. The latter may account for persistent subjective visual difficulties despite good Snellen visual acuity.

Determining the true incidence of PCMO has been difficult due to the use of different diagnostic methods (i.e. biomicroscopy, fundus fluorescein angiography-FFA, optical coherence tomography-OCT) [7] and variations in patient populations with diverse risk factors. Thus for example, the incidence of angiographic PCMO 1–2 months postoperatively has been reported as high as 20–30% and OCT PCMO may range from 4 to 41% [8, 9]. It is important to emphasize that the majority of patients with angiographic and OCT PCMO will not experience visual

M. Ugarte (✉)
Medical Retina Service, Manchester University NHS Foundation Trust, Manchester M13 9WL, UK
e-mail: marta.ugarte@manchester.ac.uk

M. Ugarte
Faculty of Biology, Medicine and Health, University of Manchester, Manchester, UK

© Springer Nature Switzerland AG 2021
C. Liu and A. Shalaby Bardan (eds.), *Cataract Surgery*,
https://doi.org/10.1007/978-3-030-38234-6_10

disturbances (i.e. subclinical PCMO) and the oedema will resolve spontaneously. Only about 1–3% of uncomplicated cases and 8% of those with surgical complications will have persistent macular oedema associated reduced vision [10, 11].

In this chapter, we will discuss the pathogenesis, methods of diagnosis, possible risk factors, as well as the current evidence to help manage PCMO.

Pathogenesis

The precise aetiology of PCMO is not fully understood. Mechanisms considered to be involved in its pathogenesis include the release of inflammatory mediators and disruption of the blood aqueous barrier (BAB) and blood retinal barrier (BRB) with the consequent increase in vascular permeability [12–16]. In the inflammation cascade, prostanoids (i.e. prostaglandins and thromboxane A2) are formed when arachidonic acid is released from the plasma membrane by phospholipase A and metabolized by the sequential actions of prostaglandin G/H synthase or cyclooxygenase. Phospholipase A and cyclooxygenase are potential targets to inhibit inflammation.

Breakdown of the BRB in retinal capillaries and/or the retinal pigment epithelium (RPE) allows serum to get into the retinal extracellular space. Since intraretinal fluid distribution is restricted by two diffusion barriers, the inner and outer plexiform layers, serum leakage from intraretinal vessels causes cysts mainly in the inner nuclear layer [12]. On the other hand, leakage from the choroid/pigment epithelium generates cyst formation in the Henle fiber layer and subretinal fluid accumulation [12].

The inflammatory mediators probably play the essential initiating role in the development of PCMO but the exact factors and events responsible for further CMO development and its chronicity have not yet been clearly identified. Contraction of the posterior hyaloid as a result of inflammation may lead to mechanical traction onto the perifoveal retinal capillaries and contribute to PCMO.

Histologically, iritis, cyclitis, retinal phlebitis and periphlebitis, as well as intracellular accumulation of fluid in Muller cells have been described [17]. Excess fluid may break through cell membranes and accumulate extracellularly. If the fluid is contained intracellularly, the condition is considered to be reversible. If the cell membranes break and fluid accumulates extracellularly, presumably, the condition then becomes irreversible.

Diagnosis

Funduscopy

On biomicroscopy, loss of the foveal depression, macular thickening and perifoveal cystic spaces can be seen. The cystic spaces can appear as yellow on funduscopy and red-free light may aid in their detection. In severe cases, swelling of the optic nerve head can be detectable. In chronic cases, the cystoid spaces may fuse, break and result in a lamellar hole [17].

Fundus Fluorescein Angiography

Angiographic CMO is diagnosed in cases with detectable leakage on FFA with hyperfluorescence of the central macula and optic disc. In the early phase of the fluorescein angiogram, retinal telangiectasias, capillary dilatation and leakage from small perifoveal capillaries are visible. In later phases, hyperfluorescence develops in the central macula with the classic petaloid pattern, and optic disc. The perifoveal petaloid hyperfluorescence represents fluorescein pooling in cystic spaces in the inner retina. Leakage and staining of the optic nerve are the result of capillary leakage. In severe cases, the cystoid spaces may have a 'honeycomb' appearance outside the immediate perifoveal region. It is important to emphasize that a decrease in visual acuity does not correlate with the extent of the leakage.

Optical Coherence Tomography

Although fluorescein angiography was considered the diagnostic gold standard for PCMO in the past, OCT is now the method of choice for diagnosis and monitoring. Its advantages include it is non-invasive and highly sensitive [12]. What is more, the thickening of macula can be effectively measured and these measurements correlate better with vision than fluorescein leakage. PCMO on OCT is characterized by loss of the foveal depression, retinal thickening, and cystic hyporeflective areas within the macula. Subretinal fluid can also be seen. In cases of persistent clinical CMO, secondary permanent complications such as lamellar hole can develop.

Extracellular fluid accumulation is the main causative factor of cyst formation. However, Müller cell swelling may also contribute to OCT-CMO development particularly in cases without significant angiographic vascular leakage.

Risk Factors

Certain anatomic and physiologic conditions disrupt the blood aqueous and blood retinal barriers and predispose to fluid accumulation within the macula after cataract surgery. The incidence of PCMO is higher with aging, in patients with diabetes mellitus [18], hypertension, leukaemia, history of retinal vein occlusion [19], recent history of uveitis [20, 21], pre-existing vitreomacular traction, epiretinal membrane [22, 23], vitreoretinal surgery [24], cataract surgery complications (e.g.

iris trauma, anterior chamber intraocular lens implant, posterior capsule rupture, vitreous disruption, vitreous loss, vitreous to the corneal wound), pseudoexfoliation [25], previous PCMO in the fellow eye, previous radiation therapy and certain medications [26–30]. Perioperative glaucoma and use of intraocular pressure lowering drops, as well as microscope light toxicity have been suggested to be risk factors for PCMO [10]. However, more recent studies did not support these findings [31].

Diabetes

The incidence of PCMO is higher in patients with diabetes mellitus with or without diabetic retinopathy [18]. Indicators of poor glycemic control such as HbA1c, severity of diabetic retinopathy and insulin dependency are all risk factors. If there is already some degree of diabetic macular edema before the cataract surgery, this should be treated prior to the operation as it rarely resolves on its own. In cases when this is not possible, intravitreal anti-inflammatory medication at the surgical time may be used.

Uveitis

Adequate pre- and post-operative control of inflammation is essential. Patients with active inflammation within 3 months of surgery have been shown to have a 6 fold increased risk of developing PCMO. Belair and Kim et al. [20] demonstrated that incidence of PCMO on OCT at 1 month post-op was 12% for eyes with uveitis and 4% for controls, at 3 months 8% and 0%, respectively (this was statistically significant). Eyes treated perioperatively with oral corticosteroids had a 7-fold reduction in PCMO.

Pediatric uveitis patients are particularly challenging as demonstrated in Sijssens et al.'s [32] publication, where they reported CMO in 3 of 19 (16%) of aphakic, and 1 of 29 (3%) pseudophakic eyes at 1 year ($P = 0.286$), and 7 of 19 (37%) and 2 of 20 (10%) cumulatively at 2 years ($P = 0.065$), of children with juvenile idiopathic arthritis-associated uveitis.

Glaucoma Medications

Topical glaucoma medication as a risk factor for PCMO is still controversial. There are multiple reports on the potential association of PCMO with the topical use of ocular hypotensive prostaglandin analogue agents (latanoprost, unoprostone, travoprost and bimatoprost) [8]. The explanation is based on the associated increase in blood aqueous disruption and inflammatory activity.

Miyake et al. [33] demonstrated in several clinical trials and cellular studies that preoperative and postoperative topical glaucoma medications, specifically latanoprost and timolol, may increase the incidence of PCMO. It appears that a commonly used preservative, benzalkonium chloride, is cytotoxic and stimulates inflammatory responses. Arcieri et al. [34] also reported the results of a randomized trial that enrolled 80 subjects, showing that aphakic and pseudophakic glaucoma patients developed more anterior chamber flare if they were randomized to take bimatoprost, latanoprost or travoprost compared to placebo ($P < 0.02$). Six of these patients developed angiographic PCMO (4 on latanoprost, $P = 0.03$), which resolved after discontinuing the prostaglandin analogues, and being treated with topical antiinflammatories.

However, in a recent retrospective comparative series by Law et al. [35], 700 eyes with glaucoma that underwent cataract surgery did not have a higher incidence of clinical PCMO compared to 553 non-glaucomatous eyes (5.14% and 5.79%, respectively, $P = 0.618$), and the use of preoperative and postoperative glaucoma medications was not associated with clinical PCMO ($P > 0.05$). It is uncertain whether the results would have differed if angiographic PCMO were the endpoint.

Differential Diagnosis

Patients with macular oedema after cataract surgery and an underlying ocular or systemic condition that predisposes to fluid accumulation in the macula may present diagnostic challenges. What is more, in some patients there may be mixed macular oedema. It is crucial to diagnose the type of macular oedema appropriately as the management may be different.

In some cases, funduscopy, FFA and OCT may help differentiate PCMO from other types of macular oedema. Certain morphological features may be associated with specific underlying pathological processes.

Pseudophakic Cystoid Macular Oedema (PCMO) Versus Diabetic Macular Oedema (DMO)

PCMO is induced by acute release of pro-inflammatory mediators, local inflammatory reaction and acute breakdown of the inner and outer BRB. In contrast, in DMO there is sustained chronic inflammation and degenerative processes leading to gradual vascular changes. These chronic processes include: (1) hyperglycaemia-related oxidative stress, (2) deposition of advanced glycation end products,

(3) impaired blood flow, (4) hypoxia, (5) pericyte loss, (6) endothelial cell loss, (7) upregulation of vesicular transport, (8) down-regulation of glial-cell derived neurotrophic factor, and to a certain degree (9) inflammation. Acute inflammation resolves quickly if the inflammatory trigger is removed. In contrast, slow, ongoing, chronic activation of the immune system will persist (Fig. 1).

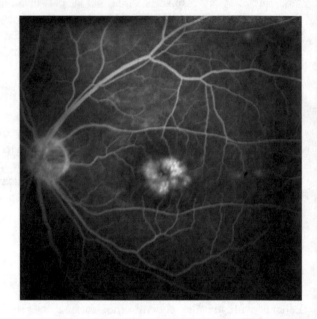

Fig. 1 Pseudophakic cystoid macular oedema: petalloid pattern of foveal hyperfluorescence and optic disc hyperfluorescence on fundus fluorescein angiography

Table 1 Morphologic features on OCT and FFA, which help differentiate pseudophakic cystoid macular oedema (PCMO) from diabetic macular oedema (DMO)

	PCMO	DMO
Layer location of cysts	Mainly inner nuclear layer	Mainly outer plexiform layer and Henle's layer
Presence of subretinal fluid	Common	Less frequent
Preserved foveal contour	Infrequent	Less frequent
Integrity of retinal layers	Common	Less frequent
Integrity of hyperreflective bands (external limiting membrane, retinal pigment epithelium, photoreceptor layer)	Common	Photoreceptor layer usually disrupted
Presence of ERM	Less frequent	Common
Presence of microaneurysms	No	Common
Presence of microfoci, hard exudates	No	Common
Presence of "hot disc" hyperfluorescence on FFA	Frequent	Infrequent

The FFA and OCT parameters [36, 37], which can help differentiate PCMO from DMO are shown in Table 1. These include: (1) macular oedema distribution, (2) the presence of microfoci and (3) the thickness of the retinal nerve fibre layer [37]. PCMO usually presents with a central MO pattern and intraretinal cystoid fluid accumulation in the central square mm of the Early Treatment of Diabetic Retinopathy Study (ETDRS) subfield, mainly cysts in the inner nuclear layer and intact hyperreflective bands. As the superficial and deep retinal capillary plexuses are located in the ganglion cell and inner nuclear layers, initially cysts appear in the INL. On the other hand, DMO usually has diffuse or focal retinal thickening and preserved foveal depression, due to focal leakage, mainly outer nuclear layer/ Henle's layer cysts, hard exudates, microfoci and disruption of the photoreceptor layers. SRF has been reported to be more common in PCMO 47–100% compared to DMO 10–35% (and seems to depend on disease duration) (Fig. 2).

Prophylaxis and Treatment

The natural history of the disease, the fact that PCMO typically resolves spontaneously with time, and the fact that presence of macular oedema with certain imaging techniques is not always correlated with loss of vision, make difficult the evaluation of any treatment modality. Further research is necessary to develop evidence-based standard algorithms for its prevention and treatment [8, 38–44].

The management is based on its pathogenesis (i.e. inflammation, blood retinal barrier disruption). In patients with chronic PCMO, a stepwise plan should be undertaken starting with topical corticosteroids and non-steroidal

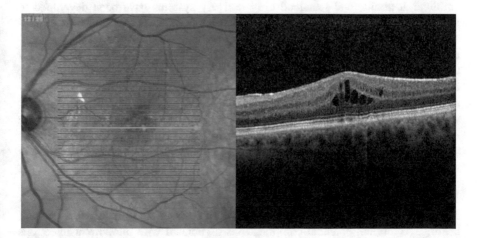

Fig. 2 Spectral domain-optical coherence tomography following uncomplicated phacoemulsification and intraocular lens implantation demonstrates newly formed typical cystoid macular oedema and mild epiretinal membrane

anti-inflammatory agents (NSAIDs). Following on to periocular (i.e, subconjunctival, sub-Tenon's, orbital floor, retrobulbar) or intravitreal injections of corticosteroids or anti-vascular endothelial growth factor (anti-VEGF) agents when topical medications have either failed or shown limited effects. PCMO refractory to medical therapy or associated with significant vitreous traction can improve with laser vitreolysis or pars plana vitrectomy.

Corticosteroids

Corticosteroids reduce inflammation by inhibiting phospholipase A2. In addition, they inhibit the migration of macrophages and neutrophils, and decrease capillary permeability and vasodilation. Topical corticosteroids (e.g. dexamethasone, prednisolone) are known to be effective in the treatment of post-cataract surgery inflammation and are used routinely on a tapering regime over a few weeks after surgery. Periocular corticosteroids (subconjunctival, sub-Tenon's, orbital floor, retrobulbar injections) have been shown to be effective in cases of PCMO refractory to topical treatment [45]. Intravitreal injections are increasingly used to manage macular edema associated with diabetic retinopathy, retinal vein occlusion and uveitis. These injections enable the delivery of corticosteroids to the retina in higher concentrations, allowing better bioavailability compared with topical administration. Jonas et al. [46, 47] demonstrated in their small prospective interventional case series that patients with PCMO benefited from intravitreal triamcinolone acetonide (IVTA) injections. Other studies have also shown beneficial effects [48, 49].

PCMO may recur even after more than one intravitreal injection of triamcinolone acetonide and sustained drug delivery systems have been developed to address this limitation. Ozurdex (Allergan, Irvine, CA) is an injectable, biodegradable intravitreal implant that provides sustained release of preservative-free dexamethasone. Ozurdex has been approved for treatment of macular edema secondary to retinal vein occlusions and non-infectious posterior uveitis. Various studies have shown beneficial effects [50–56]. A phase II study subgroup analysis investigated its efficacy in the treatment of persistent PCMO [44]. Twenty-seven patients with refractory PCMO were recruited, and randomized to receive dexamethasone implant 350 μg, dexamethasone implant 700 μg, or observation. Eight patients showed at least a 10-letter improvement at 3 months and maintained the improvement at 6 months. Another study is currently enrolling patients for a Phase II study to examine the dexamethasone implant to treat PCMO [57].

Corticosteroids use can be associated with various adverse side effects, including elevated intraocular pressure, postoperative infection, and impaired wound healing. Additional potential complications associated with intravitreal injections include sterile endophthalmitis, retinal detachment, and vitreous hemorrhage. Increased intraocular pressure in the majority of patients can be managed by observation or pressure-lowering medications [46].

Nonsteroidal Anti-inflammatory Drugs (NSAIDs)

NSAIDs inhibit COX in the inflammatory cascade. Topical administration is thought to have better ocular penetration than systemic routes [58]. The following are approved for postoperative inflammation although not for cystoid macular oedema. Ketorolac 0.4% (Acular, Allergan, Irvine, CA), diclofenac 0.1% (Voltaren, Bausch & Lomb, Tampa, FL), bromfenac 0.09% (Xibrom/Bromday, Ista Pharmaceuticals, Irvine, CA), and nepafenac 0.1% (Nevanac, Alcon, Fort Worth, TX). Nepafenac is a prodrug that is converted by intraocular hydrolases into its active form, amfenac. Nepafenac has been reported to have superior corneal penetration and posterior segment activity than other NSAIDs in rabbit models [58].

There are multiple reports on the use of these agents in the prevention and treatment of acute and chronic PCMO (both angiographic and clinical). In general, studies have proven the effectiveness of their use without clear statistical differences between the different NSAIDs or evidence to support the equivalence or superiority of topical NSAIDs with our without topical corticosteroids vs corticosteroids alone [33, 58–79].

A Cochrane review [80] found low-certainty evidence that people receiving topical NSAIDs in combination with steroids may have lower risk of poor vision due to macular oedema at 3 months after cataract surgery. Although NSAIDs may speed visual recovery in the first several weeks, there is no evidence that this practice affects long-term visual outcomes. The authors found it was unclear the extent to which this reduction had an impact on the visual function and quality of life of patients.

Topical NSAIDs are generally well tolerated. The main side effects are burning, conjunctival hyperemia, keratitis, corneal infiltrates, corneal lesions similar to those observed with other topical preparations possibly related to preservatives [81–83]. Systemic side effects, such as exacerbation of asthma [84–86], result from drainage into the nasolacrimal duct and entry into circulation. Patients with preexisting ocular surface conditions such as Sjögren's syndrome, rheumatoid arthritis, or chronic ocular surface disease should avoid NSAIDs [81, 82, 84].

Anti-VEGF Agents

VEGF is a key mediator of angiogenesis, but it also plays an important role in the inflammation, capillary permeability and BRB disruption that causes CMO. Although the biological basis for the use of anti-VEGF agents in PCMO is not established, there are some studies indicating their potential benefit.

The efficacy of intravitreal Bevacizumab (Avastin, Genentech, South San Francisco, CA), a humanized monoclonal antibody that inhibits VEGF-A, for the treatment of PCMO has been tested. Arevalo et al. [87] reported on a series of 28

eyes that received at least one 1.25 mg or 2.5 mg injection of intravitreal bevacizumab as the primary treatment of chronic PCMO. During the mean follow-up
of 8 months, 21 eyes (71%) improved best corrected visual acuity (BCVA) by 2
or more ETDRS lines. The mean baseline best corrected visual acuity and central macular thickness were 6/48 and 466 microns, which improved to 6/18 and
265 microns, respectively (both $P < 0.0001$). Eight (26%) eyes required a second
injection and 4 (13%) a third. In a 6 month follow-up study with 110 eyes, visual
and anatomic benefits were observed, although 16 (21%) eyes required a second
injection, and 6 (8%) a third one. Similar results were seen at the 24 month follow-up study, when the investigators also noted no outcome differences between
the 1.25 mg and 2.50 mg dosing.

Most other studies have focused on the treatment of chronic PCMO refractory
to other treatments. In 2008, Spitzer et al. [88] showed that 1.25 mg of intravitreal bevacizumab did not significantly improve visual outcomes in a series of 16
eyes with refractory PCMO, although there was slight decrease in retinal thickness. Arevalo et al. [89] subsequently reported a series of 36 eyes with chronic
PCMO refractory to topical, periocular, systemic and intravitreal treatments, and
showed that 26 eyes (72%) demonstrated improvement of BCVA by at least 2
ETDRS lines, and mean baseline BCVA and central macular thickness improved
from 6/60 and 500 microns, respectively, to 6/24 and 286 microns, respectively, at
12 months, after a mean of 2.7 injections per eye ($P < 0.0001$).

Another series of 10 patients that received 1.25 mg of bevacizumab also
reported promising visual and anatomic outcomes, with follow up of 6 months
[90]. "Triple therapy" with intravitreal triamcinolone, intravitreal bevacizumab
and topical NSAIDs has been shown to be effective as well [91], although the
effects of the intravitreal medications were transient.

A prospective study of 500 patients evaluated the efficacy of intraoperative
pegaptanib (Macugen, Eyetech Pharmaceuticals, New York, NY) to prevent acute
PCMO [92, 93]. Pegaptanib is a pegylated neutralizing RNA aptamer that selectively binds VEGF165, which is thought to be one of the key pathologic VEGF
isoforms. At week 4, 1 (0.4%) patient in the pegaptanib group while 11 (4.4%) in
the control group developed PCMO as seen with spectral domain OCT.

The present literature does not provide robust support for the use of anti-VEGF
treatments in the treatment of PCMO. Although there are some positive results, a
lack of randomized double-blind placebo trials limits the generalizability of these
data, and there are concerns regarding systemic toxicity in vulnerable patient populations following intravitreal antiVEGF injection, including stroke and death [94–99].

Surgery

Surgical intervention can be effective in the presence of vitreomacular traction.
Vitreolysis using the Nd:YAG laser has shown positive effects in cases of vitreous
incarceration in the cataract incision wound [100]. The rationale for performing

vitrectomy in PCMO includes the removal of vitreous adhesions and inflammatory mediators and improved access of topical medication to the posterior pole [101–103].

Miscellaneous

Carbonic Anhydrase Inhibitor (Acetazolamide)

There are some reports and small series documenting the positive effect of acetazolamide in refractory PCMO [103–106]. Oral acetazolamide may help reduce macular oedema by stimulating the RPE to pump excess fluid out of the macula. Furthermore, carbonic anhydrase inhibitors induce acidification of the subretinal space, and thereby increase fluid resorption from the retina through the RPE into the choroid. Their use may be limited by severe side effects. Topical CAIs have not yet been investigated in PCMO.

Immunomodulatory Therapy

Recent small pilot studies have started to examine subcutaneous interferon alpha (IFN-a, Imgenex, San Diego, CA) [107, 108] and intravitreal infliximab (Remicade, Centocor Ortho Biotech, Horsham, PA) with mixed results [109, 110].

Management Summary

Current guidelines for post-cataract surgery inflammation management recommend prevention as the main goal with adequate eye/patient selection and preparation, avoid iris trauma during surgery, optimal management of intraoperative complications, and treatment of postoperative inflammation in a timely manner. Many of the multiple studies performed to test the efficacy of different drugs and routes in the prophylaxis and treatment of PCMO have been poorly designed and the results are inconsistent [111]. Prospective, randomized clinical trials comparing various treatments [112] are required with standardized uveitis nomenclature, type of medication used, dosing, treatment regime and outcome measure end points (angiographic, clinical, OCT macular oedema, visual loss). Standardized reporting of CMO based on OCT may allow for more uniform quantitation of its incidence and more reliable assessment of treatment outcomes. Future studies should be large enough to detect reduction in the risk of the outcome of most interest to patients, which is chronic macular oedema leading to visual loss.

References

1. Gass JD, Norton EW. Follow-up study of cystoid macular edema following cataract extraction. Trans Am Acad Ophthalmol Otolaryngol. 1969;73(4):665–82.
2. Gass JD, Norton EW. Cystoid macular edema and papilledema following cataract extraction. A fluorescein fundoscopic and angiographic study. Arch Ophthalmol. 1966;76(5):646–61.
3. Gass JD, Norton EW. Fluorescein studies of patients with macular edema and papilledema following cataract extraction. Trans Am Ophthalmol Soc. 1966;64:232–49.
4. Irvine SR. A newly defined vitreous syndrome following cataract surgery. Am J Ophthalmol. 1953;36(5):599–619.
5. Schaub F, Adler W, Koenig MC, Enders P, Grajewski RS, Cursiefen C, Heindl LM. Impact of allergy and atopy on the risk of pseudophakic cystoid macular edema. Graefes Arch Clin Exp Ophthalmol. 2016;254(12):2417–23.
6. Ibanez HE, Lesher MP, Singerman LJ, Rice TA, Keep GF. Prospective evaluation of the effect of pseudophakic cystoid macula edema on contrast sensitivity. Arch Ophthalmol. 1993;111(12):1635–9.
7. Brar M, Yuson R, Kozak I, Mojana F, Cheng L, Bartsch DU, Oster SF, Freeman WR. Correlation between morphologic features on spectral-domain optical coherence tomography and angiographic leakage patterns in macular edema. Retina. 2010;30(3):383–9.
8. Yavas GF, Oztürk F, Küsbeci T. Preoperative topical indomethacin to prevent pseudophakic cystoid macular edema. J Cataract Refract Surg. 2007;33(5):804–7.
9. Yonekawa Y, Kim IK. Pseudophakic cystoid macular edema. Curr Opin Ophthalmol. 2012;23(1):26–32.
10. Yüksel B, Karti Ö, Kusbeci T. Topical nepafenac for prevention of post-cataract surgery macular edema in diabetic patients: patient selection and perspectives. Clin Ophthalmol. 2017;11(11):2183–90.
11. Zur D, Loewenstein A. Postsurgical cystoid macular edema. Dev Ophthalmol. 2017;58:178–90.
12. Chetrit M, Bonnin S, Mané V, Erginay A, Tadayoni R, Gaudric A, Couturier A. Acute pseudophakic cystoid macular edema imaged by optical coherence tomography angiography. Retina. 2018;38(10):2073–80.
13. Do JR, Oh JH, Chuck RS, Park CY. Transient corneal edema is a predictive factor for pseudophakic cystoid macular edema after uncomplicated cataract surgery. Korean J Ophthalmol. 2015;29(1):14–22.
14. Fleissig E, Cohen S, Iglicki M, Goldstein M, Zur D. Changes in choroidal thickness in clinically significant pseudophakic cystoid macular edema. Retina. 2018;38(8):1629–35.
15. Jarstad JS, Jarstad AR, Chung GW, Tester RA, Day LE. Immediate postoperative intraocular pressure adjustment reduces risk of cystoid macular edema after uncomplicated micro incision coaxial phacoemulsification cataract surgery. Korean J Ophthalmol. 2017;31(1):39–43.
16. Peyman GA, Canakis C, Livir-Rallatos C, Conway MD. The effect of internal limiting membrane peeling on chronic recalcitrant pseudophakic cystoid macular edema: a report of two cases. Am J Ophthalmol. 2002;133(4):571–2.
17. Michels RG, Green WR, Maumenee AE. Cystoid macular edema following cataract extraction (The Irvine-Gass Syndrome): a case studied clinically and histopathologically. Ophthalmic Surg. 1971;2:217–21.
18. Grzybowski A, Kanclerz P. Risk factors for cystoid macular edema after cataract surgery in diabetic patients. J Cataract Refract Surg. 2017;43(10):1365.
19. Cho HJ, Hwang HJ, Kim HS, Lee DW, Kim CG, Kim BY, Kim JW. Macular edema after cataract surgery in eyes with preoperative retinal vein occlusion. Retina. 2018;38(6):1180–6.
20. Bélair ML, Kim SJ, Thorne JE, Dunn JP, Kedhar SR, Brown DM, Jabs DA. Incidence of cystoid macular edema after cataract surgery in patients with and without uveitis using optical coherence tomography. Am J Ophthalmol. 2009;148(1):128–35.

21. Chu CJ, Dick AD, Johnston RL, Yang YC, Denniston AK, UK Pseudophakic Macular Edema Study Group. Cataract surgery in uveitis: a multicentre database study. Br J Ophthalmol. 2017;101(8):1132–1137.
22. Hardin JS, Gauldin DW, Soliman MK, Chu CJ, Yang YC, Sallam AB. Cataract surgery outcomes in eyes with primary epiretinal membrane. JAMA Ophthalmol. 2018;136(2):148–54.
23. Ramakrishnan S, Baskaran P, Talwar B, Venkatesh R. Prospective, randomized study comparing the effect of 0.1% nepafenac and 0.4% ketorolac tromethamine on macular thickness in cataract surgery patients with low risk for cystoid macular edema. Asia Pac J Ophthalmol (Phila). 2015;4(4):216–20.
24. Mylonas G, Sacu S, Deák G, Dunavoelgyi R, Buehl W, Georgopoulos M, Schmidt-Erfurth U, Macula Study Group Vienna. Macular edema following cataract surgery in eyes with previous 23-gauge vitrectomy and peeling of the internal limiting membrane. Am J Ophthalmol. 2013;155(2):253–259.e2.
25. Ilveskoski L, Taipale C, Holmström EJ, Tuuminen R. Macular edema after cataract surgery in eyes with and without pseudoexfoliation syndrome. Eur J Ophthalmol. 2018:1120672118799622.
26. Chu CJ, Johnston RL, Buscombe C, Sallam AB, Mohamed Q, Yang YC, United Kingdom Pseudophakic Macular Edema Study Group. Risk factors and incidence of macular edema after cataract surgery: a database study of 81984 eyes. Ophthalmology. 2016;123(2):316–23.
27. Conrad-Hengerer I, Hengerer FH, Al Juburi M, Schultz T, Dick HB. Femtosecond laser-induced macular changes and anterior segment inflammation in cataract surgery. J Refract Surg. 2014;30(4):222–6.
28. Ewe SY, Oakley CL, Abell RG, Allen PL, Vote BJ. Cystoid macular edema after femtosecond laser-assisted versus phacoemulsification cataract surgery. J Cataract Refract Surg. 2015;41(11):2373–8.
29. Henderson BA, Kim JY, Ament CS, Ferrufino-Ponce ZK, Grabowska A, Cremers SL. Clinical pseudophakic cystoid macular edema. Risk factors for development and duration after treatment. J Cataract Refract Surg. 2007;33(9):1550–8.
30. Schaub F, Adler W, Koenig MC, Enders P, Dietlein TS, Cursiefen C, Heindl LM. Combined ab interno glaucoma surgery does not increase the risk of pseudophakic cystoid macular edema in uncomplicated eyes. J Glaucoma. 2017;26(3):227–32.
31. Schaub F, Adler W, Enders P, Koenig MC, Koch KR, Cursiefen C, Kirchhof B, Heindl LM. Preexisting epiretinal membrane is associated with pseudophakic cystoid macular edema. Graefes Arch Clin Exp Ophthalmol. 2018;256(5):909–17.
32. Shorstein NH, Liu L, Waxman MD, Herrinton LJ. Comparative effectiveness of three prophylactic strategies to prevent clinical macular edema after phacoemulsification surgery. Ophthalmology. 2015;122(12):2450–6.
33. Miyake K, Ota I, Miyake G, Numaga J. Nepafenac 0.1% versus fluorometholone 0.1% for preventing cystoid macular edema after cataract surgery. J Cataract Refract Surg. 2011;37(9):1581–8.
34. Arcieri ES, Santana A, Rocha FN, Guapo GL, Costa VP. Blood-aqueous barrier changes after the use of prostaglandin analogues in patients with pseudophakia and aphakia: a 6-month randomized trial. Arch Ophthalmol. 2005;123(2):186–92.
35. Law SK, Kim E, Yu F, Caprioli J. Clinical cystoid macular edema after cataract surgery in glaucoma patients. J Glaucoma. 2010;19(2):100–4.
36. Jo EB, Lee JH, Hwang YN, Kim SM. Comparison of evaluation parameters in the retinal layer between diabetic cystoid macular edema and postoperative cystoid macular edema after cataract surgery based on a hierarchical approach. Technol Health Care. 2015;24(Suppl 1):S59–68.
37. Munk MR, Jampol LM, Simader C, Huf W, Mittermüller TJ, Jaffe GJ, Schmidt-Erfurth U. Differentiation of diabetic macular edema from pseudophakic cystoid macular edema by spectral-domain optical coherence tomography. Invest Ophthalmol Vis Sci. 2015;56(11):6724–33.

38. Guo S, Patel S, Baumrind B, Johnson K, Levinsohn D, Marcus E, Tannen B, Roy M, Bhagat N, Zarbin M. Management of pseudophakic cystoid macular edema. Surv Ophthalmol. 2015;60(2):123–37.
39. Holekamp NM. Treatment of pseudophakic CME. Ocul Immunol Inflamm. 1998;6(2):121–3.
40. Sharir M. Exacerbation of asthma by topical diclofenac. Arch Ophthalmol. 1997;115(2):294–5.
41. Warren KA, Bahrani H, Fox JE. NSAIDs in combination therapy for the treatment of chronic pseudophakic cystoid macular edema. Retina. 2010;30(2):260–6.
42. Wielders LH, Schouten JS, Aberle MR, Lambermont VA, van den Biggelaar FJ, Winkens B, Simons RW, Nuijts RM. Treatment of cystoid macular edema after cataract surgery. J Cataract Refract Surg. 2017;43(2):276–84.
43. Wielders LH, Lambermont VA, Schouten JS, van den Biggelaar FJ, Worthy G, Simons RW, Winkens B, Nuijts RM. Prevention of cystoid macular edema after cataract surgery in non-diabetic and diabetic patients: a systematic review and meta-analysis. Am J Ophthalmol. 2015;160(5):968–0.
44. Wielders LHP, Schouten JSAG, Nuijts RMMA. Prevention of macular edema after cataract surgery. Curr Opin Ophthalmol. 2018;29(1):48–53.
45. Dieleman M, Wubbels RJ, van Kooten-Noordzij M, de Waard PW. Single perioperative subconjunctival steroid depot versus postoperative steroid eyedrops to prevent intraocular inflammation and macular edema after cataract surgery. J Cataract Refract Surg. 2011;37(9):1589–97.
46. Jonas JB. Intravitreal triamcinolone acetonide: a change in a paradigm. Ophthalmic Res. 2006;38(4):218–45.
47. Jonas JB, Kreissig I, Degenring RF. Intravitreal triamcinolone acetonide for pseudophakic cystoid macular edema. Am J Ophthalmol. 2003;136(2):384–6.
48. Benhamou N, Massin P, Haouchine B, Audren F, Tadayoni R, Gaudric A. Intravitreal triamcinolone for refractory pseudophakic macular edema. Am J Ophthalmol. 2003;135(2):246–9.
49. Boscia F, Furino C, Dammacco R, Ferreri P, Sborgia L, Sborgia C. Intravitreal triamcinolone acetonide in refractory pseudophakic cystoid macular edema: functional and anatomic results. Eur J Ophthalmol. 2005;15(1):89–95.
50. Bellocq D, Korobelnik JF, Burillon C, Voirin N, Dot C, Souied E, Conrath J, Milazzo S, Massin P, Baillif S, Kodjikian L. Effectiveness and safety of dexamethasone implants for post-surgical macular oedema including Irvine-Gass syndrome: the EPISODIC study. Br J Ophthalmol. 2015;99(7):979–83.
51. Brynskov T, Laugesen CS, Halborg J, Kemp H, Sørensen TL. Longstanding refractory pseudophakic cystoid macular edema resolved using intravitreal 0.7 mg dexamethasone implants. Clin Ophthalmol. 2013;7:1171–4.
52. Dutra Medeiros M, Navarro R, Garcia-Arumí J, Mateo C, Corcóstegui B. Dexamethasone intravitreal implant for treatment of patients with recalcitrant macular edema resulting from Irvine-Gass syndrome. Invest Ophthalmol Vis Sci. 2013;54(5):3320–4.
53. Fenicia V, Balestrieri M, Perdicchi A, MauriziEnrici M, DelleFave M, Recupero SM. Intravitreal injection of dexamethasone implant and ranibizumab in cystoid macular edema in the course of irvine-gass syndrome. Case Rep Ophthalmol. 2014;5(2):243–8.
54. Garcia JM, Isaac DL, Ávila MP. Dexamethasone 0.7 mg implants in the management of pseudophakic cystoid macular edema. Arq Bras Oftalmol. 2016;79(2):113–5.
55. Khurana RN, Palmer JD, Porco TC, Wieland MR. Dexamethasone intravitreal implant for pseudophakic cystoid macular edema in patients with diabetes. Ophthalmic Surg Lasers Imaging Retina. 2015;46(1):56–61.
56. Mayer WJ, Kurz S, Wolf A, Kook D, Kreutzer T, Kampik A, Priglinger S, Haritoglou C. Dexamethasone implant as an effective treatment option for macular edema due to Irvine-Gass syndrome. J Cataract Refract Surg. 2015;41(9):1954–61.

57. Zur D, Fischer N, Tufail A, Monés J, Loewenstein A. Postsurgical cystoid macular edema. Eur J Ophthalmol. 2011;21(Suppl 6):S62–8.
58. Kim SJ, Flach AJ, Jampol LM. Nonsteroidal anti-inflammatory drugs in ophthalmology. Surv Ophthalmol. 2010;55(2):108–33.
59. Grzybowski A, Adamiec-Mroczek J. Topical nonsteroidal anti-inflammatory drugs for cystoid macular edema prevention in patients with diabetic retinopathy. Am J Ophthalmol. 2017;181:xiv–0.
60. Grzybowski A, Levitz L. Lack of evidence to support substituting nonsteroidal antiinflammatory drugs for corticosteroids to control inflammation after intraocular surgery. J Cataract Refract Surg. 2017;43(4):580.
61. Grzybowski A, Sikorski BL, Ascaso FJ, Huerva V. Pseudophakic cystoid macular edema: update 2016. Clin Interv Aging. 2016;9(11):1221–9.
62. Juthani VV, Clearfield E, Chuck RS. Non-steroidal anti-inflammatory drugs versus corticosteroids for controlling inflammation after uncomplicated cataract surgery. Cochrane Database Syst Rev. 2017;7:CD010516.
63. Kim S, Kim MK, Wee WR. Additive effect of oral steroid with topical nonsteroidal anti-inflammatory drug for preventing cystoid macular edema after cataract surgery in patients with epiretinal membrane. Korean J Ophthalmol. 2017;31(5):394–401.
64. Kim SJ, Schoenberger SD, Thorne JE, Ehlers JP, Yeh S, Bakri SJ. Topical nonsteroidal anti-inflammatory drugs and cataract surgery: a report by the American Academy of Ophthalmology. Ophthalmology. 2015;122(11):2159–68.
65. McCafferty S, Harris A, Kew C, Kassm T, Lane L, Levine J, Raven M. Pseudophakic cystoid macular edema prevention and risk factors; prospective study with adjunctive once daily topical nepafenac 0.3% versus placebo. BMC Ophthalmol. 2017;17(1):16.
66. Modjtahedi BS, Paschal JF, Batech M, Luong TQ, Fong DS. Perioperative topical nonsteroidal anti-inflammatory drugs for macular edema prophylaxis following cataract surgery. Am J Ophthalmol. 2017;176:174–82.
67. Pierru A, Carles M, Gastaud P, Baillif S. Measurement of subfoveal choroidal thickness after cataract surgery in enhanced depth imaging optical coherence tomography. Invest Ophthalmol Vis Sci. 2014;55(8):4967–74.
68. Quintana NE, Allocco AR, Ponce JA, Magurno MG. Non steroidal anti-inflammatory drugs in the prevention of cystoid macular edema after uneventful cataract surgery. Clin Ophthalmol. 2014;25(8):1209–12.
69. Shelsta HN, Jampol LM. Pharmacologic therapy of pseudophakic cystoid macular edema: 2010 update. Retina. 2011;31(1):4–12.
70. Sheppard JD. Topical bromfenac for prevention and treatment of cystoidmacular edema following cataract surgery: a review. Clin Ophthalmol. 201625;10:2099–2111.
71. Sitenga GL, Ing EB, Van Dellen RG, Younge BR, Leavitt JA. Asthma caused by topical application of ketorolac. Ophthalmology. 1996;103(6):890–2.
72. Sivaprasad S, Bunce C, Crosby-Nwaobi R. Non-steroidal anti-inflammatory agents for treating cystoid macular oedema following cataract surgery. Cochrane Database Syst Rev. 2012;(2):CD004239.
73. Sivaprasad S, Bunce C, Wormald R. Non-steroidal anti-inflammatory agents for cystoid macular oedema following cataract surgery: a systematic review. Br J Ophthalmol. 2005;89(11):1420–2.
74. Sivaprasad S, Bunce C, Patel N. Non-steroidal anti-inflammatory agents for treating cystoid macular oedema following cataract surgery. Cochrane Database Syst Rev. 2005;(1):CD004239. Review. Update in: Cochrane Database Syst Rev. 2012;2:CD004241. Cochrane Database Syst Rev. 2012;2:CD004239.
75. Steinert RF, Wasson PJ. Neodymium:YAG laser anterior vitreolysis for Irvine-Gass cystoid macular edema. J Cataract Refract Surg. 1989;15(3):304–7.
76. Tripathi RC, Fekrat S, Tripathi BJ, Ernest JT. A direct correlation of the resolution of pseudophakic cystoid macular edema with acetazolamide therapy. Ann Ophthalmol. 1991;23(4):127–9.

77. Williams GA, Haller JA, Kuppermann BD, et al. Dexamethasone posterior-segment drug delivery system in the treatment of macular edema resulting from uveitis or Irvine-Gass syndrome. Am J Ophthalmol. 2009;147(6):1048–154, 1054 e1041–2.
78. Wu L, Hernandez-Bogantes E, Roca JA, Arevalo JF, Barraza K, Lasave AF. intravitreal tumor necrosis factor inhibitors in the treatment of refractory diabetic macular edema: a pilot study from the Pan-American Collaborative Retina Study Group. Retina. 2011;31(2):298–303.
79. Yoon DH, Kang DJ, Kim MJ, Kim HK. New observation of microcystic macular edema as a mild form of cystoid macular lesions after standard phacoemulsification: Prevalence and risk factors. Medicine (Baltimore). 2018;97(15):e0355.
80. Lim BX, Lim CH, Lim DK, Evans JR, Bunce C, Wormald R. Prophylactic non-steroidal anti-inflammatory drugs for the prevention of macular oedema after cataract surgery. Cochrane Database Syst Rev. 2016;11:CD006683.
81. Aragona P, Di Pietro R. Is it safe to use topical NSAIDs for corneal sensitivity in Sjögren's syndrome patients? Expert Opin Drug Saf. 2007;6(1):33–43.
82. Aragona P, Tripodi G, Spinella R, Laganà E, Ferreri G. The effects of the topical administration of non-steroidal anti-inflammatory drugs on corneal epithelium and corneal sensitivity in normal subjects. Eye (Lond). 2000;14(Pt 2):206–10.
83. Barba KR, Samy A, Lai C, Perlman JI, Bouchard CS. Effect of topical anti-inflammatory drugs on corneal and limbal wound healing. J Cataract Refract Surg. 2000;26(6):893–7.
84. Gaynes BI, Fiscella R. Topical nonsteroidal anti-inflammatory drugs for ophthalmic use: a safety review. Drug Saf. 2002;25(4):233–50.
85. Semeraro F, Morescalchi F, Duse S, Gambicorti E, Romano MR, Costagliola C. Systemic thromboembolic adverse events in patients treated with intravitreal anti-VEGF drugs for neovascular age-related macular degeneration: an overview. Expert Opin Drug Saf. 2014;13(6):785–802.
86. Sijssens KM, Rothova A, Van De Vijver DA, Stilma JS, De Boer JH. Risk factors for the development of cataract requiring surgery in uveitis associated with juvenile idiopathic arthritis. Am J Ophthalmol. 2007;144(4):574–9.
87. Arevalo JF, Garcia-Amaris RA, Roca JA, Sanchez JG, Wu L, Berrocal MH, Maia M; Pan-American Collaborative Retina Study Group. Primary intravitreal bevacizumab for the management of pseudophakic cystoid macular edema: pilot study of the Pan-American Collaborative Retina Study Group. J Cataract Refract Surg. 2007;33(12):2098–105.
88. Spitzer MS, Szurman P, Bartz-Schmidt KU. Intravitreal bevacizumab in postoperative pseudophakic cystoid macular edema: does it really work? J Cataract Refract Surg. 2008;34(6):880; author reply 880–1.
89. Arevalo JF, Maia M, Garcia-Amaris RA, Roca JA, Sanchez JG, Berrocal MH, Wu L. Pan-American Collaborative Retina Study Group. Intravitreal bevacizumab for refractory pseudophakic cystoid macular edema: the Pan-American Collaborative Retina Study Group results. Ophthalmology. 2009;116(8):1481–7.
90. Barone A, Russo V, Prascina F, Delle Noci N. Short-term safety and efficacy of intravitreal bevacizumab for pseudophakic cystoid macular edema. Retina. 2009;29(1):33–7.
91. Shimura M, Nakazawa T, Yasuda K, Nishida K. Diclofenac prevents an early event of macular thickening after cataract surgery in patients with diabetes. J Ocul Pharmacol Ther. 2007;23(3):284–91.
92. Cervera E, Diaz-Llopis M, Udaondo P, Garcia-Delpech S. Intravitreal pegaptanib sodium for refractory pseudophakic macular oedema. Eye (Lond). 2008;22(9):1180–2.
93. Gallego-Pinazo R, Arévalo JF, Udaondo P, García-Delpech S, Dolz-Marco R, Díaz-Llopis M. Prophylaxis of pseudophakic cystoid macular edema with intraoperative pegaptanib. J Ocul Pharmacol Ther. 2012;28(1):65–8.
94. Carneiro AM, Barthelmes D, Falcão MS, Mendonça LS, Fonseca SL, Gonçalves RM, Faria-Correia F, Falcão-Reis FM. Arterial thromboembolic events in patients with exudative age-related macular degeneration treated with intravitreal bevacizumab or ranibizumab. Ophthalmologica. 2011;225(4):211–21.

95. Fung AE, Rosenfeld PJ, Reichel E. The International Intravitreal Bevacizumab Safety Survey: using the internet to assess drug safety worldwide. Br J Ophthalmol. 2006;90(11):1344–9.

96. Kemp A, Preen DB, Morlet N, Clark A, McAllister IL, Briffa T, Sanfilippo FM, Ng JQ, McKnight C, Reynolds W, Gilles MC. Myocardial infarction after intravitreal vascular endothelial growth factor inhibitors: a whole population study. Retina. 2013;33(5):920–7.

97. Kessel L, Tendal B, Jørgensen KJ, Erngaard D, Flesner P, Andresen JL, Hjortdal J. Post-cataract prevention of inflammation and macular edema by steroid and nonsteroidal anti-inflammatory eye drops: a systematic review. Ophthalmology. 2014;121(10):1915–24.

98. Ng WY, Tan GS, Ong PG, Cheng CY, Cheung CY, Wong DW, Mathur R, Chow KY, Wong TY, Cheung GC. Incidence of myocardial infarction, stroke, and death in patients with age-related macular degeneration treated with intravitreal anti-vascular endothelial growth factor therapy. Am J Ophthalmol. 2015 Mar;159(3):557–64.e1.

99. Schmier JK, Covert DW, Hulme-Lowe CK, Mullins A, Mahlis EM. Treatment costs of cystoid macular edema among patients following cataract surgery. Clin Ophthalmol. 2016;16(10):477–83.

100. Spitzer MS, Ziemssen F, Yoeruek E, Petermeier K, Aisenbrey S, Szurman P. Efficacy of intravitreal bevacizumab in treating postoperative pseudophakic cystoid macular edema. J Cataract Refract Surg. 2008;34(1):70–5.

101. Harbour JW, Smiddy WE, Rubsamen PE, Murray TG, Davis JL, Flynn HW Jr. Pars plana vitrectomy for chronic pseudophakic cystoid macular edema. Am J Ophthalmol. 1995;120(3):302–7.

102. Kumagai K, Ogino N, Furukawa M, Demizu S, Atsumi K, Kurihara H. Vitrectomy for pseudophakic cystoid macular edema. Nippon Ganka Gakkai Zasshi. 2002;106(5):297–303.

103. Ismail RA, Sallam A, Zambarakji HJ. Pseudophakic macular edema and oral acetazolamide: an optical coherence tomography measurable, dose-related response. Eur J Ophthalmol. 2008;18(6):1011–3.

104. Pendergast SD, Margherio RR, Williams GA, Cox MS Jr. Vitrectomy for chronic pseudophakic cystoid macular edema. Am J Ophthalmol. 1999;128(3):317–23.

105. Pepple KL, Nguyen MH, Pakzad-Vaezi K, Williamson K, Odell N, Lee C, Leveque TK, Van Gelder RN. Response of inflammatory cystoid macular edema to treatment using oral acetazolamide. Retina. 2018. https://doi.org/10.1097/IAE.0000000000002044.

106. Ticly FG, Lira RP, Zanetti FR, Machado MC, Rodrigues GB, Arieta CE. Prophylactic use of ketorolac tromethamine in cataract surgery: a randomized trial. J Ocul Pharmacol Ther. 2014;30(6):495–501.

107. Deuter CM, Gelisken F, Stübiger N, Zierhut M, Doycheva D. Successful treatment of chronic pseudophakic macular edema (Irvine-Gass syndrome) with interferon alpha: a report of three cases. Ocul Immunol Inflamm. 2011;19(3):216–8.

108. Maleki A, Aghaei H, Lee S. Topical interferon alpha 2b in the treatment of refractory pseudophakic cystoid macular edema. Am J Ophthalmol Case Rep. 2018;10:203–5.

109. Wolf EJ, Braunstein A, Shih C, Braunstein RE. Incidence of visually significant pseudophakic macular edema after uneventful phacoemulsification in patients treated with nepafenac. J Cataract Refract Surg. 2007;33(9):1546–9.

110. Wu L, Arevalo JF, Hernandez-Bogantes E, Roca JA. Intravitreal infliximab for refractory pseudophakic cystoid macular edema: results of the Pan-American Collaborative Retina Study Group. Int Ophthalmol. 2012;32(3):235–43.

111. Grzybowski A. Re: Kessel et al.: post-cataract prevention of inflammation and macular edema by steroid and nonsteroidal anti-inflammatory eye drops: a systematic review (Ophthalmology. 2014;121:1915–24). Ophthalmology. 2015;122(2):e16–7.

112. https://clinicaltrials.gov/ct2/show/NCT01284478Ozurdex for Combined Pseudophakic Cystoid Macular Edema and Diabetic Macular Edema After Cataract Surgery. Accessed 29th September 2018.

Prophylaxis and Treatment of Endophthalmitis

Andrzej Grzybowski and Magdalena Turczynowska

Epidemiology of Endophthalmitis

Endophthalmitis is one of the most serious complications of ophthalmic surgery. It may cause severe visual acuity impairment, or even loss of the eye [1]. It can be divided into several categories depending upon the etiologic agent, the onset of symptoms, or the degree of inflammation. Postoperative endophthalmitis is defined as a serious inflammation due to an infectious process from bacteria or fungi that enter the eye during the perioperative period. Although any type of eye surgery could cause endophthalmitis, the highest incidence was observed after secondary IOL implantation [2]. Polypropylene loop supports have been associated with a greater chance of infection, as bacterial adherence to polypropylene exceeds that for other materials [3]. According to various studies, the incidence for endophthalmitis after cataract surgery in several European countries varies between 0.03 and 0.7% [4–16]. In 2012, the European Registry of Quality Outcomes for Cataract and Refractive Surgery (EUREQUO), has set the maximum acceptable value of incidence for postoperative endophthalmitis after cataract extractions at the level 0.05% [17]. Over the years, many improvements in technology, techniques, and procedures of cataract surgery have significantly reduced the incidence of postoperative endophthalmitis (POE). The most recent reports confirmed low incidence of POE, under 0.1% [18]. Endophthalmitis classically presents with severe acute ocular inflammation, decreased vision and

A. Grzybowski
Department of Ophthalmology, University of Warmia and Mazury, Olsztyn, Poland

Institute for Research in Ophthalmology, Foundation for Ophthalmology Development, Poznan, Poland

M. Turczynowska (✉)
Stefan Żeromski Specialist Municipal Hospital, Cracow, Poland
e-mail: m.turczynowska@gmail.com

pain 4–7 days after surgery. Depending on the causative organism it can develop very early—even 1 day after surgery in case of high-virulence microorganisms [19]. Acute-onset POE is most often caused by coagulase-negative staphylococci (CNS). In contrary, chronic postoperative endophthalmitis (caused by less virulent fungi or *Propionibacterium acnes*) can take several months to develop. The etiology of postoperative endophthalmitis is highly dependent on multiple geographical factors, and varies in different countries. Bacterial virulence level is the most important prognostic factor predictive of the final visual result. Streptococcal strains are often virulent, producing exotoxins, thus associated with poor visual outcome. The patient's periocular flora remains the most common source of sporadic postoperative infection.

The symptoms of POE may vary according to its severity. The most common include eye redness, pain, ocular discharge, blurred vision, and lid swelling [19]. It has been proved that surgical complications are related with higher incidence of postoperative endophthalmitis [4]. According to the ESCRS study, a higher risk of infection includes patients with clear corneal incisions (vs. scleral tunnel incisions), those with complications at the time of surgery (wound leak, capsular or zonular complication) and those without intracameral injection of cefuroxime. However, several large case series found no greater likelihood of infection with corneal versus other types of incisions [20]. After all, careful watertight incision construction and closure is obligatory, because the incidence of infection undoubtfully increases with wound leak. Also the type of IOL was considered as a risk factor, with the higher probability of endophthalmitis for silicone intraocular lens versus other materials [4], however this evidence is not consistent. Other factors associated with increased rates of endophthalmitis include prolonged surgical time, immunodeficiency, active blepharitis, lacrimal duct obstruction, inferior incision location, incomplete removal of lenticular cortex, male gender, older age, previous intraocular injections, and less experienced surgeons [20, 21]. Risk factors of postoperative endophthalmitis are presented in Table 1.

Table 1 Risk factors for postoperative endophthalmitis

Preoperative:	Older age
	Diabetes mellitus
	Blepharitis
	Use of corticosteroids
	Active systemic infection
Intraoperative:	No antiseptics/Failure to use topical PVI preparation
	Prolonged surgery
	Posterior capsular rupture (with/without vitreous loss)
Postoperative:	Noncompliance with treatment
	Wound leak
	Hypotony

Prophylaxis

Prophylaxis patterns against infectious postoperative endophthalmitis differ in several countries. This includes topical antibiotics before surgery, 5% povidone iodine to the conjunctival sac, skin disinfection with 10% povidone iodine, eyelid draping, antibiotics in the irrigating solutions, as an intracameral injection at the close of surgery, as subconjunctival injections, or applied topically after surgery [20]. According to the Cataract and Anterior Segment Preferred Practice Pattern Panel, the use of a 5% solution of povidone iodine in the conjunctival sac is strongly recommended to prevent infection. There is also mounting evidence that injecting intracameral antibiotics as a bolus at the conclusion of surgery is an efficacious method of endophthalmitis prophylaxis. The evidence supporting subconjunctival antibiotic prophylaxis is relatively weak, it is also associated with many risks that include pain, globe perforation, hemorrhage, and intraocular toxicity from subconjunctival leakage through the incision. As an alternative to intracameral or subconjunctival injection, topical antibiotic instillation may be more protective when initiated on the day of surgery instead of on the first postoperative day, however, it does increase antibiotic resistance. Due to the lack of sufficient evidence it is impossible to recommend any specific antibiotic drug or method of delivery for endophthalmitis prophylaxis. However, increasing evidence supports now the role of intracameral antibiotics [21].

Due to very low endophthalmitis rates after cataract surgery it is difficult to verify prophylactic algorithms. In 2013 the European Society of Cataract and Refractive Surgeons (ESCRS) has published guidelines on prevention and treatment of postoperative endophthalmitis [22]. These recommendations include performing surgical procedures in specially prepared operating rooms (proper air flow design, sterile and/or single-used equipment), hand washing with an antiseptic soap solution, mask, gown, and sterile gloves. Antisepsis of the periocular skin area, cornea, and conjunctival sac should be performed with topical povidone-iodine. The 5–10% povidone-iodine solution should be left in place at the skin surface for at least 3 min. In case of any contraindications (allergy or hyperthyroidism), the 0.05% solution of chlorhexidine may be used instead. ESCRS guidelines for prophylaxis of POE are listed in Table 2. It is preferred to use povidone-iodine

Table 2 ESCRS recommendations for prophylaxis of postcataract endophthalmitis

specially prepared operating theaters • proper air-flow design • sterile and/or single-used equipment
washing hands with an antiseptic soap solution
mask, gowning and sterile gloves
draping to cover eyelashes and lid margins
antisepsis of the periocular skin area, cornea and conjunctival sac with povidone–iodine
intracameral injection of 1 mg cefuroxime in 0.1 ml saline (0.9%) at the end of surgery

solution not containing any detergent as it can irreversibly coagulate the cornea. Administration of lidocaine gel prior to povidone iodine appears to diminish its antimicrobial efficacy. Application of povidone-iodine remains the only technique supported by level II evidence to reduce the incidence of endophthalmitis [23]. Even lower povidone iodine concentrations may be useful for the prevention of endophthalmitis. For ocular surface washing, the safe and highly bactericidal concentrations range from 0.05 to 5.0%. Repeated washing of the ocular surface with 0.25% povidone iodine every 20–30 seconds during ophthalmic surgeries was shown to be effective in eliminating the conjunctival flora, and minimizing the passage of bacteria into intraocular compartment [24]. Its use is simple, safe for the cornea, effective and inexpensive. Moreover, there have been no reports on resistance to PVI nor anaphylaxis in topical ophthalmic use, and it does not induce resistance or cross-resistance to antibiotics [25].

In 2007 the ESCRS published the results of the prospective study on perioperative prophylaxis of postoperative endophthalmitis. The study showed that intracameral injection of cefuroxime reduced fivefold the risk for contracting endophthalmitis following phacoemulsification cataract surgery [4]. In 2012 a specific commercial cefuroxime sodium at the necessary concentration (0.1 mg/mL) for intracameral use (Aprokam®) received approval by the European Medicines Agency (EMA) and was introduced to European market. By now it is officially approved for intracameral prophylaxis of postoperative endophthalmitis after cataract surgery in most European countries. Cefuroxime has a broad-spectrum of action, and covers most gram-positive and gram-negative organisms commonly associated with postoperative infectious endophthalmitis: Staphylococci and Streptococci (except methicillin resistant Staphylococcus aureus, MRSA; methicillin-resistant Staphylococcus epidermidis, MRSE; and Enterococcus faecalis), gram-negative bacteria (except Pseudomonas aeruginosa), and P. acnes. Until now, many other retrospective studies have also reported that intracameral injection of cefazolin, cefuroxime, or moxifloxacin have reduced the incidence of post-cataract endophthalmitis.

In many countries, where intracameral cefuroxime is not commercially available, surgeons opt for off-label, broad-spectrum fluoroquinolones. The number of reports regarding the safety of intracameral administration of moxifloxacin has increased [26–32]. The study published by Matsuura et al. has shown that intracameral moxifloxacin (50–500 mg/mL) administration 3-fold reduced the risk of endophthalmitis. In this study, intracameral moxifloxacin administration did not result in severe complications, such as toxic anterior segment syndrome or corneal endothelial cell loss [33]. In 2019, Melega et al. have published results of randomized controlled trial demonstrating safety and efficacy of intracameral moxifloxacin in post-cataract endophthalmitis risk reduction [34]. In a recently published study, Haripriya et al. statistically compared POE rates with and without intracameral moxifloxacin prophylaxis for phacoemulsification versus manual small-incision cataract surgery (M-SICS), and for a subgroup of eyes complicated by posterior capsule rupture (PCR) or requiring secondary surgery.

It was the largest series to date (of 2,062,643 consecutive eyes). The study has shown, that intracameral moxifloxacin was associated with a 3.5-fold POE rate reduction both overall and for M-SICS, and a 6-fold POE rate reduction for phacoemulsification [35].

Moxifloxacin has many advantages compared to cefuroxime as an antibiotic for intracameral injection. It offers a broader activity spectrum and a concentration-dependent action mechanism. Cefuroxime is time-dependent drug; therefore, as medication turnover after intracameral administration is rapid, moxifloxacin may be more effective than cefuroxime. Moxifloxacin also seems to be a better choice in patients with a documented IgE-mediated reaction to penicillin, when use of cephalosporins should be avoided, due to cross-reactivity between penicillins and cephalosporins (This is not true for Cefuroxime which has a different side-chain and has no cross-reactivity with Penicillin unlike the third generation Cephalosporins). Furthermore, commercial moxifloxacin (Vigamox) is preservative free, can be diluted and used directly for intracameral administration; complicated preparation procedures are not necessary [33].

Many practitioners also used intracameral vancomycin as prophylaxis against POE during routine cataract surgery [36]. However, a rare but visually devastating complication, hemorrhagic occlusive retinal vasculitis (HORV), has been recently reported. It is a complication of cataract surgery in which vancomycin prophylaxis was used. Presentation is delayed, with a mean onset of symptoms 8 days after the procedure, and it is associated with retinal hemorrhages, vascular nonperfusion and venous sheathing [37, 38]. Although the precise cause still remains unknown, this condition is thought to represent a delayed immune reaction similar to vancomycin-induced leukocytoclastic vasculitis. Despite treatment with high-dose corticosteroids, antiviral medication, and early vitrectomy in many patients, visual outcomes were poor in this series [37, 38]. Based on above finding, the use of vancomycin for endophthalmitis prophylaxis is now strongly discouraged [21]. It should be emphasized, that all of the studies assessing the effectiveness of intracameral antibiotics in POE prophylaxis were based on endophthalmitis rate greater than 0.05%. It is not clear if it is possible to achieve similar results with lower endophthalmitis rate.

The use of topical antibiotics preoperatively and/or postoperatively does not have any specific benefit over the use of povidone iodine or chlorhexidine preoperatively and over intracameral antibiotics injected at the close of surgery [22]. It is also difficult to obtain perfect patient compliance with drop regimens, as they remain complex and can be difficult for patients to understand (especially older ones, those with dementia or cognitive difficulties). Moreover, the high cost of some of the prescribed agents may encourage patients not to fill all of the prescriptions. The consequence of noncompliance are complications after surgery, and also development of antibiotic resistance. Nowadays, there have been proposed some new approaches that reduce the need for topical therapy. They include intracameral injection, sustained or slow-release drug delivery mechanisms, and the recently introduced "Dropless cataract surgery," which involves intravitreal injection of single-use, compounded combination of antibiotics and corticosteroids

[39]. Unlike direct intracameral antibiotic injection, there are no corresponding studies to support the efficacy of placing antibiotics in the irrigation bottle, as in this case the intraocular antibiotic concentration and duration are unpredictable.

Intravenous antibiotics do not penetrate effectively in a non-inflamed eye, and thus are not recommended. Certain oral fluoroquinolone antibiotics penetrate the blood/ocular barrier adequately to reach levels above the minimum inhibitory concentrations for many organisms inside the eye, and oral antibiotics that penetrate well into the eye may be used selectively [20]. Oral antibiotic prophylaxis is recommended only in cases of coexisting severe atopic disease and lid margins colonization with Staphylococcus aureus [22].

The evidence supporting subconjunctival antibiotic prophylaxis is relatively weak. As an alternative to intracameral injection, topical antibiotics may be used. It is recommended to initiate therapy on the day of surgery instead of on the first postoperative day. Due to the lack of sufficiently large prospective clinical trials, nowadays, there is insufficient evidence to recommend a specific antibiotic drug or method of delivery for endophthalmitis prophylaxis. However, increasing evidence supports the role of intracameral antibiotic use.

Diagnosis and Treatment

Accurate diagnosis of POE and immediate treatment are crucial to achieve optimal clinical results with recovery of useful vision. The differential diagnosis includes toxic anterior segment syndrome (TASS), retained lens material in the anterior chamber or vitreous, vitreous hemorrhage, postoperative uveitis, and viral retinitis. Table 3 summarizes the differentiating features between infectious endophthalmitis and TASS. In case of any doubt, even when the cultures are negative, patients should always be regarded as having infectious endophthalmitis and immediately treated.

Clinical diagnosis of endophthalmitis requires further microbiological exams: gram stain, culture, or PCR. The samples for culture should be obtained from aqueous and vitreous. 0.1–0.2 mL of aqueous should be aspirated via limbal paracentesis during the anterior chamber tap using a 25-gauge needle. Vitreous samples might be obtained by either needle tap, vitreous biopsy, or pars plana vitrectomy (PPV).

Published in 1995 the Endophthalmitis Vitrectomy Study (EVS) recommended vitrectomy for patients with light perception only [1], however more recent studies have shown that early vitrectomy is beneficial also for patients with better visual acuity [40–42]. According to ESCRS guidelines, vitrectomy performed by a vitreoretinal surgeon remains a gold standard of treatment of acute POE, as it allows obtaining larger sample of vitreous, and at the same time removes bacterial load in the vitreous [22]. The decision whether or not to perform surgery should be taken each time individually, taking into account rather the clinical appearance and course, than the presenting vision alone. In case vitrectomy is not possible to

Table 3 Characteristics of Endophthalmitis vs TASS

	Endophthalmitis	TASS
Cause	Bacterial, fungal, or viral infection	Noninfectious reaction to toxic agent present in BSS solution/ Antibiotic injection/Endotoxin/ Residue Gram stain and culture negative
Onset	4–7 days	12–24 h
Signs/symptoms	• Significantly decreased VA • Pain • Lid swelling with edema • Conjunctival injection, hyperemia • Marked AC inflammatory response with hypopyon	• Blurry vision • Pain (mild to moderate) • Diffuse corneal edema • Dilated, irregular • Nonreactive pupil • Increased IOP • Mild to severe AC reaction with cells, flare, hypopyon, fibrin
Vitreous involvement	• Vitreous involvement present	• Signs and symptoms limited to anterior chamber (no vitreous involvement)
Treatment	• Intravitreal and topical antibiotics • Vitrectomy in selected cases	• Intensive corticosteroids

perform immediately, the vitreous biopsy with a vitreous cutter, not with a syringe and needle should be performed. Subsequently, antibiotics should be injected intravitreally and repeated as necessary according to the clinical response at intervals of 48–72 h. Just after collecting samples of infected vitreous, intravitreal injection of antibiotics should be performed.

According to ESCRS guidelines, a first choice combination of antibiotics is vancomycin 1 mg in 0.1 mL and ceftazidime 2.25 mg in 0.1 ml. Amikacin 400 μg in 0.1 mL and vancomycin 1 mg in 0.1 mL remain second choice option. Each drug should be injected from separate syringe and 30 G needle. At the same time, 400 μg of preservative-free dexamethasone may also be injected into the vitreous. In case of severe acute purulent endophthalmitis, additional systemic antibiotic therapy with the same drugs used for intravitreal injections should be considered for 48 h, with optional systemic therapy with corticosteroids (prednisolone 1 or even 2 mg/kg/day) [22].

References

1. Endophthalmitis Vitrectomy Study Group. Results of the Endophthalmitis Vitrectomy Study. A randomized trial of immediate vitrectomy and of intravenous antibiotics for the treatment of postoperative bacterial endophthalmitis. Arch Ophthalmol. 1995;113(12):1479–96.
2. Aaberg TM Jr, Flynn HW Jr, Schiffman J, Newton J. Nosocomial acute-onset postoperative endophthalmitis survey. A 10-year review of incidence and outcomes. Ophthalmology. 1998;105(6):1004–10.

3. Patwardhan A, Rao GP, Saha K, Craig EA. Incidence and outcomes evaluation of endophthalmitis management after phacoemulsification and 3-piece silicone intraocular lens implantation over 6 years in a single eye unit. J Cataract Refract Surg. 2006;32:1018–21.
4. Endophthalmitis Study Group, European Society of Cataract & Refractive Surgeons. Prophylaxis of postoperative endophthalmitis following cataract surgery: results of the ESCRS multicenter study and identification of risk factors. J Cataract Refract Surg. 2007;33(6):978–88.
5. Romero P, Méndez I, Salvat M, Fernández J, Almena M. Intracameral cefazolin as prophylaxis against endophthalmitis in cataract surgery. J Cataract Refract Surg. 2006;32(3):438–41.
6. Yu-Wai-Man P, Morgan SJ, Hildreth AJ, Steel DH, Allen D. Efficacy of intracameral and subconjunctival cefuroxime in preventing endophthalmitis after cataract surgery. J Cataract Refract Surg. 2008;34(3):447–51.
7. Garat M, Moser CL, Martín-Baranera M, Alonso-Tarrés C, Alvarez-Rubio L. Prophylactic intracameral cefazolin after cataract surgery: endophthalmitis risk reduction and safety results in a 6-year study. J Cataract Refract Surg. 2009;35(4):637–42.
8. García-Sáenz MC, Arias-Puente A, Rodríguez-Caravaca G, Bañuelos JB. Effectiveness of intracameral cefuroxime in preventing endophthalmitis after cataract surgery Ten-year comparative study. J Cataract Refract Surg. 2010;36(2):203–7.
9. Barreau G, Mounier M, Marin B, Adenis JP, Robert PY. Intracameral cefuroxime injection at the end of cataract surgery to reduce the incidence of endophthalmitis: French study. J Cataract Refract Surg. 2012;38(8):1370–5.
10. Friling E, Lundström M, Stenevi U, Montan P. Six-year incidence of endophthalmitis after cataract surgery: Swedish national study. J Cataract Refract Surg. 2013;39(1):15–21.
11. Rodríguez-Caravaca G, García-Sáenz MC, Villar-Del-Campo MC, Andrés-Alba Y, AriasPuente A. Incidence of endophthalmitis and impact of prophylaxis with cefuroxime on cataract surgery. J Cataract Refract Surg. 2013;39(9):1399–403.
12. Beselga D, Campos A, Castro M, Fernandes C, Carvalheira F, Campos S, Mendes S, Neves A, Campos J, Violante L, Sousa JC. Postcataract surgery endophthalmitis after introduction of the ESCRS protocol: a 5-year study. Eur J Ophthalmol. 2014;24(4):516–9.
13. Rahman N, Murphy CC. Impact of intracameral cefuroxime on the incidence of postoperative endophthalmitis following cataract surgery in Ireland. Ir J Med Sci. 2015;184(2):395–8.
14. Lundström M, Friling E, Montan P. Risk factors for endophthalmitis after cataract surgery: predictors for causative organisms and visual outcomes. J Cataract Refract Surg. 2015;41(11):2410–6. 5 Epidemiology of Endophthalmitis and Treatment Trend in Europe 54.
15. Creuzot-Garcher C, Benzenine E, Mariet AS, de Lazzer A, Chiquet C, Bron AM, Quantin C. Incidence of acute postoperative endophthalmitis after cataract surgery: a nationwide study in France from 2005 to 2014. Ophthalmology. 2016;123(7):1414–20.
16. Daien V, Papinaud L, Gillies MC, Domerg C, Nagot N, Lacombe S, Daures JP, Carriere I, Villain M. Effectiveness and safety of an intracameral injection of cefuroxime for the prevention of endophthalmitis after cataract surgery with or without perioperative capsular rupture. JAMA Ophthalmol. 2016;134(7):810–6.
17. Lundström M, Barry P, Henry Y, Rosen P, Stenevi U. Evidence-based guidelines for cataract surgery: guidelines based on data in the European Registry of Quality Outcomes for Cataract and Refractive Surgery database. J Cataract Refract Surg. 2012;38(6):1086–93.
18. Flynn HW, Batra NR, Schwartz SG, Grzybowski A. Differential Diagnosis of Endophthalmitis. In: Flynn HW, Batra NR, Schwartz SG, Grzybowski A, editors. Endophthalmitis in clinical practice. Cham, Switzerland: Springer International Publishing AG; 2018. p. 19–40.
19. Endophthalmitis Vitrectomy Study Group. Results of the Endophthalmitis Vitrectomy Study. Arch Ophthal. 1995;113(12):1479–96.
20. Keay L, Gower EW, Cassard SD, et al. Postcataract surgery endophthalmitis in the United States: analysis of the complete 2003 to 2004 Medicare database of cataract surgeries. Ophthalmology. 2012;119:914–22.

21. Olson RJ, Braga-Mele R, Chen SH, Miller KM, Pineda R, Tweeten JP, Musch DC. Cataract in the adult eye preferred practice pattern®. Ophthalmology. 2017;2(124):P1–119.

22. ESCRS guidelines on prevention and treatment of endophthalmitis following cataract surgery [webpage on the Internet]. The European Society for Cataract and Refractive Surgeons; 2013. http://www.escrs.org/endophthalmitis/guidelines/ENGLISH.pdf.

23. Schwartz SG, Flynn HW Jr, Grzybowski A, et al. Intracameral antibiotics and cataract surgery: endophthalmitis rates, costs, and stewardship. Ophthalmology. 2016;123:1411–3.

24. Shimada H, Nakashizuka H, Grzybowski A. Prevention and treatment of postoperative endophthalmitis using povidone-iodine. Curr Pharm Des. 2017;23(4):574–85.

25. Grzybowski A, Kanclerz P, Myers WG. The use of povidone-iodine in ophthalmology. Curr Opin Ophthalmol. 2018;29(1):19–32.

26. Espiritu CRG, Caparas VL, Bolinao JG. Safety of prophylactic intracameral moxifloxacin 0.5% ophthalmic solution in cataract surgery patients. J Cataract Refract Surg. 2007;33:63–8.

27. Kim S-Y, Park Y-H, Lee Y-C. Comparison ofthe effect of intracameral moxifloxacin, levofloxacin and cefazolin on rabbit corneal endothelial cells. Clin Exp Ophthalmol. 2008;36:367–70.

28. Lane SS, Osher RH, Masket S, Belani S. Evaluation of the safety of prophylactic intracameral moxifloxacin in cataract surgery. J Cataract Refract Surg. 2008;34:1451–9.

29. O'Brien TP, Arshinoff SA, Mah FS. Perspectives on antibiotics for postoperative endophthalmitis prophylaxis: potential role of moxifloxacin. J Cataract Refract Surg. 2007;33:1790–800.

30. Arbisser LB. Safety of intracameral moxifloxacin for prophylaxis of endophthalmitis after cataract surgery. J Cataract Refract Surg. 2008;34:1114–20.

31. Matsuura K, Suto C, Akura J, Inoue Y. Bag and chamber flushing: a new method of using intracameral moxifloxacin to irrigate the anterior chamber and the area behind the intraocular lens. Graefes Arch Clin Exp Ophthalmol. 2013;251:81–7.

32. Haripriya A, Chang DF, Ravindran RD. Endophthalmitis reduction with intracameral moxifloxacin prophylaxis: analysis of 600 000 surgeries. Ophthalmology. 2017;124:768–75.

33. Matsuura K, Miyoshi T, Suto C, Akura J, Inoue Y. Efficacy and safety of prophylactic intracameral moxifloxacin injection in Japan. J Cataract Refract Surg. 2013;39(11):1702–6.

34. Melega MV, Alves M, Lira RPC, et al. Safety and efficacy of intracameral moxifloxacin for prevention of post-cataract endophthalmitis: randomized controlled clinical trial. J Cataract Refract Surg. 2019;45(3):343–50.

35. Haripriya A, Chang DF, Ravindran RD. Endophthalmitis reduction with intracameral moxifloxacin in eyes with and without surgical complications: Results from 2 million consecutive cataract surgeries. J Cataract Refract Surg. 2019;45(9):1226–33.

36. Chang DF, Braga-Mele R, Henderson BA, Mamalis N, et al. Antibiotic prophylaxis of postoperative endophthalmitis after cataract surgery: Results of the 2014 ASCRS member survey. J Cataract Refract Surg. 2015;41:1300–5.

37. Witkin AJ, Shah AR, Engstrom RE, et al. Postoperative hemorrhagic occlusive retinal vasculitis: expanding the clinical spectrum and possible association with vancomycin. Ophthalmology. 2015;122:1438–51.

38. Witkin AJ, Chang DF, Michael Jumper J, Charles S, Eliott D, Hoffman RS, Mamalis N, Miller KM, Wykoff CC. Vancomycin-associated hemorrhagic occlusive retinal vasculitis. Ophthalmology. 2017;124:583–95.

39. Lindstrom RL, Galloway MS, Grzybowski A, Liegner JT. Dropless cataract surgery: an overview. Curr Pharm Des. 2017;23(4):558–64.

40. Kuhn F, Gini G. Ten years after … are findings of the Endophthalmitis Vitrectomy Study still relevant today? Graefes Arch Clin Exp Ophthalmol. 2005;243(12):1197–9.

41. Kuhn F, Gini G. Vitrectomy for endophthalmitis. Ophthalmology. 2006;113:714.

42. Grzybowski A, Turczynowska M, Kuhn F. The treatment of postoperative endophthalmitis: should we still follow the endophthalmitis vitrectomy study more than two decades after its publication? Acta Ophthalmol. 2018;96(5):e651–4.

Posterior Capsule Opacification

Matthew McDonald

Introduction

Half of global blindness is caused by cataract [1]. This light scattering reduction in transparency of the lens is only amenable by means of surgery, which may initially restore high visual quality. Unfortunately, posterior capsule opacification (PCO), the most common complication of cataract surgery, develops in a significant proportion of patients which can lead to vision loss.

PCO arises after a number of weeks to many years. Occurring in up to half of patients post-operatively, younger patients or those with inflammatory ocular conditions are at highest risk. After a cataract procedure, when the intra-ocular lens (IOL) is inserted into the lens capsule, lens epithelial cells on the anterior capsule remain despite the rigors of surgical trauma. This resilient group of cells then colonise the previously cell-free posterior capsule as a form of wound healing response. A thin cover of cells is insufficient to affect the light path, but subsequent changes to their extracellular matrix and cellular organisation give rise to light scatter (particularly through capsule wrinkling) and clinically significant visual deterioration. A fibroblastic transformation takes place, causing capsular fibrosis or Elschnig pearls (a morphological subtype of PCO—*see topic below*). If these changes are sufficiently severe, corrective laser surgery is required (specifically using the Nd:YAG laser) which is both expensive and entails risk (e.g. corneal oedema, iritis, lens dislocation, macular oedema).

Economic analysis of the burden of PCO shows that in the United States alone, Nd:YAG laser capsulotomy procedures cost $158,000,000 USD in 2003 [2]. Square-edge IOL design (e.g. AMO Tecnis), lowered the above sum from even higher in previous years. Current figures in 2020 will be higher due to population rise and ageing population, despite significant advancements in IOL design (Figs. 1 and 2).

M. McDonald (✉)
Department of Ophthalmology, University of Auckland, Auckland, New Zealand
e-mail: drmattmcd@gmail.com

Humane Research Trust, Norfolk and Norwich University Hospital Trust, Norwich, UK

© Springer Nature Switzerland AG 2021
C. Liu and A. Shalaby Bardan (eds.), *Cataract Surgery*,
https://doi.org/10.1007/978-3-030-38234-6_12

Fig. 1 Posterior capsule opacification. Appearance of fibrotic morphological subtype at slit lamp view. *Reproduced with permission from Eyerounds.org, University of Iowa, USA. Author: Doan, A.*

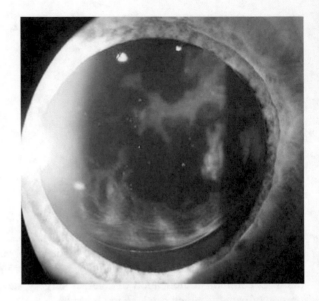

Fig. 2 Posterior capsule opacification. Appearance on retroillumination at slit lamp view. *Reproduced with permission from Eyerounds. org, University of Iowa, USA. Author: Doan, A.*

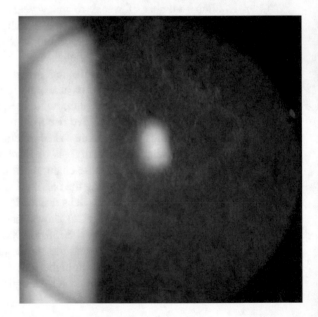

Biological Processes Behind PCO

Posterior capsule opacification (PCO) is a fibrotic disorder with a complex pathophysiology. In sequence of key events:

1. Survival of lens epithelial cells post-surgical trauma
2. Proliferation of lens epithelial cells
3. Migration from the anterior capsule and equatorial regions to the posterior capsule, encroaching upon the visual axis
4. Transdifferentiation to myofibroblast phenotype
5. Extracellular matrix (ECM) deposition
6. Extracellular matrix contraction (leading to characteristic 'wrinkling' seen on the posterior capsule under high magnification).

Understanding the biochemical mechanisms regulating these events increases our knowledge of PCO and aids the development of strategies to prevent or treat it.

Fibrosis, generally speaking, is a pathological process which disrupts a tissue's architecture by excessive fibroconnective tissue, typically in response to a reparative or reactive response to a cellular insult [3, 4]. From metabolic malfunction, ischaemia, degeneration, or autoimmune inflammatory processes, the cellular infiltration involved in these processes leads to proliferation and transdifferentiation of a cellular phenotype (e.g. epithelial cells) to activated fibroblasts, called myofibroblasts, which contribute to 'excessive' production of extra-cellular matrix (ECM), leading to contraction and disruption of tissue architecture [3].

Cell Survival, Proliferation, and Growth Factor Signalling

PCO begins with the trauma of surgical instrumentation within the eye. The population of lens epithelial cells which remain after IOL implantation, predominantly on the anterior lens capsule and equatorial region, orchestrate the subsequent wound-healing response of PCO through cellular signaling.

The blood-aqueous barrier is breached through surgery, causing the release of cytokines and growth factors. As this occurs, lens cells release matrix metalloproteases, MMPs, which cleave capsule-bound growth factors (Figs. 3, 4 and 5).

Each fibrotic process in the eye shares fundamental factors that propagate the wound-healing response and subsequent pathology. Thrombin, HGF (hepatocyte growth factor), EGF (epidermal growth factor), PDGF (platelet-derived growth factor), FGF (fibroblast growth factor) all lead to survival, proliferation, and migration, while FGF also enables cellular differentiation to myofibroblast phenotype. Transforming growth factor-beta (TGF-β) remains the key player for transdifferentiation and matrix contraction, which signals through its well-recognised *smad* signaling pathway. TGF-β2, in particular, induces transdifferentiation to myofibroblast phenotype. It will also influence matrix deposition and contraction (TGF-β1 subtype), while PDGF stimulates fibronectin, glycosaminoglycans (GAG), and hyaluronic acid production in fibroblasts. However, there are other, possibly unknown, factors and differential signaling mechanisms behind matrix

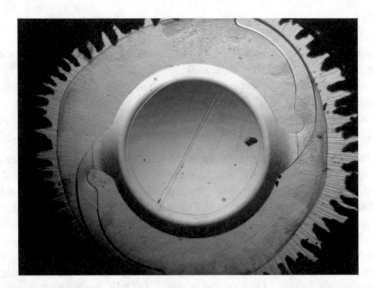

Fig. 3 Phase-contrast microscope view of an in vitro bag-zonular-ciliary body complex isolated from donor globes, suspended in culture medium, with an IOL inserted to study the effects of PCO. The image above illustrates residual lens epithelial cells in the equatorial regions with a silhouette of the ciliary body, lens zonules, and lens capsule containing the IOL. *Image taken with Professor I. M. Wormstone, University of East Anglia, UK*

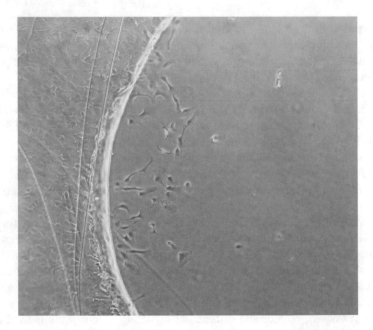

Fig. 4 Phase-contrast microscope view. The same in vitro bag-zonular-ciliary body complex isolated from donor globes from Fig. 3, in greater magnification along the rhexis edge, shows lens epithelial cell migration across the posterior capsule over the rhexis edge, encroaching upon the visual axis in the early stages of PCO. *Image taken by author with Professor I. M. Wormstone, University of East Anglia, UK*

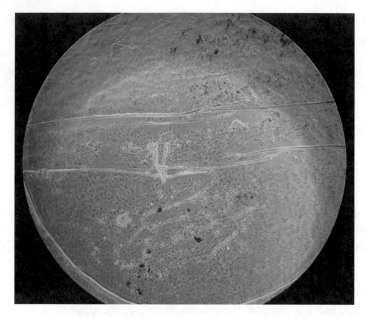

Fig. 5 Phase-contrast microscope view in Professor I. M. Wormstone's laboratory, *University of East Anglia, UK.* This in vitro bag-zonular-ciliary body complex (identical culture to Figs. 3 and 4, but four weeks later) illustrates well established PCO, with lens epithelial cell proliferation and subsequent development of extracellular matrix contraction ('furrowing' of capsule), obstructing the visual axis

contraction which is the end result of advanced lens epithelial cell proliferation and gives rise to the end stage of PCO.

Recent studies have cast the net further to identify more compounds involved in fibrosis, such as VEGF [6]. It has been proven that an active VEGF-A signalling system is functioning in the lens in all stages of development [7]. Assessment of medium from human lens capsular bag cultures have demonstrated high levels of VEGF relative to other growth factors and potentially mediated by IL-10. In fact, levels were >10 fold more than detected for basic FGF [8]. It has been proven that treatment of cells with TGF-β, EGF, PDGF, and IL-6 induce VEGF mRNA production, suggesting that paracrine or autocrine release of these compounds works with hypoxic conditions in regulating VEGF, which is known to bind to heparin sulphate proteoglycans (HSPGs) on the lens capsule, facilitating PCO changes over time.

A recent study shed light on other growth factors, such as interleukins IL-1ra, IL-8, IL-10, IL-12(p70 subtype), IL-15, IP-10 (interferon-γ-inducible protein 10), MCP-1 (monocyte chemoattractant protein-1), and MIP-1β (macrophage inflammatory protein-1 beta) [6]. Many of these cytokines have been associated with cellular proliferation and other fibrotic conditions.

The extra-cellular matrix and saturation of growth factors typically exists in a closed environment with traditional 'in-the-bag' IOLs. Irrigation of the capsular bag when left open facilitates 'aqueous wash' which is accomplished with new 'open-bag' IOL designs, limiting PCO development to such an extent that its progression is directly related to how far apart the capsules are from one another (not only for cellular proliferation, but also for markers of transdifferentiation) [6]. This in-vitro study with a fully open capsular bag (all edges reflected flat in culture medium) prevented PCO altogether, further supporting the idea that PCO is driven through concentrated growth factor signaling in a closed system.

Epithelial to Mesenchymal Transition

In epithelial to mesenchymal transition (EMT), which all fibrotic processes share, epithelial cells experience a multitude of biochemical and morphological changes, disconnecting themselves from their basal surface and basement membrane to migrate, resist apoptosis, and produce ECM components. The resulting mesenchymal cell leaves the epithelial layer from which it originated and turns myofibroblastic [9].

In PCO, there is loss of E-cadherin from epithelial cells, a key event in EMT, causing a transition to a mesenchymal phenotype which enables migration across the posterior capsule, obscuring the visual axis. This occurs with an upregulation of N-cadherin, Vimentin, and α-SMA (alpha-smooth muscle actin), an important marker for fibroblast-myofibroblast conversion and a marker of matrix contraction [9–12]. Factors that bind to the E-cadherin promoter to inhibit its transcription include the zinc finger proteins, Snail and Slug signalling pathway (Snail1 and Snail2), which induces EMT with zinc finger E-box-binding (ZEB1/2) and Smads to promote Wnt signalling and α-SMA expression [9]. These early points in EMT destabilise communication between epithelial cells as gap junctions are compromised and desmosomes interrupted (Fig. 6). Groups of actin microfilaments form the basis of the contractile apparatus of myofibroblasts which terminate in the fibronexus (mature focal adhesions). This adhesion complex uses transmembrane integrins to connect intracellular actin to extracellular fibronectin domains. This results in a mechanotransduction system (converting mechanical stimulus to biochemical activity) which transmits forces created by stress fibres to the encompassing extracellular matrix, resulting in contraction and disruption to tissue organisation [13].

Elschnig Pearls

Elschnig pearls are a morphological subtype of PCO and remain an important cause behind post-operative visual decline (Fig. 7). This regenerative subtype of PCO is thought to be an attempt at lens fibre production from residual lens

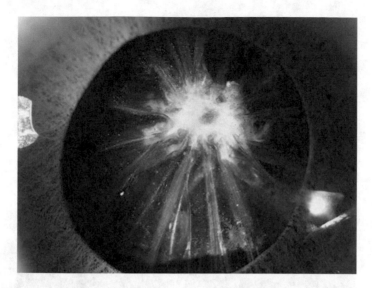

Fig. 6 Slit lamp view. This patient received an iris-sutured posterior chamber IOL which was chosen due to zonular weakness. Iris pigment deposition is noticeable on the anterior lens capsule with dramatic capsular phimosis one month post-op and radial folds. This was later treated with Nd:YAG anterior capsulotomy. *Reproduced with permission from Eyerounds.org, University of Iowa, USA. Authors: Vislisel, J., Critser, B.*

epithelial cells, but this is debated. Due to lack of normal lenticular pressure, remaining lens epithelial cells form globular and spherical shapes, either basally elongated with microvilli or completely smooth on microscopy. In 1993, Sveinsson and colleagues published an article on the ultrastructure of Elschnig pearls to understand their aetiology [14]. Their group documented nuclei which range from oval-shape to lobulated with the occasional vesicular body. They rapidly change, often enlarging then disappearing before reappearing again. Thought to be caused by osmotic variation and apoptosis following years of cell migration and proliferation, these dynamic changes remain an area of further research. Clinically, Elschnig pearls behave like cysts, but they contain material with a higher refractive index than neighbouring tissue, which means they could be filled with lens fibre material and unsaturated lipids [15]. Interestingly, a transmission electron microscope (TEM) has been used to examine Elschnig pearls on a Millipore filter [16]. This group of researchers theorised that Elschnig pearls are biophysical products of lens fibre degradation of *no* cellular origin. In support of this theory, formations similar to these have been found in some forms of cataract.

Nd:YAG capsulotomies [*see section on 'Treatment of PCO' below*] in eyes with this form of PCO shed light on their behaviour, leading to an increased rate of disappearance around capsulotomy margins. This is thought to be due to less contact pressure between the IOL and posterior capsule, which typically facilitates migration. Or perhaps they fall into the vitreous cavity after migrating over the capsulotomy margin? The force behind the Nd:YAG's laser shockwave is another possible

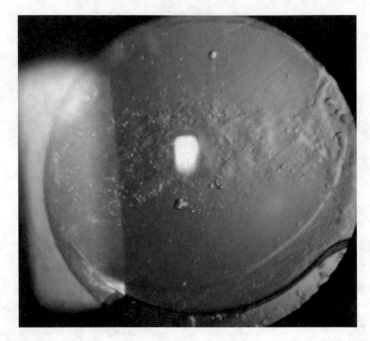

Fig. 7 Elschnig Pearls. Slit lamp view. *Reproduced with permission from Eyerounds.org, University of Iowa, USA. Author: Bhatti, S., of Bhatti Eye Clinic*

mechanism behind their disappearance. Pearls that do remain on the capsulotomy margin have been termed "pearl strings", which remain particularly stubborn and proliferate further over time. Whichever theory (or combination thereof) may be correct, it is important to focus on preventing them in the first instance (Fig. 7).

Prevention of PCO

Historically, Nishi [17] reported that PCO incidence was reduced by closer apposition of the IOL to the posterior capsule status post implantation. Nishi and colleagues found that the posterior chamber lens suppressed the migration of LECs toward the centre of the capsule and also suppressed development of a ring-shaped opacity at the site of contact between the posterior capsule and the anterior capsule rim. Fixation of the posterior chamber lens within the bag enhanced these suppressive effects. This represents the no-space, no-cell theory. The posterior convexity of the IOL (particularly with square-edge design) and posterior vaulting of the IOL with resultant pressure on the posterior capsule due to anteriorly angulated haptics has helped. There is a competing theory advocating an 'open bag' approach which argues separation of the anterior and posterior capsule allows for dilution of growth factors which prevents PCO from developing altogether [*further detail under 'IOL Design'*].

IOL Material

Biconvex and planoconvex polymethylmethacrylate (PMMA) IOLs were found to have a beneficial effect on PCO in early studies [18–20]. Additional benefits were observed when utilising silicone plate haptic IOLs [21] and biomaterials such as Alcon AcrySof material (hydrophobic acrylic). The 'sandwich' theory, originally hypothesised by Dr. Linnola, states that an IOL composed of bioadhesive material will stick firmly to the posterior capsule, preventing anything more than a monolayer of lens epithelial cells from proliferating. As such, research ensued to study the bioadhesive properties of different IOL materials [22]. Hydrophobic acrylic lenses produced the strongest results (bound strongest to fibronectin on the lens capsule), followed by PMMA IOLs, silicone, and lastly hydrophilic acrylic IOLs. Interestingly, collagen type IV, which is found to be associated with anterior capsule phimosis and fairly aggressive fibrotic change, had a predilection for silicon IOLs.

IOL Design

PCO rates further declined with the introduction of square edge optics of the posterior surface, which allow a sharp bend on the capsule, making it difficult for LECs to migrate under the optic ('**sandwich theory**'). With square-edge design, rates of PCO declined despite choice of material. However, scanning electron microscope studies have shown that hydrophobic acrylic still have the sharpest lens edges [23]. Efforts have since focused on creating the best edges possible to exert a maximal force to prevent cellular migration. Despite these square edge designs, these edges may eventually be breached, resulting in victory for lens epithelial cell migration.

Contrary to the sandwich theory (lens capsule 'shrink wrap' over an IOL), the **open-bag theory** of PCO supports the idea that with greater space between the anterior and posterior capsule, greater inhibition of PCO occurs. A study in Scientific Reports supports such a theory [6]. Separation of the anterior and posterior capsule increases levels of aqueous humour, 'washing out' growth factors which lead to their dilution (these are normally upregulated following the traumas of cataract surgery, as mentioned previously). Another theory, which supports bulkier designs, shows that mechanical stretch and compression of the lens capsule in all regions results in a general (albeit mechanical) inhibitory effect. This may hold true for the FluidVision IOL (Powervision Inc.), which has fluid-filled haptics allowing for up to five dioptres of accommodation in patients, provided their lens capsules do not fibrose. Silicon oil in large haptic components flow back and forth between the optic to dynamically modify IOL curvature and therefore spherical power (Fig. 8).

The Zephyr® IOL (Anew Optics, Inc.) is unique in that it supports the theory of open-bag design with complete separation of anterior and posterior capsule from the optic, which suggests a tight seal against the posterior capsule is not

Fig. 8 Fluidvision
IOL. *Images courtesy of*
Powervision, Inc., Belmont,
California, USA

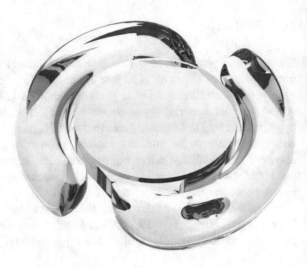

necessarily essential for PCO prevention. Endocapsular flow is facilitated through its design. Eventually, full inhibition of fibrosis and maintenance of an open-bag may prove essential for accommodative IOLs which restore the natural physiology of lens/lens capsule behaviour.

Capsular Tension Rings and Endocapsular Equator Rings

Capsular tension rings (CTRs) have been employed historically to maintain an open bag design and to 'stretch' the lens capsule, preventing wrinkling in PCO. Hara et al. [24], published long term data advocating the use of endocapsular equator rings ("E-Rings"), which separate the anterior capsule from the posterior capsule with an IOL implanted in the middle. This reduced PCO rates dramatically, with none of their patients requiring YAG capsulotomy by 7 years (compared to 45% YAG rate in control group).

Capsular tension rings, which differ from E-rings, have also been used in patients with weak zonules and have also proven modestly effective in PCO prevention. Small incision phacoemulsification with the insertion of an IOL in complicated cataract cases was made significantly safer with the advent of capsular tension rings (CTRs) [25]. Indications for CTRs are any condition compromising zonular integrity [26].

These include (and are not limited to):

- Marfan's syndrome
- Homocysteinuria
- Syphilis
- Congenital ectopia lentis
- Zonular trauma

- Marchesani's syndrome
- Scleroderma
- Porphyria
- Hyperlysinemia
- Hyperlipoproteinemia
- Sulfite oxidase deficiency.

Contraindications include compromised capsular bag integrity, in addition to posterior capsule rupture (beware posterior polar cataracts). CTRs may be implanted before or after phacoemulsification. Early trials inserted CTRs after hydrodissection (resulting in cortical cleaving), prior to phacoemulsification. Although every patient is unique and surgeons have their own preferences, it is more common today to dial a CTR into place (using forceps or the Geuder AG injector) after phacoemulsification [26] (Figs. 9 and 10).

Importantly, capsular tension rings also lead to less anterior capsule fibrosis (increased risk with intraocular inflammation, small rhexis, weak zonules) (Fig. 11).

Inhibition of Cell Growth Using Chemical Agents

In 1988, a study pioneered the evaluation of pharmacologic agents in relation to the in vitro inhibition of LEC proliferation and migration in PCO [27]. The research determined that drugs were capable of inhibiting LEC growth and/or migration and were efficacious in the prevention of PCO (thapsigargan, in particular) [28].

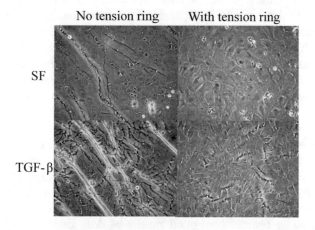

Fig. 9 Phase-contrast microscopy (10x magnification) showing coverage of the central posterior capsule of human donor eyes at endpoint (day 28), in both serum-free (SF) medium (top row) and with the addition of TGF-β2 (bottom row), in the presence (right side) and absence of CTR (left side). No CTR showed more furrowing of the lens capsule compared to intervention, which would prove clinically significant. *Images courtesy of Professor C. Liu and Professor I. M. Wormstone, University of East Anglia, UK*

No tension   With tension

SF

TGF-β

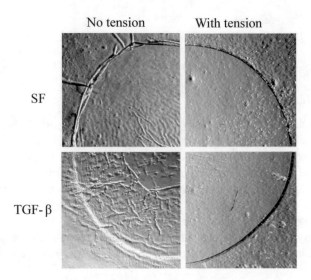

Fig. 10 Low-power phase-contrast microscopy shows coverage of the posterior capsule (in representative quarters) of human donor eyes at endpoint (day 28), in both serum-free (SF) medium (top row) and with the addition of TGF-β (bottom row), in the presence (right side) and absence of CTR (left side). As shown previously in higher magnification, no CTR showed more furrowing of the lens capsule compared to intervention, which would prove clinically significant. *Images courtesy of Professor C. Liu and Professor I. M. Wormstone, University of East Anglia, UK*

A number of pharmacological agents have been previously proposed to inhibit lens cell growth that leads to PCO, including 5-fluorouracil, daunomycin, doxorubicin, methotrexate, axitinib (pan-VEGFR inhibition), and even distilled water, most of which have been tested on cell cultures [6]. At the clinical level, there are two predominant methods of applying the desired agent to target cells; supplementation of the irrigation medium and treatment of IOL surfaces. The primary complication associated with any method of drug delivery is toxicity to other tissues, specifically the corneal endothelium.

Equatorial cells are the least accessible cells to irrigation due to their location and protection from residual fibres, but they are dynamic cells in the initial stages of cell growth following surgery. The rapid rate of progression across the capsule suggests these bow region cells remain in high abundance and future attempts should consider localised delivery of drugs to this particular cell population.

The IOL offers a more controlled means of drug delivery and by utilising the haptic component in addition to the main IOL body, cytotoxic agents can be applied directly to the equatorial cells. The nature of drug attachment should be sufficiently strong to prevent significant leakage into surrounding tissues, yet sufficiently weak to permit accumulation by the contiguous cells.

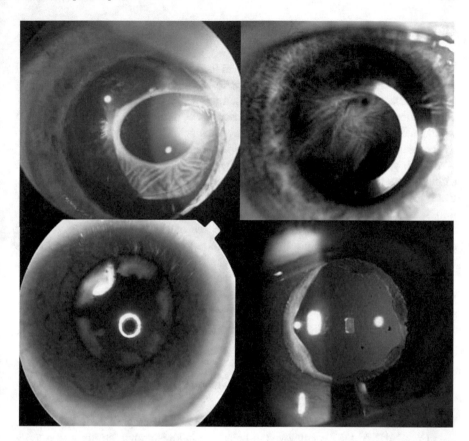

Fig. 11 Clinical photographs at slit lamp examination of the anterior capsule before and after radial Nd:YAG anterior capsulotomy. The top row demonstrate pre-laser anterior capsule fibrosis with the bottom row showing post-laser treatment for each eye. This is a more advanced Nd:YAG laser technique which requires no posterior offset when aiming the laser. *Images courtesy of Professor C. Liu*

Thapsigargin has been chosen in the past as a cytotoxic agent to be delivered via IOLs because it is a hydrophobic substance that adheres well to plastic. It has also been shown in previous experiments with tissue-cultured rabbit lens cells that growth could be inhibited by exposure to nanomolar concentrations of thapsigargin. Thapsigargin is readily transferred from the IOL through the cell membrane and accumulates on the endoplasmic reticulum. The early effects of inactivation of the endoplasmic reticulum appear to be a loss of the cell's ability to divide or synthesise proteins. The exposure ultimately ends in the death of all cells within the lens capsule. However, with loss of cells in the lens capsule, there is occasionally loss of IOL stability. Without the classic PCO 'shrink wrap' effect on an IOL, the IOL may continue to move freely in the lens capsule (depending on its design, of course).

Closed Capsular Bag Irrigation

In 2003, Maloof developed a method using an irrigation device made from biomedical grade silicon that would allow the surgeons to reseal the capsular bag after targeting lens epithelial cells during human cataract surgery [29]. The extension arm has a vacuum channel that applies suction to a ring that passes through the phacoemulsification wound and provides an irrigation and outflow channel. The tool is short and folds easily for insertion through a 3.2–3.5 mm incision using Kelman–McPherson forceps.

In their study, there was no leakage of dyes into the chamber, confirming it was a closed system. Slit lamp biomicroscopic examination was performed at day 1, week 1 and 3 and 6 months. The 6-month follow-up examination showed a reduction in anterior capsule opacification in comparison to control groups. A follow-up at 1 year continued to confirm a reduced degree of anterior capsule fibrosis and capsular phimosis in the study groups compared to the control group. PCO was not seen in the majority of the treatment eyes.

However, investigation of a definitive technique and product for sealed capsular irrigation continues as none have ever made it into common practice as of yet.

Treatment of PCO

Neodymium : Yttrium-Aluminium-Garnet (Nd:YAG) Laser

When PCO occurs to such an extent that the visual axis is compromised, the Nd:YAG laser ($Y_{2.97}Nd_{0.03}Al_5O_{12}$) is employed to create a window through the fibrous posterior capsule. This solid-state laser emits a focused wavelength of low divergence at 1064 nm (1% Nd doping). For other applications this may be frequency-doubled or -tripled.

The Nd:YAG laser is photo disruptive, which means it is pigment independent, using high energy in a small spot for a brief duration (highly concentrated) which causes localised temperature increase to 15,000 degrees Celsius. Its acoustic shockwave breaks through tissue and is directed backward, toward the ophthalmologist/operator, meaning the laser must be focused just *posterior* to the capsule (250–350 μm Offset) using a helium neon aiming beam.

Preoperative Assessment

- BCVA
- Glare test
- Pinhole
- Intraocular pressure (IOP)
- Thorough slit lamp examination (anterior and posterior segment post-dilation).

Contraindications for YAG Capsulotomy

- Corneal pathology affecting transparency, such as scars, oedema, or infiltrates
- Aqueous pathology such as cells/flare, or hyphaema.

Pre- and Post-Operative

Prior to treatment, an ophthalmologist may apply topical anaesthetic and a coupling agent, such as 2.5% hydroxypropyl methylcellulose, to accommodate an Abraham YAG lens which helps form a seal against the cornea, force the eyelids apart, and focus the laser at a precise magnification. However, this will differ between surgeons and many may choose not to use a capsulotomy lens for this procedure. Pressure lowering drops (e.g. apraclonidine or brimonidine) and steroids may also be administered post-treatment to control inflammation and potential IOP rise. This will also vary according to surgeon preference.

Capsulotomy Techniques

A YAG posterior capsulotomy typically begins with an initial energy of around 1 mJ, with 250–350 μm posterior offset and a fixed spot size and duration. It is key to avoid the IOL and anterior hyaloid face. Pearl-type PCO phenotypes require less energy (e.g. 1 mJ starting energy) than dense, fibrous PCO phenotypes (e.g. 2.5 mJ starting energy). After an initial firing shot with the laser, tissue response is gauged. Energy may then be increased by 0.3–0.5 mJ each time. Each break must be continuous with the previous one as the surgeon aims each shot. Many shape approaches to capsulotomies exist, such as forming a cross (cruciate), bucket handle, square, or circle. Many surgeons prefer the cruciate shape as this limits detachment of capsular tissue into the vitreous. Otherwise the patient may complain of increased floaters post-operatively. It is best to avoid large capsulotomies in patients with a high axial length, as this is associated with increased rate of complication. Total laser energy is also an important contributor to complications, which ranges in incidence from 2 to 12%. It is best to also avoid localised areas of dense fibrotic change with the YAG capsulotomy.

*Refer to Fig. 11 for the radial Nd:YAG laser approach to **anterior** capsule fibrosis. No posterior offset is used in this variation to preserve the surface of the IOL (this prevents pitting and dislocation).*

Complications of YAG Laser Therapy

- Intra-ocular pressure increase *(most common)*
- Corneal oedema
- Uveitis
- Iritis
- Pitting of the IOL
- Glare
- IOL decentration or dislocation to vitreous
- Cystoid macular oedema
- Retinal tears and detachment (including macular holes).

Future of PCO Prevention

Our understanding of PCO has deepened considerably since its description, but there is still much to learn about this pathophysiological process. Our knowledge of the processes that underpin PCO is crucial to success (e.g. growth factor activation, lens capsule properties, and surgical factors). Fortunately there are a variety of in vitro models of PCO to facilitate this process. A combination of

IOL design and drug delivery methods may prevent PCO altogether in the future. Using the lens as a drug delivery system by either incorporating the drug into a slow release gel (for long-term inhibition) or as nanoparticles contained on the lens haptics, for example, are current areas of research. Alternatively, injecting a pharmacological drug before lens implantation may produce encouraging results in preventing PCO. Drug-eluting lenses with innovative designs and new materials may be the future of cataract surgery. The permeability of the lens capsule should be an important area of study to understand how it handles and contains pharmaceutical compounds. In the meantime, it is prudent to further investigate the biochemical processes underpinning PCO to greater enhance our understanding and technology.

References

1. McCarty CA, Taylor HR. The genetics of cataract. Invest Ophthalmol Vis Sci. 2001;42(8):1677–8.
2. Cleary G, Spalton DJ, Zhang JJ, Marshall J. In vitro lens capsule model for investigation of posterior capsule opacification. J Cataract Refract Surg. 2010;36:1249–52.
3. Eldred JA, Dawes LJ, Wormstone IM. The lens as a model for fibrotic disease. Philos Trans R Soc Lond B Biol Sci. 2011;366(1568):1301–19.
4. Friedlander M. Fibrosis and diseases of the eye. J Clin Invest. 2007;117(3):576–86.
5. Laurent GJ, McAnulty RJ, Hill M, Chambers R. Escape from the matrix: multiple mechanisms for fibroblast activation in pulmonary fibrosis. Proc Am Thorac Soc. 2008;5(3):311–5.
6. Eldred JA, McDonald M, Wilkes H, Spalton D, Wormstone IM. Growth factor restriction impedes progression of wound healing following cataract surgery: identification of VEGF as a putative therapeutic target. Sci Rep. 2016;6 (Article number: 24453).
7. Shui YB. Vascular endothelial growth factor expression and signaling in the lens. Invest Ophthalmol Vis Sci. 2003;44(9):3911–9.
8. Dawes LJ, Duncan G, Wormstone IM. Age-related differences in signaling efficiency of human lens cells underpin differential wound healing response rates following cataract surgery. Invest Ophthalmol Vis Sci. 2013;54(1):333–42.
9. Kalluri R, Weinberg RA. The basics of epithelial-mesenchymal transition. J Clin Invest. 2009;119(6):1420–8.
10. Leask A, Abraham DJ. TGF-beta signaling and the fibrotic response. FASEB J. 2004;18(7):816–27.
11. Saika S, Yamanaka O, Sumioka T, Miyamoto T, Miyazaki K, Okada Y, Kitano A, Shirai K, Tanaka S, Ikeda K. Fibrotic disorders in the eye: targets of gene therapy. Prog Retin Eye Res. 2008;27(2):177–96.
12. Terrell A. β1-integrin may regulate egr1 (early growth response 1) within the lens. University of Delaware. 2013;7–11(62):91–108.
13. Gabbiani G. The myofibroblast in wound healing and fibrocontracetive diseases. J Pathol. 2003;200:500–3.
14. Sveinsson O. The ultrastructure of Elschnig's pearls in a pseudophakic eye. Acta Ophthalmol (Copenh). 1993;71(1):95–8.
15. Brown N. Visibility of transparent objects in the eye by retroillumination. Br J Ophthalmol. 1971;55(8):517–24.

16. Jongebloed WL, Kalicharan D, Los LI, van der Veen G, Worst JG. A combined scanning and transmission electron microscope investigation of human (secondary) cataract material. Doc Ophthalmol. 1991;78(3–4):325–34.

17. Nishi O. Incidence of posterior capsule opacification in eyes with and without posterior chamber intraocular lenses. J Cataract Refract Surg. 1986;12(5):519–22.

18. Apple DJ, Solomon KD, Tetz MR, Assia EI, Holland EY, Legler UF, Tsai JC, Castaneda VE, Hoggatt JP, Kostick AM. Posterior capsule opacification. Surv Ophthalmol. 1992;37(2):73–116.

19. Hansen SO, Solomon KD, McKnight GT, Wilbrandt TH, Gwin TD, O'Morchoe DJ, Tetz MR, Apple DJ. Posterior capsular opacification and intraocular lens decentration. Part I: Comparison of various posterior chamber lens designs implanted in the rabbit model. J Cataract Refract Surg. 1988;14(6):605–13.

20. Martin RG, Sanders DR, Van der Karr MA, DeLuca M. Effect of small incision intraocular lens surgery on postoperative inflammation and astigmatism. A study of the AMO SI-18NB small incision lens. J Cataract Refract Surg. 1992;18(1):51–7.

21. Cumming JS. Postoperative complications and uncorrected acuities after implantation of plate haptic silicone and three-piece silicone intraocular lenses. J Cataract Refract Surg. 1993;19(2):263–74.

22. Linnola R, Werner L, Pandey S et al. Adhesion of fibronectin, vitronectin, laminin, and collagen type IV to intraocular lens materials in pseudophakic human autopsy eyes. Part 1: Histological sections. J Cataract Refract Surg. 2000;26:1792–806.

23. Nanavaty M, Spalton D, Boyce J et al. Edge profile of commercially available square-edged intraocular lenses. J Cataract Refract Surg. 2008;34:677–86.

24. Hara T, Narita M, Hashimoto T, Motoyama Y, Hara T. Long-term study of posterior capsular opacification prevention with endocapsular equator rings in humans. Arch Ophthalmol. 2011;129(7):855–63.

25. Friedman N. Capsular tension rings: a short- or long-term solution? 2008. http://www.ophthalmologyweb.com/Featured-Articles/20010-Capsular-Tension-Rings-A-Short-or-Long-Term-Solution/. Accessed June 2018.

26. Fine H. The capsular tension ring: indications for use. Cataract Refract Surg Today. 2004;32–34.

27. McDonnell PJ, Krause W, Glaser BM. In vitro inhibition of lens epithelial cell proliferation and migration. Ophthalmic Surg. 1988;19(1):25–30.

28. Wormstone IM, Liu CS, Rakic JM, Marcantonio JM, Vrensen GF, Duncan G. Human lens epithelial cell proliferation in a protein-free medium. Invest Ophthalmol Vis Sci. 1997;38(2):396–404.

29. Maloof A, Neilson G, Milverton EJ, Pandey SK. Selective and specific targeting of lens epithelial cells during cataract surgery using sealed- capsule irrigation. J Cataract Refract Surg. 2003;29(8):1566–8.

Market Forces, Premium Cataract Surgery and Managing the Unhappy Patient

Sophie J. Coutts and Allon Barsam

Funding and Size of the Market

Within the United Kingdom, the National Health Service (NHS) provides cataract surgery at no cost to the patient providing they are a resident of the UK. Within this service there are waiting lists and consultant led care pathways. There is however neither certainty nor choice of a named consultant surgeon performing the operation. In large teaching hospitals it is highly likely that an ophthalmologist-in-training rather than a consultant will perform the surgery either under supervision or unsupervised. Most trusts only allow use of a monofocal intraocular lens (IOL) although some trusts do have the option of toric lenses for higher astigmatism only. The NHS has been founded on the principle of being free at the point of service so any co-payment scheme involving paying for extra care such as premium lenses is against its ethos and not allowed. The maximum waiting time of 18 weeks is achieved for 90–95% of patients.

Private sector cataract surgery in the UK offers a service where patients either directly pay their chosen surgeon (self-pay) and clinic/hospital or if the patient pays for a private insurance policy, the insurance provider pays the patient's chosen surgeon a surgery fee with the facility fee going to the clinic or hospital. This insured pathway normally requires initiating via a General Practitioner (Family Medicine Physician) or Optometric referral, on condition that both the surgeon and the clinic/hospital are registered and recognized/"approved" by the insurance company. This gives the patient a guarantee of consultant continuity at all stages of the process. Normally there is a faster time frame for this private care pathway than with the NHS. The private care pathway also guarantees the patient complete

S. J. Coutts (✉)
North East London NHS Treatment Centre, London, UK
e-mail: sjcoutts@doctors.org.uk

A. Barsam
Ophthalmic Consultants of London, London, UK

© Springer Nature Switzerland AG 2021
C. Liu and A. Shalaby Bardan (eds.), *Cataract Surgery*,
https://doi.org/10.1007/978-3-030-38234-6_13

219

choice of surgeon for self-pay surgery and some choice of surgeon for insured surgery. The reason there is not total choice of surgeon in the insured sector is because some consultants choose not to be recognised by certain insurers as they find the renumeration not worthwhile. Furthermore, some insurance companies will suspend or refuse recognition of consultants often on account of the insurance companies policies on surgical or diagnostic fees. This service also gives the surgeon and patient the choice of premium lens implants, such as toric and presbyopic lenses allowing greater spectacle independence. However, the extra fee for premium lenses is not funded by most insurance companies and instead is passed to the patient as an additional cost. The same is true of adjuvants to conventional phacoemulsifcation surgery such as femtosecond laser surgery (femto-phaco).

In continental Europe most countries have a universal health care system. However, many residents purchase private health insurance cover. Germany for example, operates a policy of "sickness funds" with citizens contributing in proportion to their income. Additional services can be bought or statutory health cover can be opted out and complete private coverage sought. However cataract surgery with premium IOLs similar to the UK, are paid for via private insurance or self funded.

The United States of America operates with no universal health cover such as the NHS for patients of all ages and economic circumstance. There are no nationwide medical facilities open to the general public but local government owned medical facilities such as county hospitals do exist. Residents require health insurance cover which people buy on their own or obtain via their or a family member's work employer, this covers conventional cataract surgery but premium IOLs are not included in this and patients pay the extra fee for such lenses.

The health systems of Canada and Australia are hybrid systems. Both have a universal health care system for residents paid for via taxes and called public healthcare insurance (medicare). This covers elective cataract surgery not with premium lenses and often with a long wait for treatment. A higher proportion of residents take supplementary private insurance and in Australia the government actively encourages private insurance, offering rebates on insurance costs. Premium lenses if with medicare or private medical insurance providers are not covered and termed 'out of pocket' cataract surgery costs paid for by the patient [1].

The global cataract surgery devices market in 2016 was valued at US$6.8 billion and by 2023 is expected to reach US$8.5 billion. The phacoemulsification systems to remove cataracts, IOLs, instruments and ophthalmic viscoelastic devices all used in surgery are classed as cataract surgery devices [2].

This market growth is however impeded by the low income or developing world economies where cataract surgery is less dependent on phacoemulsification. Instead manual or small incision cataract surgery (SICS)/extra capsular cataract extraction (ECCE) predominate the field and accordingly premium lenses take a backstage position.

Within the developing world the availability of SICS has revolutionised cataract surgery. Despite private and government institutional provision there remains a massive shortfall in provision of eye care and cataract services to many of their populations. Sadly cataracts remain a leading cause of blindness in these regions.

Patient Expectations and Consent for Premium Cataract Surgery

Premium IOL decisions require a specific consultation to determine patient suitability and expectations for vision. A patient happy wearing reading spectacles after cataract surgery could have conventional monofocal IOL surgery and those who want reading spectacle independence can be consulted on premium lens options.

There are three conventional viewing distances of near, intermediate, and far. Whilst a monofocal IOL allows for a single correction at far, some patients prefer spectacle independence from reading at near or at an intermediate distance. Near distance is the zone where images are focused for near tasks commonly between range 30 cm (3.0 Dioptres) to 40 cm (2.5 Dioptres), such as for book reading. Intermediate distance is within the range 50 cm (2 Dioptres) to 100 cm (1 Dioptre) and is the focus used for facial recognition, computer use and reading the mobile phone. A presbyopic IOL can accommodate for all of these focal points to achieve the best patient satisfaction. With increasing reliance on close vision for hand held electronic devices and computer use permeating almost every element of modern life and work, presbyopic IOL solutions are gaining in popularity with patients.

Spectacle free vision however doesn't always necessitate use of a presbyopic correcting IOL. Monovision is an option in patients who want a degree of spectacle independence but are either not expressing a desire to have a presbyopic IOL or initial consultation deems them unsuitable candidates for a presbyopic IOL. Monovision is the planned insertion of an IOL for the non-dominant eye to be myopic in the region of −2.00 to −2.50 Dioptres and so allow near vision, and the dominant eye corrected to emmetropia for distance vision. Whilst it may take 3–4 weeks for patients to adapt to monovision, with greater tolerance in patients already using contact lens monovision, it is used on a case specific basis as it brings concerns of altered depth perception and reduced stereopsis post procedure and is only tolerated in 2/3 of patients. Mini-monovision conversely corrects one eye for far vision and the other eye for intermediate with only a slight undercorrection in the region of −1.00 Dioptres of myopia. Mini-monovision however does not rely on recognition of a dominant eye, gives intermediate vision such as for recognition of faces and has a patient tolerance of more or less 100%. When aiming for spectacle independence, it is important to explain that only 90% or so will achieve full independence. A further procedure may be necessary for fine tuning any refractive surprise. Finally, those receiving multifocal implants needs to be warned of glare and halos, and requiring higher luminance for reading [3].

At initial consultation it is important to understand the patient's visual needs and ask about their vocation, activities and the probability of tolerance for glare and haloes. Those who have a profession involving frequent night driving or who have glare at night are unlikely to be suitable for presbyopic IOLs. In addition patients with significant maculopathy such as epiretinal membranes or lamellar holes may not tolerate presbyopic IOLs. Multifocal IOLs are also relatively contraindicated in those with glaucoma and early dementia.

All patients should be advised on post operative concerns such as glare, halo, quality of vision, residual refractive error and to reduce these, the possibility of a surface enhancement procedure after cataract surgery. Those not pre-warned on such may see any concern as a complication they were not aware of preoperatively.

Patients with >2.50 Diopters of cylindrical correction pre-operatively should be consulted on the option of being fitted with a monofocal or presbyopic toric intraocular lens, This option of a toric IOL then expands the consent process to include the risk of post-operative IOL rotation and in such an event the possibility for further surgery to reposition the IOL. Patients with a cylindrical correction of <1.50 Diopters can be consented on limbal relaxing incisions at the time of surgery which may be single or paired, and positioned where the cornea is steeper, to a length as long in clock hours as the cornea is steep in dioptres. Patient consent for LRIs includes complications such as globe perforation, reduced corneal sensation, dry eye, induction of irregular astigmatism and cylindrical axis shift.

Post premium IOL insertion it is important to re-evaluate a patient, assessing for satisfaction with near, intermediate and distance vision before proceeding to second eye surgery, remembering that patients do best with bilateral presbyopic IOL implantation. The second eye cataract surgery is usually within one month of first eye surgery. Immediately sequential bilateral cataract surgery is an option to improve bilateral adaptation.

Patient understanding of acceptable and expected surgical outcomes is needed for the achievement of optimal results. Those patients with unrealistic visual post operative expectations or excessive complaints regarding spectacles or contact lenses may be unsuitable candidates for presbyopic IOLs.

In general all cataract surgery and specifically premium IOL surgery cases require careful patient selection and counselling. The same precise surgical technique used in conventional monofocal cataract surgery is also required with premium lenses. However a presbyopic IOL needs precise centration for the best optical effect and visual results, this can be achieved with a well centred capsulorrhexis and good zonular integrity.

Managing the Unhappy Patient After Cataract Surgery

After cataract surgery with monofocal IOLs unhappy patients have issues centred around unexpected refractive errors (so enforcing the importance of preoperative biometry checks), aberrations such as negative or positive dysphotopsias, late IOL dislocations and cases where the operation had intraoperative complications.

The primary reason for an unhappy patient after premium cataract surgery is when uncorrected vision goals are not met. These patients require attention to detail from a surgical, pharmacological and psychological perspective, with six common causes at fault:

(1) Consecutive Treatment

– Immediately sequential bilateral cataract surgery
  Patients preoperatively need to be aware full functionality is achieved only after second eye IOL is placed. The importance of having both eyes completed is critical for the success of the procedure along with providing for an adequate neuroadaptation period.
– Delayed sequential bilateral cataract surgery
  The second IOL choice may be predicated on the patient's response to the first surgery and if extremely dissatisfied with the first eye, consecutive surgery is not advised until the first eye is optimised.

(2) Cylinder and residual refractive error

Presbyopic IOL patients are sensitive to very small refractive errors. Any astigmatism greater than 0.50 D in a symptomatic patient should be treated. Limbal relaxing incisions (LRI) can be useful for less than 1.50 D of cylinder, and for more than 1.50 D of cylinder surface ablation or laser in situ keratomileusis (LASIK) provides more accurate results.

Patients receiving toric IOLs should have full correction of their preoperative corneal astigmatism, though if there has been a rotation of the IOL the cylindrical refraction may not be fully corrected. The mechanisms behind this are thought to be continued expansion of the haptics destabilizing the desired IOL position, wound leak, leaving the eye overinflated and not at physiological intraocular pressure or retained viscoelastic around the haptics. Toric IOL rotation of 1 degree away from desired axis results in 3.5% loss of cylindrical correction, with 7% loss in correction for 3.5 degrees rotation and a 34% loss for 10 degrees rotation. In the case of 10 degrees rotation the toric IOL requires repositioning and if proceeding to sequential cataract surgery with a toric IOL a capsular tension ring used. With toric IOLs the surgeon should have a low tolerance for inserting a capsular tension ring, especially if the IOL seems mobile, in cases of axial myopia or in conditions where lens repositioning is restricted by for example a poorly dilating pupil.

(3) Capsular opacification (For details see PCO chapter)

Presbyopic IOLs cause glare and can reduce contrast sensitivity with possible capsular opacity magnifying these issues. Depending on the patient's complaint and mesopic/scotopic pupil size presbyopic IOL patients may require a larger capsulotomy than normal. However it is important to be certain that the posterior capsule is the issue, as once opened, safe IOL exchange will be more challenging.

(4) Cystoid macular oedema (CMO) See CMO chapter for details

Patients who have conventional cataract surgery with no risk factors and no cap-sular rupture, have up to a 70% chance of having macular thickening on optical coherence tomography (OCT) and a 12% chance of having visually significant CMO without the use of a topical NSAID. In addition, the loss of contrast sensitiv-ity associated with a presbyopic IOL is made much worse by CMO. Once the nor-mal architecture of the retina is lost, that visual quality is degraded for life. Snellen visual acuity will improve, but contrast sensitivity will be permanently reduced. The best way to look for CMO after cataract surgery is with OCT. In addition, OCT is a very effective screening tool preoperatively for epiretinal membranes (ERM) and lamellar macular holes. Presbyopic IOL patients will not tolerate the lenses if they have significant maculopathy. Topical nonsteroidal anti-inflammatory agents should be used perioperatively in eyes with ERM to decrease the risk of cystoid macular oedema and improve retinal function. Many sources recommend using a topical NSAID four times a day for 3 days preoperatively and continue it for 4–6 weeks post-operatively to help prevent CMO. For those patients with first eye post-operative CMO when they are listed for second eye cataract surgery prophylactic topical NSAID should be a must and a baseline OCT taken [4].

(5) Corneal and ocular surface disease

The tear film is the most important refracting surface of the eye, with mild disrup-tion impacting quality of vision. It is reported that topical cyclosporine use in dry eye multifocal IOL patient gave improved contrast sensitivity in the cyclosporine treated eye versus the other eye receiving just artificial tears [5].

(6) Centration of the pupil relative to the IOL

If the IOL in its capsular bag is not centred behind the pupil the patient will com-plain of glare or halo. Dysphotopsias are thought to be the result of an optical aberration where light reflects off the IOL edge onto the retina and can be experi-enced after cataract surgery with both monofocal and premium lenses. Glare and haloes are termed positive dysphotopsia and temporal shadow effects or dark areas in visual field are negative dysphotopsias.

Negative dysphotopsia can be experienced after in the bag IOL implantation with suspected causes being IOL design (square edge as opposed to round), cor-neal incision scars, anterior capsulotomy size and distance of the IOL from the iris. Positive dysphotopsia is more common in the case of presbyopic lenses and overall in post cataract patients. This is largely because of the shift in IOL material to acrylic from lower refractive index PMMA or silicone lenses and a move to square edged haptics from round edge design, the former concentrating stray light on to the retina as a positive dysphotopsia [6].

A systematic approach which addresses the six above factors is required when treating such dysphotopsia patients and in particular those with presbyopic IOLs. Post operative patients with presbyopic IOLs are advised on a period of neuroad-aptation to the lens, usually 3 months, especially in cases of dysphotopsia.

In correcting for premium lens post operative error, a misaligned toric IOL can be rotated. In presbyopic IOL cases post operative astigmatism should be half a dioptre or less, any more can be corrected with LRIs. Higher cylindrical astigmatism can be corrected with corneal refractive procedures of LASIK or photorefractive keratectomy (PRK).

For both presbyopic and monofocal IOLs with refractive errors or 'refractive surprise' LASIK or piggyback IOLs can be used. IOL exchange should be avoided as it is traumatic and provides a less predictable refractive outcome. IOL exchange may prove necessary for those who cannot tolerate multifocal IOLs after several months or a year of adaptation. Some surgeons advocate earlier exchange for fear of capsular phimosis and shrink wrapping making for difficult explanation of the original lens.

Treatment in such cases is expedited as soon as it is safe for the patient. Commonly LRIs can be performed as soon as 6 weeks following surgery. Patients who require LASIK or PRK can also be treated as soon as six weeks following presbyopic IOL surgery, however in most cases it is advisable to wait at least 3 months for stable refraction before considering corneal refractive procedures. Also it is important to consider any concern as a possible psychological issue and that the lens is not the right choice for the patient's eye [7].

Most importantly patients who are unhappy after cataract surgery should never feel abandoned and advised that a solution will be sought. In the case of presbyopic IOL intolerance, patients should be told that in a worst case scenario an IOL exchange for a monofocal IOL is almost always an alternative.

In conclusion, there are options which need consideration to improve visual outcomes in patients with monofocal and presbyopic IOLs. It is important to investigate and treat organic problems first before assuming that neuroadaption will improve the issue, and so ultimately make an unhappy patient a happy post operative patient.

References

1. Zhang X, Lee P, Thompson T, et al. Health insurance coverage and use of eye care services. Arch Ophthalmol. 2008;126(8):1121–6.
2. Cataract surgery devices market: global industry trends, share, size, growth, opportunity and forecast 2018–2023. IMARC Services Pvt. Ltd., 2018:1–89.
3. Labiris G, Giarmoukakis A, Patsiamanidi M, Papadopoulos Z, Kozobolis VP. Mini-monovision versus multifocal intraocular lens implantation. J Cataract Refract Surg. 2015;41(1):53–7.
4. Rosetti L, Autelitano A. Cystoid macular oedema following cataract surgery. Current Opin Ophthalmol. 2000;11:65–72.
5. Donnenfeld ED, Solomon R, Roberts CW, Wittpenn JR, McDonald MB, Perry HD. Cyclosporine 0.05% to improve visual outcomes after multifocal intraocular lens implantation. J Cataract Refract Surg. 2010;36:1095–100.
6. Henderson B, Geneva II. Negative dysphotopsia: a perfect storm. J Cataract Refract Surg. 2015;41:2291–312.
7. Donnenfeld ED, Nattis A, Rosenberg E, Barsam A. Refractive intraocular lenses, managing unhappy patients. In: Hovanesian JA, editor. Refractive surgery: best practices and advanced technology. Slack Incorporated; 2017:215–24.

Carbon and Cataracts: How to Make Your Service Sustainable

John Buchan, Cassandra Thiel and Peter Thomas

Introduction

There are certain things about current human behaviour that we can say with abso-
lute certainty will not be continued into the future. Fossil fuel powered motor cars
are not a long-term part of the future for humanity; neither are the current cataract surgical practices found in high-income settings such as in Europe and North
America. We are not, as yet, facing up to this reality, but will be required to do so
imminently.

Cataract surgery is one of the most frequently performed surgical procedure
globally each year, and with more than one in three of the 36 million blind people on earth being blind due to cataract (2015 estimate), there is a requirement
for the current surgical activity to increase markedly [1]. Planning for the progressively greater burden of health care on global resources is now centring around the
necessity for services to be sustainable in perpetuity, in keeping with the direction of the United Nations who set Sustainable Development Goals (SDG) as the
over-arching international strategic agenda.

This chapter aims to set out the case for change, and detail practical and
evidence-based interventions to promote the development of sustainable cataract
services.

J. Buchan (✉)
London School of Hygiene and Tropical Medicine, International Centre for Eye Health,
London, UK
e-mail: john.buchan1@nhs.net

C. Thiel
Department of Population Health, Division of Healthcare Delivery Science & Department of
Ophthalmology, NYU Grossman School of Medicine, New York University, New York, USA
e-mail: Cassandra.Thiel@nyulangone.org

P. Thomas
Moorfields Eye Hospital NHS Foundation Trust, London, UK

© Springer Nature Switzerland AG 2021
C. Liu and A. Shalaby Bardan (eds.), *Cataract Surgery*,
https://doi.org/10.1007/978-3-030-38234-6_14

The Triple Bottom Line

Estimation of the "costs" of providing cataract services cannot be thought of merely in terms of the direct financial costs. A key concept in the health economics of sustainability is the Triple Bottom Line (TBL) (Fig. 1).

The use of the TBL in service delivery planning recognises that there is a finite financial resource allocated to health care, but there is also a finite social and human resource, and a finite environmental resource. If we constantly run services that draw too heavily on any one of these three components of the TBL, we will at some point, collectively run out of credit and face the negative consequences of failing to live within our means.

The environmental impact can be quantified using a technique called Life Cycle Analysis or Life Cycle Assessment (LCA), with standards set out in ISO 14040. LCA quantifies the resources used and emissions generated across the life cycle of a product or process—including raw material extraction, product and component manufacturing, use phase, reuse phases (if they exist), end of life or disposal, and all transportation steps in between. Environmental impact is most frequently equated with Greenhouse Gas emissions (GHGs) that cause global warming or climate change. In LCA, these emissions are represented in units of carbon dioxide equivalents (CO_2e). However, LCA can be used to estimate many types of environmental emissions, including air pollutants, smog forming emissions, water emissions causing eutrophication or acidification, toxic emissions, and even land use changes.

LCA evaluation of healthcare services as a whole shows them to be a major consumer of resources, emitting 10% of GHGs in the US, 7% in Australia, and 5% in the UK and Canada, with a substantial portion of emissions originating

Fig. 1 The triple bottom line for sustainable eye health care

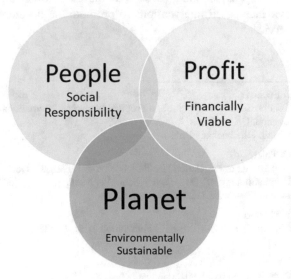

in operating rooms [2–6]. A report released in 2019 estimates global healthcare emissions (excluding those of African countries) result in 4.4% of the world's total GHGs [7]. If global healthcare were a country, it would be the 5th largest carbon emitter in the world.

> **TBL: Social Costs**—a financially and environmentally sustainable service might be configured, but if it were dependant on working hospital staff intensively whilst paying little attention to engagement and morale of the team members, or on child labour in a low-income country producing surgical instruments, this would not represent a sustainable solution.

What We Do Know? The Case for Change

Patients' Safety and Population Health

The negative impact of climate change on health worldwide has been estimated in terms of the disability adjusted life years (DALY) caused [8]. In the same way as a health care intervention can be shown to add quality adjusted life years (QALY), interventions that reduce the per case CO_2e emissions of cataract surgery can reduce the number of DALY caused by environmental impact. There is, therefore, a patient safety issue around running unsustainable cataract services.

Climate changing emissions are not the only concerning triple bottom line issue, modern supply chains lead to ethical and environmental issues in the communities involved in the supply chains. The UK's National Health Service (NHS) discovered child labour was involved in the manufacturing of surgical instruments at sites in Pakistan. In the suburbs of Chicago, USA, a factory that sterilises single-use supplies for surgical procedures closed after the community discovered that the Ethylene Oxide (EtO) used in sterilization was likely causing higher rates of cancer in residents living near the factory site. This factory was within their legal limits for EtO emissions, yet community pressure forced this particular site to close [9, 10]. Though it may seem a success for this community, EtO is still used as the primary sterilizer for all single-use sterile surgical supplies. Which communities still bear the burdens of producing these important, sterile medical supplies? At the other end of the product life cycle, electronic wastes, some of which are related to medical instrumentation, have also been found to increase cancer rates in communities where e-waste is being disassembled and discarded [11].

In addition to these population-level issues, healthcare providers are becoming more concerned with our patients' exposures during treatment. Organisations such as *Healthcare Without Harm* are advocating for the removal of certain toxic ingredients from medical products, building construction and furnishings. These include formaldehyde and other fire repellents commonly found in furnishings; Volatile Organic Compounds often found in carpeting, paint and other finishes; mercury, which can still be found in thermometers; and PVC and other phthalate-containing plastics which can leach hormone-mimicking compounds into patient bloodstreams. These are particularly concerning for our smallest patients in neonatal intensive care units.

Inter-generational and Inter-national Justice

Equity issues can be seen across the medical supply chain. Pakistan manufactures most of the US and UK's stainless-steel surgical instruments, and South East Asia is a major site for single-use surgical supply manufacturing. Many of these workers cannot access affordable, quality care for themselves and their families. The US and other developed countries are sending expired or unused supplies abroad as it is against US regulation to use it in US hospitals. While this may temporarily benefit poorer hospitals in need of supplies, it is ethically ambiguous. Such practices have also led to the dumping of broken or old medical equipment in locations not able to fix or maintain the equipment.

On the issue of climate change, the largest contributors to greenhouse gas emissions are high income countries. In contrast, by virtue of geographical distribution and organisational reserves to cope, the worst affected by climate change are low- and middle-income countries. This creates an inter-national injustice. The same dynamic can be described between generations, where the current decision makers and beneficiaries in high income settings are perpetuating unsustainable healthcare delivery practices, the negative consequences of which will be borne by those currently too young to have any influence over the choices being made, or benefit from them.

Opportunities for Change

Recent research has begun to assess the footprint of cataract care. One study in the UK analysed the carbon footprint of phacoemulsification [12]. Morris, et al. included building energy use; staff and patient travel; procurement of pharmaceuticals, disposable medical supplies, paper and food; Information Technology support, waste disposal, and water consumption. The largest portion of GHGs (54% or 98 kg CO_2e) came from the procurement of supplies, which are largely single use and disposable. The next biggest source of emissions (36% or 66 kg CO_2e) was in energy use for the theatre. This included the heating, ventilation, and air conditioning; lighting; and plug loads from equipment (electricity draw from the machines themselves).

However, phacoemulsification can be performed differently based on surgeon, surgical facility, and even country. Recent research shows a dramatic difference in the environmental footprint and financial costs of individual cataract surgery in different locations. This variation in the environmental costs is unrelated to outcomes, suggesting opportunities for improvement are possible without sacrificing quality of care.

Case Study of Aravind Eye Care System

Though there are many successful, high volume cataract surgical facilities, one in particular has been well studied in terms of its environmental footprint. Aravind Eye Care System in Southern India was founded in 1976. It has grown into 7 Tertiary hospitals and a network of secondary care hospitals and primary eye clinics; a system that provides over 450,000 surgical procedures per year. Aravind's mission is to end needless blindness in the local population. To achieve this, Aravind has built their operating theatres around efficiency (Fig. 2).

Using a technique called task shifting, surgeons only perform cut-to-close duties while in the operating theatre. Appropriately trained mid-level ophthalmic

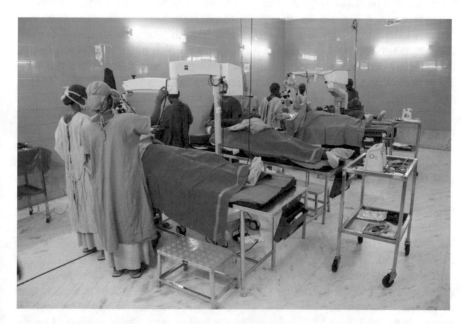

Fig. 2 A typical operating theatre at Aravind Eye Care System in Southern India. Here, two surgeons operate on four beds. Aravind's efficiency methods may look radically different from western approaches, but Aravind is able to achieve excellent quality outcomes while performing surgeries at 1/10th the cost and 1/20th the carbon emissions when compared to the USA and the UK

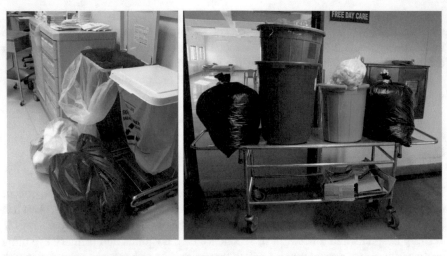

Fig. 3 Left, Waste from 1 phacoemulsification in the USA. Right, Waste from 93 phacoemulsifications performed during one day at Aravind Eye Care System's Pondicherry Hospital

professionals (MLOPs) prepare patients, apply the eye shield post operatively, and escort patients in and out of theatre. To maximise the use of the surgeon's time, there are two beds per surgeon. One bed is being operated on, while the other is being prepped. A surgeon can then go back and forth between the patients on each bed until the end of the surgical list, performing as many as 10 cataract operations an hour. Each bed is assigned a MLOP as a scrub nurse who is responsible for ensuring properly sterilized, reusable instruments and supplies are ready for the next case. Reusable instruments are removed from each bed following surgery and sterilized via 'sequential same day sterilization' technique in an autoclave. Essentially, instruments are run through the full sterilization cycle but are not allowed to dry in the autoclave. Because these instruments will be used immediately back in theatre, there are no risks to the patient, and this enables Aravind to maintain fewer instrument trays for their fast surgeons. Aravind's surgical team uses reusable gowns, masks, and caps which are laundered at the end of the surgical list. They do not rescrub between cases, instead using a sterilizing gel on their hands as they switch between patients.

Financially, Aravind is a profitable hospital where 2/3 of surgical procedures are delivered for free or reduced cost and 1/3 are delivered at a market rate of about US$250 per phacoemulsification operation. This is less than a tenth the cost of a phacoemulsification in the US, which reduces the financial barriers and promotes equity of access to surgery [13, 14]. As for outcome quality indicators such as posterior capsule rupture and endophthalmitis, Aravind achieves comparable outcomes to the US and UK, if not slightly better, most easily explained by the fact that higher-volume surgeons report lower complication rates [15, 16].

A study of their per-phaco carbon footprint revealed that Aravind generates 5% of the GHGs as the same procedure conducted in the UK [17]. A UK phaco is equivalent to driving a car 500 km, whereas a phaco provided by Aravind Eye Care systems in India is equivalent to driving the same car 23 km [15]. Aravind achieves this in a variety of ways, including the process streamlining and task shifting mentioned above, as well as standardisation of process and instrumentation, maximizing the reuse of supplies, and minimizing waste (Fig. 3).

The Need for Context Specific Benchmarking

The detailed examples of CO_2e costs for individual pathways that have been created, provide us with international comparators and potential benchmarks [12]. However, the impact of regulatory and cultural context and the dominant surgical technique employed [18] make it difficult for those in high-income, low-sustainability settings to make the transition to more sustainable practices.

For example, regardless of how sustainable and demonstrably safe the practice of re-using surgical gowns and gloves (with inter-operative disinfection of the gloves by, for example, washing in 100% alcohol) for multiple cases on a cataract list is—the regulatory frameworks in most high-income settings would prevent adoption of this practice. Even the practice of autoclaving unwrapped instrument sets between cases in theatre, which was historically common practice in high-income settings and has not been shown to be associated with any increased risk of patient harm compared to more energy intensive sterilisation options, is frequently prohibited in cataract surgical services [19]. Changing to a more evidence-based approach to surgical safety is clearly necessary, but national regulatory change is difficult for individual organisations to achieve.

Local audit cycles, taking the benchmark of an institution's own per case CO_2e consumption would permit every institution to improve from where they currently stand. Although such audits are not as yet routine practice, a tool called Eyefficiency (Fig. 4) has been developed to permit audit of environmental impact of cataract surgery by individual surgical units. The tool collects data at two levels: unit level data which includes information about staffing, clinical pathways, instrument use, waste handling, travel of patients and staff; and operating-list level data which captures time-and-motion data to establish theatre practice, productivity, and efficiency. The two data sources can be combined to allow analysis of a unit's efficiency, costs, and carbon footprint. To promote improvement in sustainability, a unit can compare itself with others either nationally or globally. This comparison is seen as an important driver for local practice change and identification of wasteful processes. The division into list and unit level data also illustrates the need for cooperation between clinical staff and hospital management who have different and complementary means by which they can influence practice.

Fig. 4 The Eyefficiency
apps allow time-and-motion
studies to be performed
on cataract operating
lists. The data collected
is enriched with casemix,
staffing, operational,
and practical questions
that contribute towards
a detailed sustainability
assessment (performed on the
Eyefficiency.org website)

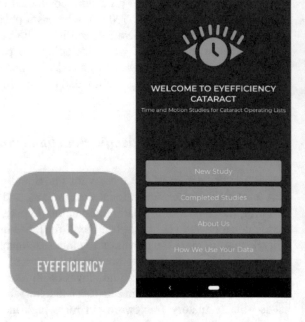

Common Approaches for More Sustainable Cataract Care

Despite regional variation in custom and regulation, there are a few common approaches any surgical facility can take to begin tackling sustainability in cataract care. One standard framework is, in this order: (1) rethink, (2) reduce, (3) reuse, and (4) recycle. Rethinking the process is an important first step in minimising emissions. Rethinking requires not just the surgeon's best effort, but everyone needed to provide quality cataract surgery—the clinical team (nurses, anaesthetists, surgeons, trainees, assistants), administration, housekeeping and building services, engineering and maintenance teams, procurement officers, and even the patient. All are required to effectively provide care currently, and all will be needed to redesign care in a fully sustainable way.

A Culture of Sustainability

Communication of sustainability and sustainability-driven care goals is a good first step towards TBL cataract surgery. This increases engagement of all stakeholders and raises awareness of environmental, equity, and cost issues. Auditing tools such as Eyefficiency can help boost engagement on this topic and also establish baseline data with which to track improvements. A process of cyclical auditing, by which practice is re-assessed and re-benchmarked at defined intervals, would help to keep sustainability prominent in the thoughts of practitioners. Other local services, through teaching sessions or simply due to proximity via shared staff and clinical space, are then more likely to become aware of sustainability issues and potential solutions they may also adopt. Owing to the relatively high staff turnover of many units, particularly driven by regular changeover of trainee surgeons, regional spread of better practice can be encouraged. Focusing on sustainable cataract services is also likely to impact other clinical areas, and this is already seen to be happening with glaucoma services also starting to ask whether they can reduce their environmental footprint [20].

Process Improvements

The provision of cataract care is highly variable. Unnecessary care, exemplified by excessive pre- and post-operative investigation and review, is common and has been shown not to increase patients safety [21]. These tests create emissions from staff and patient travel, overhead energy use, and clinical supplies used. Pre- and post-operative review is a particular area of unjustified variation [22]. Eliminating unnecessary steps in the care pathway can eliminate these emissions. Many units persist with a practice of multiple post-operative reviews (e.g. 1-day, 1-week, and 1-month follow-up) for a standard cataract operation, driven by a combination of unchallenged traditional beliefs and incentives for encounter-based compensation. By whole-pathway redesigns, many hospitals have dramatically reduced peri-operative hospital visits, [23] although no UK eye department was found to be offering true "one-stop cataract lists" in a 2016 UK survey of cataract services (https://www.rcophth.ac.uk/wp-content/uploads/2018/10/RCOphth-Way-Forward-Cataract.pdf). Devolution of post-operative follow-up to community services, for example local optometry practices, has also become common practice. With the correct governance in place, this allows safe care while drastically reducing the number of patients who need to travel longer distances into hospital (in one case, only 2.95% of patients who underwent uncomplicated surgery required review in hospital) [24].

Procurement Reduction

Reduction in consumption is of greatest benefit. Procurement of consumables is the largest part of the CO_2e generation from surgery. Rationalisation of surgical packs may permit reduced consumption by identifying unnecessary items. Some reduction will require a change of surgical technique for some surgeons, such as arm covers for theatre chairs if those surgeons who use these are prepared to progress to operating without. Similarly, surgeons may agree to align their practice such that either the cystotome or the capsulorrhexis forceps can be dispensed with—as either item can be used to do capsulorrhexis on its own. Items such as these could be removed from routine packs—but be available single wrapped in case needed in exceptional circumstances. The same would be true for spear swabs, eye shields, and a separate blade for paracentesis (where a keratome can equally be used for both main incision and paracentesis) or changing the taps in your scrub room to reduce energy and water use [25]. Even small incremental changes, evolution not revolution, are worthwhile because of the scale of cataract surgical needs with a total of around 500,000 operations annually in the UK alone.

Reduce Needless Waste

A 2019 study illuminated the quantity of physical waste generated from unused pharmaceutical in cataract surgery (via phaco) in 4 centres in the USA. Up to 99% of eye drops by volume were unused and wasted between cases [26]. In 2 of the 4 sites, the cost of these unused drugs totalled over $190,000 US per month—enough to cover over 50 cataract operations at each location. Much of this waste is due to unnecessarily large packaging and restrictive reuse or multi-use policies. Even though some bottles were labelled multi-dose, they were required to be thrown out, and likewise, drugs that the patient would need to use after the surgery were thrown out and purchased by the patient in a pharmacy following surgery all because they were not labelled with the patient's name prior to the patient entering the operating theatre. Essentially, there is no evidence-based practice for a large amount of this costly waste [27, 28]. Standardisation between surgeons can also reduce the waste of unused, pre-packaged supplies, while increasing buying power.

Defensive medical practices need to be addressed. Because medico-legal systems internationally frequently compare the practice of the clinician being investigated to the majority practice typified by the behaviour of a "reasonable person", adherence to national or local practices provide some level of protection to individual clinicians. If national level recommendations can migrate to more evidence-based approaches, this then mitigates the need for wasteful defensive practices. For example, where an anaesthetic injection is felt to be unavoidable—the anaesthetic may come in a 10- or 20-ml vial, but only 3–4 ml of that may be used in the block. Retaining the residual anaesthetic for use on subsequent patients has not been demonstrated to represent any risk, yet anecdotally, new vials are often utilised for each patient. The environmental and financial costs of such practices put patients at quantifiable risks, however these risks are frequently not considered [27, 28].

Productivity and Sustainability

As the CO_2e costs are "per case" estimates—perhaps the biggest opportunity for immediate improved CO_2 efficiency is in more cases per list. This would reduce the overhead energy burdens per case but may not affect supply use for each case unless the procurement issues are tackled first. The UK healthcare regulatory body *Monitor* recommends that every hospital should be able to turn around one cataract case per half hour, whereas the national mode is 6 cases per 4 hour list [22]. Moving from 6 cases per list to 8 will reduce the financial costs per case but also the carbon costs as there is a substantial element of fixed carbon costs which are incurred exactly the same regardless of productivity—such as building related heating/lighting costs.

Recycling, the Last Resort but a Big Engager

Recycling operating theatre wastes can be difficult due to concerns about contamination as well as the specialised plastics that are sometimes found in hospitals (for example "blue wrap"). With changes to countries' recycling import policies, waste from developed countries may not even be recycled, leading to increased emissions from transporting garbage across the world before ultimately landfilling or incinerating it. Recycling is the least effective tool to reduce emissions like GHGs; however, because waste is such a visible component of our GHG footprint, it can be a wonderful engagement tool to bring various stakeholders on board to sustainability.

What Don't We Know?

Variation in Care

Sitting in the operating theatre of different surgeons, you will have noticed that each seems to have a specific way of doing things. This variation in practice at the individual level influences the carbon footprint of care. There is also variation between facilities. Based on location, staff and patients may have to travel further, may travel by train or bus, or may have to drive. Different buildings will be more energy efficient, and procurement teams may enable greater specialisation for individual surgeons—thus reducing standardisation and increasing potential waste of supplies. Without knowing how much variation exists in care pathways, we don't know where the main opportunities lie. That is, we do not know how much cost and carbon savings could be generated by attacking the various components of the pathway, from number of staff, increasing patient throughput, decreasing packaging, reducing the number of pre or post-surgical visits, etc. Phrased as a research question, "What are the major opportunities for CO_2 equivalent reduction in HIC that can be realised without compromising actual safety?"

Acceptability of Significant Changes to Care Models

In the UK, independent treatment centres that focus on a single procedure already pursue aggressive cost-saving strategies in order to support high volume operating lists in non-hospital premises. In other countries, cataract surgery is the preserve of high-volume specialist cataract surgeons. It is quite possible that these models could offer significant sustainability benefits. Provision of the majority of cataract surgery by a small number of high-volume surgeons in non-hospital locations, however, would encounter significant resistance from ophthalmologists in the UK where most ophthalmologists are cataract surgeons even if sustainability benefits could be clearly demonstrated. High volume centres are also often criticised on other fronts, most notably a lack of effort in training the next generation of surgeons which could threaten the sustainable availability of surgical expertise.

Regulatory Barriers and Infection Control

Clearly infection control is a top priority when addressing sustainability in care pathways. It would be far less sustainable all around to have to fix a complicated surgery than to do it correctly the first time. That said, many infection control guidelines and practices have questionable effect on actual infection control but do seem to drive up the cost and emissions of care. [Examples: gloves for vaccination delivery, what kind of cap to use in the OT, sterilizing instrument trays for same day use, etc.] Regulations are shown to be major barriers to addressing unused pharmaceutical waste in the US, but what other regulations need to be shifted to encourage more sustainable practice without compromising quality outcomes [19]? What will need to be done to ensure safety if cataract surgery in high-income countries shifted away from single-use plastics and toward all reusable products [29]?

Summary

The case for the need for change in the way we deliver cataract services to make them sustainable seems compelling, and some opportunities for change are within the grasp of every ophthalmologist or eye department. However, taking these opportunities will require hard work for individuals and organisations. Not least the effort required to bring on board colleagues who prefer the status quo, or those charged with local and national *health and safety* regulations who feel a strong necessity to enforce practices that increase *perceived safety*. As environmental degradation is increasingly accepted as one of the most pressing threats to health in the 21st century, then changes to practice should become more easily accepted that act to combat that threat and provide a safer future for everyone.

References

1. Flaxman SR, Bourne RRA, Resnikoff S, et al. Global causes of blindness and distance vision impairment 1990–2020: a systematic review and meta-analysis. Lancet Glob Health. 2017;5(12):e1221–34.
2. Eckelman MJ, Sherman JD. Estimated global disease burden from US health care sector greenhouse gas emissions. Am J Public Health 2017;(0):e1–e3.
3. Eckelman MJ, Sherman J. Environmental impacts of the U.S. health care system and effects on public health. PLoS ONE. 2016;11(6):e0157014.
4. Malik A, Lenzen M, McAlister S, McGain F. The carbon footprint of Australian health care. Lancet Planet Health. 2018;2(1):e27–35.
5. Sustainable Development Unit. Carbon Footprint update for NHS in England 2015: National Health Services (NHS), 2016.
6. Eckelman MJ, Sherman JD, MacNeill AJ. Life cycle environmental emissions and health damages from the Canadian healthcare system: an economic-environmental-epidemiological analysis. PLOS Med. 2018;15(7):e1002623.
7. Karliner J, Slotterback S, Boyd R, Ashby B, Steele K. Health care's climate footprint: how the health sector contributes to the global climate crisis and opportunities for action: healthcare without harm ARUP; 2019.
8. Eckelman MJ, Sherman JD. Estimated global disease burden from US health care sector greenhouse gas emissions. Am J Public Health. 2018;108(S2):S120–2.
9. Hawthorne M. Sterigenics is leaving Willowbrook, eliminating key source of cancer-causing ethylene oxide in Chicago's western suburbs. Chicago Tribune. 2019 9/30/2019.
10. Colledge Michelle. Information regarding sterigenics international in Willowbrook, IL. Chicago, IL: US Department of Health and Human Services; 2018.
11. Wang J, Chen S, Tian M, et al. Inhalation cancer risk associated with exposure to complex polycyclic aromatic hydrocarbon mixtures in an electronic waste and urban area in South China. Environ Sci Technol. 2012;46(17):9745–52.
12. Morris DS, Wright T, Somner JE, Connor A. The carbon footprint of cataract surgery. Eye (Lond). 2013;27(4):495–501.
13. Hong-Gam Le JRE, Venkatesh R, Srinivasan A, Kolli A, Haripriya A, Ravindran RD, Ravilla T, Robin AL, Hutton DW, Stein JD. A sustainable model for delivering high-quality efficient cataract surgery in Southern India. Health Affairs. 2016;35(10):1783–90.
14. Hutton DW, Le H-G, Aravind S, et al. The cost of cataract surgery at the Aravind Eye Hospital, India. Investig Ophthalmol Vis Sci 2014;55(13):1289.
15. Thiel CL, Schehlein E, Ravilla T, et al. Cataract surgery and environmental sustainability: waste and lifecycle assessment of phacoemulsification at a private healthcare facility. J Cataract Refract Surg. 2017;43(11):1391–8.
16. Bell CM, Hatch WV, Cernat G, Urbach DR. Surgeon volumes and selected patient outcomes in cataract surgery: a population-based analysis. Ophthalmology. 2007; 114(3):405–10.
17. Morris DS, Wright T, Somner JEA, Connor A. The carbon footprint of cataract surgery. Eye. 2013;27:495–501.

18. Venkatesh R, van Landingham SW, Khodifad AM, et al. Carbon footprint and cost-effectiveness of cataract surgery. Curr Opin Ophthalmol. 2016;27(1):82–8.
19. Chang DF, Mamalis N, Ophthalmic Instrument Cleaning and Sterilization Task Force. Guidelines for the cleaning and sterilization of intraocular surgical instruments. J Cataract Refract Surg. 2018;44(6):765–73.
20. Namburar S, Pillai M, Varghese G, Thiel C, Robin AL. Waste generated during glaucoma surgery: a comparison of two global facilities. Am J Ophthalmol Case Rep. 2018;12:87–90.
21. Keay L, Lindsley K, Tielsch J, Katz J, Schein O. Routine preoperative medical testing for cataract surgery. Cochrane Database Syst Rev. 2019;1:CD007293.
22. Buchan JC, Amoaku W, Barnes B, et al. How to defuse a demographic time bomb: the way forward? Eye (Lond). 2017;31(11):1519–22.
23. Tey A, Grant B, Harbison D, Sutherland S, Kearns P, Sanders R. Redesign and modernisation of an NHS cataract service (Fife 1997–2004): multifaceted approach. BMJ (Clin Res Ed). 2007;334(7585):148–52.
24. Voyatzis G, Roberts HW, Keenan J, Rajan MS. Cambridgeshire cataract shared care model: community optometrist-delivered postoperative discharge scheme. Br J Ophthalmol. 2014;98(6):760–4.
25. Somner JE, Stone N, Koukkoulli A, Scott KM, Field AR, Zygmunt J. Surgical scrubbing: can we clean up our carbon footprints by washing our hands? J Hosp Infect. 2008;70(3):212–5.
26. Tauber J, Chinwuba I, Kleyn D, Rothschild M, Kahn J, Thiel CL. Quantification of the cost and potential environmental effects of unused pharmaceutical products in cataract surgery. JAMA Ophthalmol. 2019;Online early.
27. Lee P. Challenging considerations regarding waste and potential environmental effects in cataract surgery. JAMA Ophthalmol. 2019.
28. Tauber J, Chinwuba I, Kleyn D, Rothschild M, Kahn J, Thiel CL. Quantification of the cost and potential environmental effects of unused pharmaceutical products in cataract surgery. JAMA Ophthalmol. 2019.
29. Steyn A, Ivey A, Cook C, Stevens D, Thiel C, Chang DF. Reuse in cataract theatres. South African Ophthalmol J. 2018;13(4):8–9.

Afterword

Modern cataract surgery can be a life-changing procedure (usually for the better). There are so many nuances and skills needed to determine a good outcome, that knowledge alone is insufficient to ensure success. Professor Liu's book not only provides up to date and thorough knowledge and information but also looks at strategies to improve practical skills as well as patient related factors such as their experience and critically, their safety. It also covers important topics such as modern teaching and training—so important to ensure that the ever-increasing skills required of modern surgeons are transferrable to the next generation. One such member of this up and coming generation of eye surgeons is Ahmed Shalaby Bardan who is Professor Liu's immediate past Fellow and co-editor and who has also done a brilliant job of ensuring that this new book is up to the standard which we all hope to attain.

Christopher's extensive experience, coupled with his wise choice of authors, has resulted in a detailed, thorough and complete collection of expertise relating to the world's commonest operation and provides trainees and established surgeons alike with a must-have reference.

Larry Benjamin FRCS(Ed) FRCOphth DO
Immediate past-president UKISCRS
President Ophthalmic section Royal Society of Medicine
Honorary President Moorfields Association
October 2020

C. Liu and A. Shalaby Bardan (eds.), *Cataract Surgery*,
https://doi.org/10.1007/978-3-030-38234-6

Index

Printed in the United States
by Baker & Taylor Publisher Services